ESSENTIALS OF

NEUROPHYSIOLOGY

Titles in the Series

Ackermann
Essentials of Human Physiology

Atwood, MacKay
Essentials of Neurophysiology

Moore
Essentials of Human Embryology

Romero-Sierra
Essentials of Neuroanatomy

ESSENTIALS OF
NEUROPHYSIOLOGY

HAROLD L. ATWOOD, PH.D.

Professor and Chairman
Department of Physiology
University of Toronto
Toronto, Ontario, Canada

W.A. MACKAY, PH.D.

Associate Professor
Department of Physiology
University of Toronto
Toronto, Ontario, Canada

1989
B.C. DECKER INC
TORONTO • PHILADELPHIA

Publisher

B.C. Decker Inc
3228 South Service Road
Burlington, Ontario   L7N 3H8

B.C. Decker Inc
320 Walnut Street
Suite 400
Philadelphia, Pennsylvania   19106

Sales and Distribution

United States and Puerto Rico
The C.V. Mosby Company
11830 Westline Industrial Drive
Saint Louis, Missouri   63146

Canada
McAinsh & Co. Ltd.
2760 Old Leslie Street
Willowdale, Ontario   M2K 2X5

Australia
McGraw-Hill Book Company Australia Pty. Ltd.
4 Barcoo Street
Roseville East 2069
New South Wales, Australia

Brazil
Editora McGraw-Hill do Brasil, Ltda.
rua Tabapua, 1.105, Itaim-Bibi
Sao Paulo, S.P. Brasil

Colombia
Interamericana/McGraw-Hill de Colombia, S.A.
Apartado Aereo 81078
Bogota, D.E. Colombia

Europe
McGraw-Hill Book Company GmbH
Lademannbogen 136
D-2000 Hamburg 63
West Germany

France
MEDSI/McGraw-Hill
6, avenue Daniel Lesueur
75007 Paris, France

Hong Kong and China
McGraw-Hill Book Company
Suite 618, Ocean Centre
5 Canton Road
Tsimshatsui, Kowloon
Hong Kong

India
Tata McGraw-Hill Publishing Company, Ltd.
12/4 Asaf Ali Road, 3rd Floor
New Delhi 110002, India

Indonesia
P.O. Box 122/JAT
Jakarta, 1300 Indonesia

Italy
McGraw-Hill Libri Italia, s.r.l.
Piazza Emilia, 5
I-20129 Milano MI
Italy

Japan
Igaku-Shoin Ltd.
Tokyo International P.O. Box 5063
1-28-36 Hongo, Bunkyo-ku,
Tokyo 113, Japan

Korea
C.P.O. Box 10583
Seoul, Korea

Malaysia
No. 8 Jalan SS 7/6B
Kelana Jaya
47301 Petaling Jaya
Selangor, Malaysia

Mexico
Interamericana/McGraw-Hill de Mexico, S.A. de C.V.
Cedro 512, Colonia Atlampa
(Apartado Postal 26370)
06450 Mexico, D.F., Mexico

New Zealand
McGraw-Hill Book Co. New Zealand Ltd.
5 Joval Place, Wiri
Manukau City, New Zealand

Panama
Editorial McGraw-Hill Latinoamericana, S.A.
Apartado Postal 2036
Zona Libre de Colon
Colon, Republica de Panama

Portugal
Editora McGraw-Hill de Portugal, Lda.
Rua Rosa Damasceno 11A–B
1900 Lisboa, Portugal

South Africa
Libriger Book Distributors
Warehouse Number 8
''Die Ou Looiery''
Tannery Road
Hamilton, Bloemfontein 9300

Southeast Asia
McGraw-Hill Book Co.
348 Jalan Boon Lay
Jurong, Singapore 2261

Spain
McGraw-Hill/Interamericana de Espana, S.A.
Manuel Ferrero, 13
28020 Madrid, Spain

Taiwan
P.O. Box 87–601
Taipei, Taiwan

Thailand
632/5 Phaholyothin Road
Sapan Kwai
Bangkok 10400
Thailand

United Kingdom, Middle East and Africa
McGraw-Hill Book Company (U.K.) Ltd.
Shoppenhangers Road
Maidenhead, Berkshire
SL6 2QL England

Venezuela
McGraw-Hill/Interamericana, C.A.
2da. calle Bello Monte
(entre avenida Casanova y Sabana Grande)
Apartado Aereo 50785
Caracas 1050, Venezuela

Essentials of Neurophysiology

ISBN 1–55664–055–2

Library of Congress catalog card number: 88–51491

10   9   8   7   6   5   4   3   2   1

CONTENTS

INTRODUCTION

This review is intended as a study guide to significant points in neurophysiology for those who have completed a course in the subject; it is also useful as a "map" for those who intend to embark on a study of the nervous system.

The orientation is toward basic principles as they apply to human neurophysiology. Many of the principles are derived from experiments with various species of animals and linked to the human nervous system. Neuroanatomy has been included as a necessary component of the material relating to the central nervous system.

We organized the material into self-contained Units with connecting cross-references to other relevant material. The Units have been grouped into Sections which cover broad topics. The student can pick out and review particular Units at will or read through an entire Section to get an overview of the general topic under consideration. The figures and tables carry much of the message and are a good starting point for review or preview of a Unit. An Index provides further aid in finding subjects of interest, and a Glossary has been included to help with general technical terms. Where alternative nomenclature or classifications exist, we have tried to select the simplest and most widely applicable.

Many figures and tables were adapted from excellent text books currently available or from journal articles. Credit for these are given with each figure or table, so that the student who wishes to pursue a topic in more detail can consult the appropriate source.

Mastery of the field of neurophysiology and related neuroscience requires substantial effort, akin to obtaining the Black Belt in judo, and one should not expect to become well-rehearsed after a single exposure. In addition, most of the topics presented here are still being actively researched, so that "final answers" often are not available. In spite of these difficulties, modern research has led to a general picture of the nervous system's control of behavior and of the cellular mechanisms that sustain neural operation. The principles and details presently known provide the starting point for understanding normal function and disease in the nervous system. This review attempts to chart what we feel are the significant concepts and facts for those who need this knowledge as a step towards further basic or clinical work.

We acknowledge help in preparing this review from the following individuals:

Marianne Hegstrom-Wojtowicz, who assisted us in a major way with preparation and adaptation of illustrations, correspondence, and proof-reading;

Evan Atwood, who provided a number of new illustrations and adaptations;

Jean Bilyk and Anna Fleming, who word-processed the manuscript, and Alma Cull, who helped with this aspect and in other ways too numerous to mention; and

Walter Bailey and his associates, for constant advice and encouragement along the way.

Harold L. Atwood
William A. MacKay
November, 1988

1

THE NERVOUS SYSTEM AND NERVE CELLS

UNIT 1
HOW THE COMPONENTS FIT TOGETHER

In the first part of this review (Units 1 to 76), we outline the properties of the components of the peripheral and central nervous systems and discuss general properties of effectors and sensory receptors.

Nerve cells (neurons). Conduct information to and from the rest of the body and within the central nervous system. Neurons located entirely within the central nervous system are **interneurons** (also called **projection** or **local circuit** neurons, depending on their distribution); those leading to the central nervous system from sensory receptors are **afferent neurons**; those leading from the central nervous system to effectors are **efferent neurons.**

Glial cells. Numerous small cells associated with neurons. **Oligodendro-cytes** provide myelin sheath for neurons within the central nervous system; **Schwann cells** have a similar function in the peripheral nervous system. **Astro-cytes** support and separate neurons and blood vessels (see Unit 30).

Blood-brain barrier. Capillaries limit the materials entering and leaving the central nervous system (see Unit 2).

Sensory receptors. Specialized nerve endings, often combined with other cells to form **sense organs**; designed to respond to a particular stimulus such as light, sound, or mechanical change (see Unit 62).

Effectors. Specialized cells innervated (or influenced) by efferent neurons or substances released into the blood by central neurons; designed to produce well-defined actions or response. **Muscles,** innervated by efferent motor neurons, and **smooth muscles,** innervated by the autonomic nervous system, are prominent examples (see Unit 52-61).

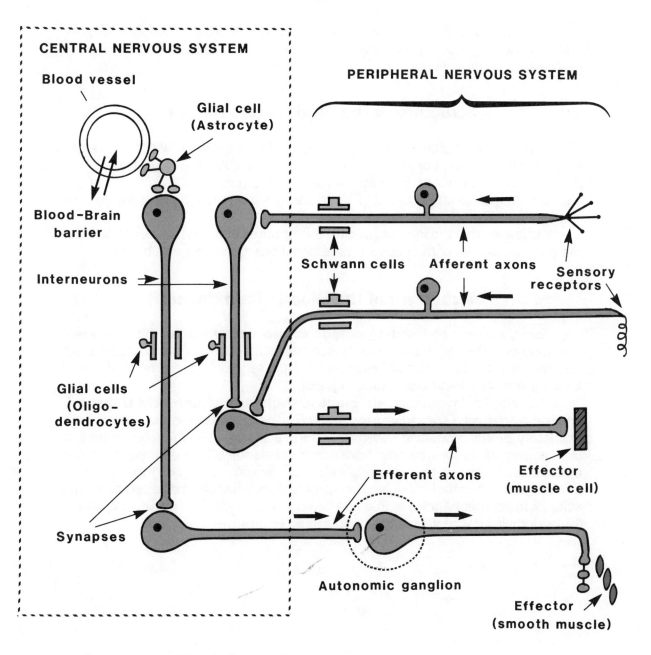

Figure 1 Nerve cells, their targets, and their companions.

UNIT 2
BLOOD-BRAIN BARRIER

Exchange of materials between the central nervous system and the rest of the body is tightly regulated. This protects the central nervous system from changes in its chemical environment.

Structure of the Blood-Brain Barrier

Capillaries in the brain are composed of **endothelial cells**, which are tubular in form, with abutting edges connected by impermeable **tight junctions** (Figs. 2A and 2B). A secreted **basement membrane** maintains the shape of the capillary. In addition, processes of brain **astrocytes** surround and support the capillary (see Fig. 2A).

It is known that the inner and outer membranes of the *endothelial cells* are the main regulators of the passage of material between brain and blood.

Mechanism of the Blood-Brain Barrier

Water, oxygen, and carbon dioxide diffuse rapidly across the interposed membranes of the endothelial cells. Most other materials are excluded, but specialized **transport molecules** and **pumps** allow passage of specific molecules, and ions between brain and blood (see Fig. 2B).

Of particular importance are **glucose transport, amino acid transport, and ion transport**. Glucose transport supplies the central nervous system with its obligatory energy-producing substrate. Amino acids are used in protein synthesis and as precursors for neuronal transmitter substances. Two different transport molecules are known to transport "essential" amino acids (i.e., those not produced by brain metabolism). One transport molecule handles large neutral amino acids, and another handles acidic and basic amino acids. The **sodium pump** of the endothelial cell regulates the brain's ionic environment.

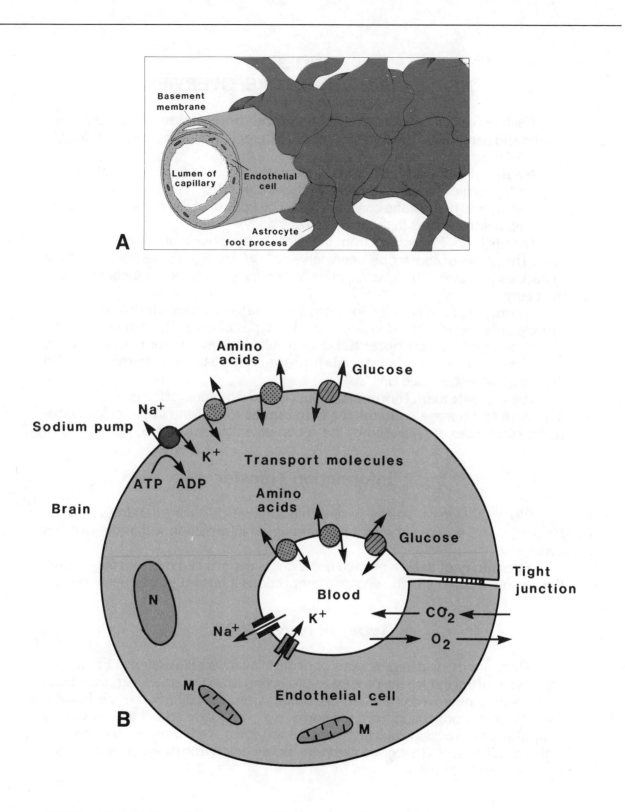

Figure 2 *A,* Brain capillary and astrocyte support. *B,* Exchange across the endothelial cell membranes. N, cell nucleus; M, metochondrion. (*A,* Adapted from Goldstein GW, Betz AL. The blood-brain barrier. Sci Am 1986; 255:77.)

UNIT 3
NERVE CELL STRUCTURE: OVERVIEW

Each nerve cell consists of a **neuronal cell body (soma)** and projections (axons and dendrites). The functions of the different parts of the neuron (Fig. 3A) are as follows.

Neuronal cell body, or soma. Contains the cell nucleus (genetic material), endoplasmic reticulum (protein synthesis), and Golgi apparatus (processing of secretory and membrane components). The control of the nerve cell's growth and metabolism resides in the neuronal cell body.

Dendrites. Projections from the soma that receive input from other nerve cells. The points of contact between nerve cells where signals are transferred are **synapses** (see Unit 32). Synaptic input at dendrites controls electrical activity of the neuron.

Axon. A process projecting from the soma to target cells (other nerve cells, muscle cells, glands, blood vessels, or other types of cell). The axon carries the electrical signal (**action potential**) that results in activation of the target cells. Also, the axon **transports materials** from the soma to the axon terminals, and in the reverse direction (see Unit 26).

Presynaptic axon terminals. Specialized structures at the end of the axon that store and release **transmitter substances** to activate target cells. Transmitter substances are released by the action potential (see Unit 33).

Information Transfer

Electrical signals usually pass within a nerve cell from dendrites to axon terminals. The synapses control the passage of information within the nervous system.

Specificity of action of each nerve cell is determined by its location within the nervous system and the synaptic connections it has with other nerve cells.

Types of Nerve Cells

There are many different types of neuron; a few are illustrated in Figure 3B. Most are **multipolar** (many processes projecting from the soma, e.g., vertebrate motoneuron, neurosecretory neuron, brain pyramidal cell). Some are **bipolar** (two processes projecting from the soma, e.g., vertebrate retinal bipolar cell) or **unipolar** (one process projecting from the soma, e.g., vertebrate sensory neuron, with a single process that gives rise to an axon leading from a sense organ to the central nervous system).

Myelinated and Unmyelinated Axons

Many vertebrate axons have a **myelin sheath** (mostly lipid material) which enhances the speed of electrical impulse transmission (see Unit 18). Others (usually smaller) have a thin glial sheath, but lack the specialized myelin layer; they conduct impulses more slowly.

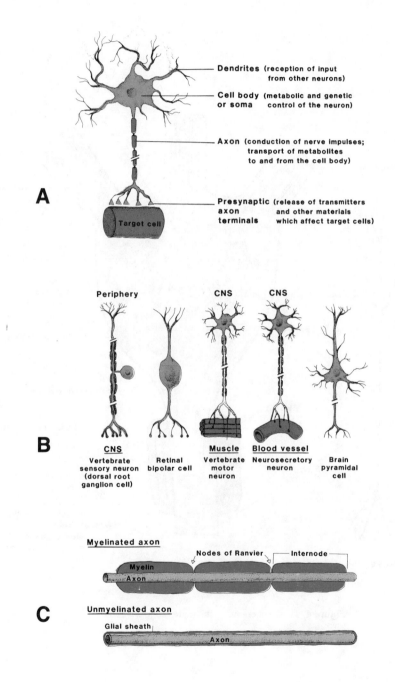

Figure 3 *A*, Functional divisions of a neuron; *B*, Representative types of neurons; and *C*, Myelinated and unmyelinated axons. (*B*, Modified after Kandel ER, Schwartz JH. Principles of neural science. New York: Elsevier, 1985:23.)

UNIT 4
NERVE CELL STRUCTURE: CELLULAR COMPONENTS

The functions of the nerve cell depend upon properties of its surface **membrane** and upon activities of **nucleus** and **cytoplasmic (neuroplasmic) components** (Fig. 4A).

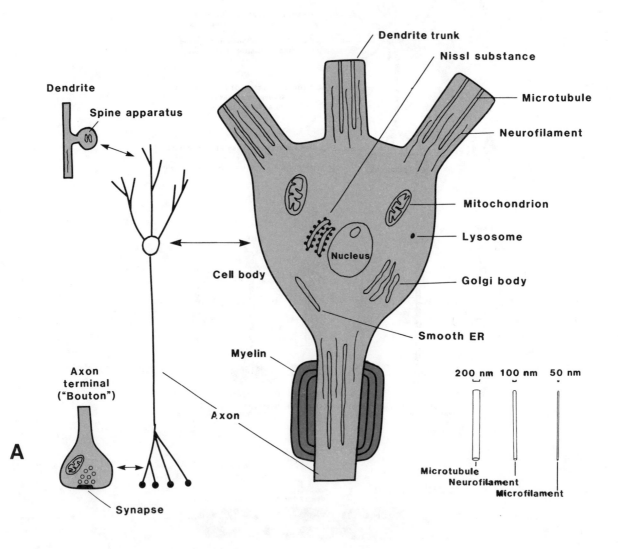

Figure 4 *A*. Components of the neuron. *Figure continues.*

The Neuronal Membrane

The surface **membrane** is composed of a lipid bilayer with attached proteins and carbohydrates (Fig. 4B). Lateral movement of lipids and proteins can occur, but some proteins are anchored in place by cytoplasmic filaments. This gives rise to regional specialization of the neuron's surface.

The **lipid bilayer** restricts movement of water, ions, and proteins into or out of the cell.

Membrane proteins may form channels for passage of ions, pumps, transport systems for specific materials, or receptors.

Carbohydrate parts of membrane glycoproteins protrude into the extracellular space and form a thin layer at the cell surface **(glycocalyx)**. Glycoproteins may serve as adhesion molecules or as "recognition molecules" that act to establish specific cell-to-cell contacts between neurons and their targets.

The Nucleus

The main role of the nucleus is to control synthesis of specific proteins. The genetic material (DNA and associated proteins) is regulated to initiate synthesis of specific proteins needed by the cell.

The Neuroplasm

The neuroplasm contains organelles that perform essential functions for the cell.

Mitochondria.   Responsible for **aerobic metabolism**, i.e., production of the high-energy phosphate compound adenosine triphosphate (ATP) by the enzymes of the citric acid cycle. ATP is produced by oxidation of pyruvate, which is derived from glucose. Nerve cells are highly dependent upon oxygen and glucose supplies.

Mitochondria also store calcium; they function as a low-affinity, high-capacity calcium reservoir.

Endoplasmic reticulum (smooth ER).   Functions in secretion, storage of calcium, and axoplasmic transport.

The **Golgi apparatus** accepts proteins manufactured by the cell that are to be exported, forms protein-containing vesicles, and releases them into the neuroplasm. Some are then carried by axoplasmic transport to the axon terminals (see Unit 26).

Smooth ER throughout the neuron binds calcium and maintains the internal concentration at a low level (0.1 μM). Prolonged elevation of intracellular calcium levels leads to the death of the neuron.

Ribosomes.   Composed of protein and ribonucleic acid (RNA) exported from the nucleus to function in **protein synthesis**. Clusters of ribosomes **(polyribosomes)** are also found. Most of the proteins formed by free ribosomes and polyribosomes remain within the cell.

Rough endoplasmic reticulum (rough ER) is endoplasmic reticulum with attached ribosomes. Most of the proteins formed by rough ER are exported from the cell.

Nissl substance is an accumulation of rough ER and polyribosomes near the nucleus in nerve cells. It produces neuron-specific proteins.

Lysosomes.   Membrane-bound structures containing hydrolytic enzymes that degrade cellular proteins as well as materials taken into the cell.

The neuron also contains **calcium-activated proteases**—enzymes that degrade cellular proteins when the calcium concentration is elevated (hence the requirement for long-term maintenance of low levels of intracellular calcium).

Microtubules, Neurofilaments, and Microfilaments.   Microtubules (composed of the protein **tubulin** and **microtubule-associated** proteins, or MAPs) are involved in axoplasmic transport and in regulating the shape of neuronal processes.

Neurofilaments (composed of fibrous proteins) probably regulate the shape of neuronal processes.

Microfilaments (some of which contain the protein **actin**) regulate movement of materials within the surface membrane, serve as anchors for membrane structures, and form part of the "cytoskeleton" which limits and regulates movement of intracellular organelles.

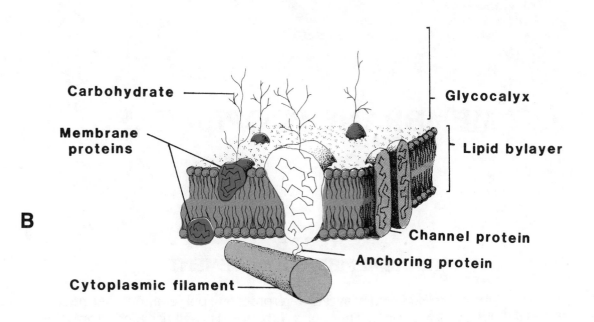

B

Carbohydrate

Membrane proteins

Glycocalyx

Lipid bylayer

Channel protein

Anchoring protein

Cytoplasmic filament

Figure 4 (*continued***)** *B*, General membrane structure. (*A*, Modified after Shepherd GM. The synaptic organization of the brain. New York: Oxford University Press, 1979:17 and Shepherd GM. Neurobiology. New York: Oxford University Press, 1983:61. *B*, Adapted from Fawcett DW. The Cell. Philadelphia: WB Saunders, 1981:5.)

2

MEMBRANE PROPERTIES

UNIT 5
TRANSMEMBRANE MOVEMENT

The cell membrane's lipid bilayer is waterproof and only sparingly permeable to materials on either side. The cell's **interior** is well isolated from the **extracellular environment**. But since materials have to enter and leave the cell if the cell is to survive and function, several different mechanisms have evolved to *control* and *regulate* transmembrane traffic of materials.

1. **Diffusion.** Materials can **diffuse** through the membrane's lipid bilayer if they are lipid-soluble. The more lipid-soluble molecules diffuse through more rapidly.
2. **Leakage channel.** Any transmembrane passages (formed by transmembrane proteins) can serve as sites for **diffusion** of mobile molecules, such as water.
3. **Active transport.** An ATP-powered pump. **Active transport** (movement of material against a concentration gradient) is mediated by specialized proteins that use the energy of ATP to bind and transport particular substances. (*Example*: Na^+-K^+ pump)
4. **Carrier-mediated diffusion (facilitated diffusion).** A specialized membrane molecule attracts and carries particular substances across the membrane.
5. **Exchange transport (co-transport).** Gradient-dependent exchange. **Exchange transport** utilizes the transmembrane ionic gradients to move particular substances into or out of the cell. (*Example*: Na^+-Ca^{++} exchange)
6. **Voltage-gated channel.** **Transmembrane voltages** can open (or close) channels for particular ions. (*Example*: Na^+ channel of nerve membrane)
7. **Ion-gated channel.** **Ions** (usually Ca^{++} within the cell) control channels for particular ions. (*Example*: Ca^{++}-gated K^+ channel)
8. **Ligand-gated channel.** **Ligands** (transmitter substances or drugs) can open or close channels for particular ions. (*Example*: Acetylcholine-operated channels)

9. **"Second messenger" gated channel.** **Ligands** (transmitter substances, drugs, or hormones) can control channels for particular ion species by activating intracellular "second messenger" systems which alter channel properties. (*Example*: Cyclic adenosine monophosphate-controlled K$^+$ channels of nerve cells)

10. **Pinocytosis and exocytosis.** Vesicles are formed to take up or extrude large molecules, respectively. These processes require metabolic energy.

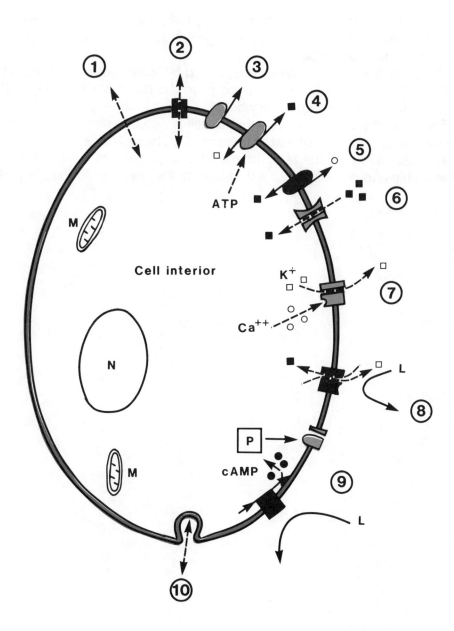

Figure 5 Movement of materials across the cell membrane. N, cell nucleus; M, mitochondrion; cAMP, cyclic adenosine monophosphate; P, cAMP-dependent protein kinase and substrate proteins; L, ligand. Numbers indicate the different types of transmembrane movement as listed on the opposite page.

UNIT 6
RESTING POTENTIAL

The **resting potential** can be measured by inserting a small glass capillary pipette through the membrane without damaging it (Fig. 6A). Then a voltage-reading meter connected to electrodes *inside* and *outside* the membrane shows a reading of $^-90$ mV (to $^-60$ mV, depending on the type of cell).

Charge Separation

The resting potential is due to separation of positive and negative charges at the membrane (Fig. 6B). No new charge is created; rather, charges already present in solution are separated.

In aqueous solution, charges are carried by **ions**. Normally, the number of negatively charged ions (e.g., Cl^-) is equal to the number of positively charged ions (e.g., Na^+) in the system as a whole.

The concentration of ions inside the cell is equal to that outside the cell, so there is no net movement of **water** by osmosis. The cell does not shrink or swell.

The separation of charge at the membrane represents a tiny fraction of the total available and is confined to a thin layer at the membrane (see Fig. 6B).

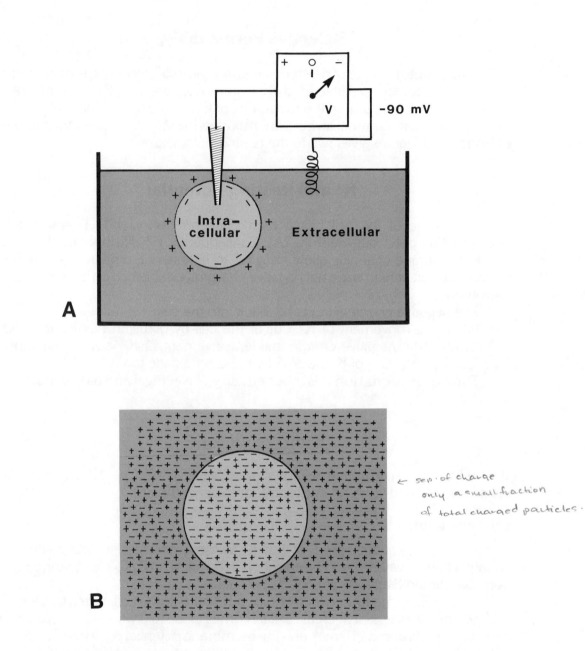

Figure 6 *A*, Measuring the resting potential. *B*, Charge separation. (*B*, Modified after Kandel ER, Schwartz JH. Principles of neural science. New York: Elsevier, 1985:50.)

UNIT 7
RESTING POTENTIAL AND SELECTIVE ION PERMEABILITY

Selective Permeability

Ions in solution are of different sizes and carry different charge distributions. Membrane channels available for **diffusion of ions** are selectively permeable to different ions, depending on the properties of the ions and the channel.

At rest, most mammalian cells are more permeable to K^+ **ions** than to other **cations**. This feature gives rise to the resting potential.

K^+ and Resting Potential

The inside of the cell has a high concentration of K^+. There is a low concentration of K^+ outside (Fig. 7A). Consequently, K^+ diffuses out of the cell.

If membrane channels allow *only* K^+ to diffuse out, negative counter-ions (anions) are left behind and a net negative charge is established on the inside of the membrane.

The negative charge attracts K^+ back into the cell.

When the movement of K^+ out of the cell by diffusion has established a sufficiently large negative charge inside, movement of K^+ out by diffusion is balanced by attraction of K^+ back in by the electrostatic force.

The **Nernst equation** describes equality of electrical and diffusional forces for K^+.

$$E\,(mV) = -61 \log \frac{C_i}{C_o}$$

Where E = transmembrane electrical potential at 37° C, $C_i = K^+$ concentration inside the cell, and $C_o = K^+$ concentration outside the cell.

Observations

The Nernst equation predicts that the transmembrane electrical gradient (E) should change when the concentration ratio of K^+ (C_i/C_o) is changed. The potential should decrease when C_i/C_o is smaller.

C_i/C_o can be made smaller by *raising* K^+ outside the cell. When this is done, the membrane potential decreases. It becomes close to 0 when $C_o = C_i$ (Fig. 7B; here, C_i for K^+ is about 110 mM, and the membrane potential is 0 when C_o for K^+ is 110 mM).

However, the membrane potential in nerve cells does not strictly obey the equation when external K^+ is low (see Fig. 7B). This suggests that the membrane is not *exclusively* permeable to K^+ under these conditions.

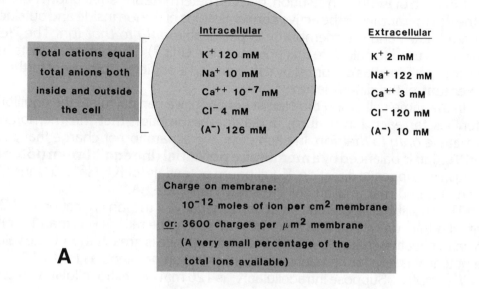

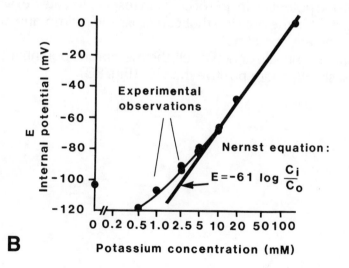

Figure 7 *A*, An idealized vertebrate cell. *B*, The Nernst equation and reality.

UNIT 8
EQUILIBRIUM POTENTIALS FOR IONS

For each of the ions in solution, one can determine an "equilibrium potential" for the cell membrane, if the active concentrations of the ion inside and outside the cell are known and the membrane is permeable *only to that ion*. The Nernst equation is used to calculate this potential (see Unit 7). The potential exists when charge separation has occurred by diffusion and is sufficient to prevent further **net movement** of the diffusible ion.

In the same cell, using the Nernst equation, we can calculate the equilibrium potentials for each ion in turn, under the assumption that the membrane is permeable *only to that ion*. In each case, the separation of charge that occurs by **diffusion** is balanced by a **membrane potential** (the **equilibrium potential**) acting in the opposite direction. Equilibrium potentials for K^+, Na^+, Cl^-, and Ca^{++} for an idealized mammalian cell are shown in Figure 8A.

The equilibrium potential for an ion is negative if the ion is a cation and C_i/C_o is greater than unity. The sign becomes reversed if the ratio is less than 1, or if the ion has a negative charge, as does Cl^-. When valence is greater than 1, the value of the potential is less for an equivalent concentration gradient, as for Ca^{++}.

Example: Suppose intracellular K^+ is 120 mM and extracellular K^+ is 2 mM. Then

$$E_K = -61 \log \frac{120}{2} = -108 \text{ mV}$$

This calculated potential (inside of cell with respect to outside) will actually be measured *only* if K^+ is the only ion that can cross the membrane and no forces other than diffusion are operating.

In a mammalian muscle or nerve cell, the membrane potential is found to be close to E_{Cl} and slightly more positive than E_K (Fig. 8B).

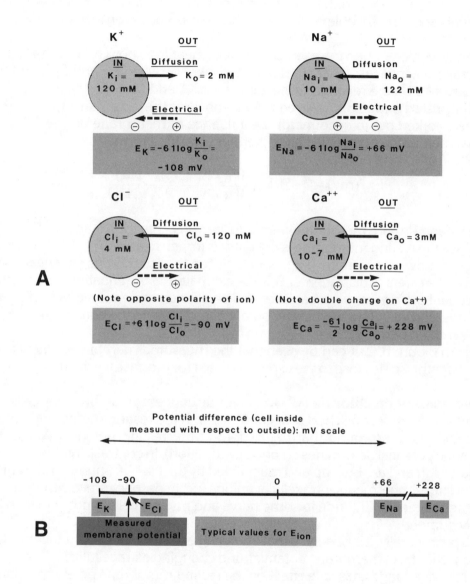

Figure 8 *A,* Diffusion and electrical forces at equilibrium potentials for individual ions. *B,* Road map of ionic equilibrium potentials.

UNIT 9
HOW PERMEABILITY TO MORE THAN ONE ION
INFLUENCES MEMBRANE POTENTIAL

A "first principles" argument.   The equilibrium potential for a single ion is realized *only* when the membrane is permeable to that ion *and to no other.* If the membrane is permeable only to K^+, the membrane potential sits at E_K (Fig. 9, 1). If the membrane is permeable only to Na^+, the membrane potential sits at E_{Na} (Fig. 9, 5).

What happens when the membrane is permeable to both K^+ and Na^+? The membrane potential assumes a value somewhere between E_K and E_{Na}, and the value depends on the relative permeabilities for K^+ and Na^+ (Fig. 9, 2-4).

Simplified equation.   An equation (known as the Goldman equation) that has been worked out to account for the influence of membrane permeability on the final membrane potential is given here in simplified form.

$$E_m \text{ (mV)} = -61 \log \frac{(P_K \cdot K_i + P_{Na} \cdot Na_i)}{(P_K \cdot K_o + P_{Na} \cdot Na_o)}$$

where P_K and P_{Na} are membrane permeability constants for K^+ and Na^+.

Since the resting membrane is not entirely impermeable to Na^+, this ion with its large positive equilibrium potential displaces the membrane potential away from E_K. The extent of displacement can be estimated by the equation, which takes into account the relative permeabilities and equilibrium potentials of K^+ and Na^+.

General rule: The membrane potential is closest to the equilibrium potential of the most permeant ion.

From Figure 9, 2, it can be seen that the measured membrane potential of -90 mV for the cell is close to the expected result for the case in which $P_{Na} = 0.01$ P_K.

A comment on chloride (Cl^-).   Chloride concentrations in many cells are low and are rapidly established in accordance with the resting membrane potential. Thus, it is often found that E_{Cl} is right at the resting potential (since the membrane potential determines chloride distribution). In contrast, intracellular K^+ levels are high and are built up and maintained by the Na^+-K^+ pump and by high levels of large, impermeant intracellular anions (proteins, phosphate compounds, and other materials. Chloride in some nerve and muscle cells is not known to be actively pumped.

Experimentally, it is observed that changing extracellular Cl^- produces only a transient change in membrane potential, and changing extracellular Na^+ or Ca^{++} over fairly wide ranges has little effect on the resting membrane potential. Changing extracellular K^+ alters the membrane potential in approximate agreement with the Nernst equation. Thus, the strongest *immediate* force contributing to the membrane potential is the transmembrane gradient of K^+.

Chloride is not considered important in setting up nerve and muscle resting and action potentials, but it is important in certain types of synaptic transmission (see Units 43 and 44).

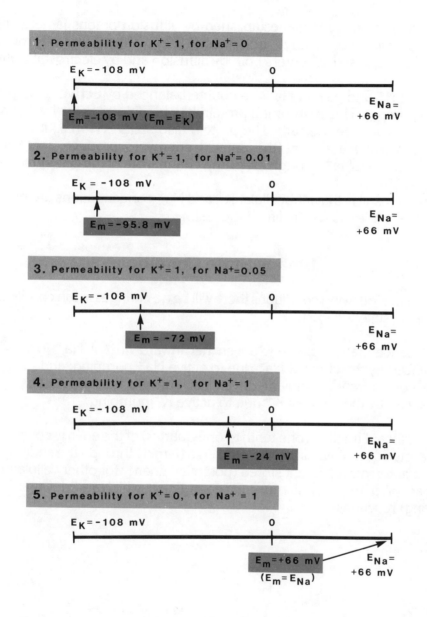

Figure 9 How membrane potential is affected by changes in membrane permeability for K⁺ and Na⁺.

UNIT 10
ROLE OF ACTIVE TRANSPORT

The Cell Is Not in Equilibrium for K$^+$ and Na$^+$

The membrane potential established by diffusion of ions is not sufficiently negative to prevent net loss of K$^+$ from the cell (Fig. 10A). It is also very much more negative than E_{Na}, so Na$^+$ enters both by diffusion and by electrostatic attraction (Fig. 10B).

Loss of K$^+$ and gain of Na$^+$ are counterbalanced by **active transport** (the "sodium pump"). This membrane protein has binding sites for Na$^+$ (inside the cell) and K$^+$ (outside the cell). The protein also splits ATP (i.e., it has ATPase enzymatic activity) and uses the derived energy to produce conformational changes that move Na$^+$ through the pump channel out of the cell, and K$^+$ into the cell (Fig. 10C).

The net result is that intracellular K$^+$ and Na$^+$ concentrations are maintained at near-constant levels for the life of the cell.

Steady-State Condition

Under the following conditions there will be no changes in ion concentrations, and a steady state will exist:

1. The concentration gradient-driven net inward flux of Na$^+$ ions is exactly balanced by the efflux of Na$^+$ due to active Na$^+$ pumping; and
2. The concentration gradient-driven net outward flux of K$^+$ ions is exactly balanced by the influx of K$^+$ due to active K$^+$ pumping.

A significant fraction (one-tenth to one-quarter) of the energy consumed by a cell is devoted to maintaining ionic gradients (largely through the sodium pump). The ionic gradients represent stored (potential) energy for other cellular activities such as action potentials and muscular contraction, which are "downhill" (energy-dissipating) reactions.

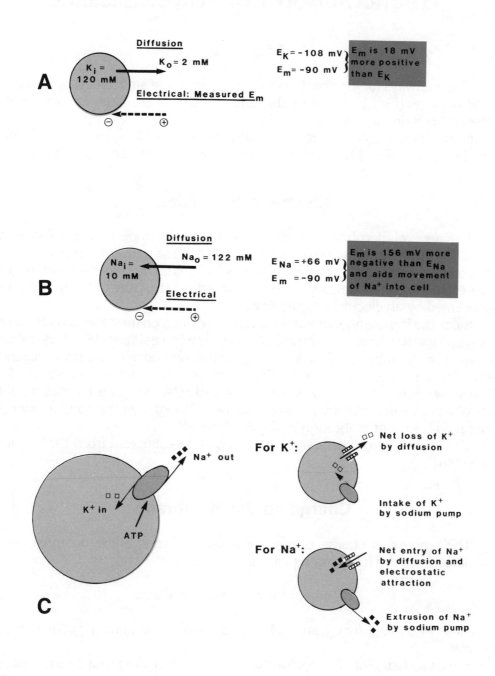

Figure 10 *A,* Leakage of K^+ out of a cell due to nonequilibrium. *B,* Leakage of Na^+ into a cell due to nonequilibrium. *C,* The counterbalancing role of the sodium pump.

UNIT 11
ELECTRICAL MODEL OF NERVE MEMBRANE

Channels

The pathways for ion flow through the membrane are formed by transmembrane proteins (Fig. 11A). The **channels** so formed are large enough to allow water and certain ions to pass.

In the resting nerve membrane, there are substantial numbers of channels available for K^+ (Fig. 11B), and smaller numbers for Na^+ and Cl^- (Fig. 11C).

Electrical Properties

The general membrane structure is largely lipid, impermeable to water and ions. It has the properties of an electrical capacitor and can store electrical charge (created by separation of positive and negative ions). Thus, an electrical model of the membrane can be developed, in which the lipid structure of the membrane is represented by an electrical **capacitor** (C_m).

Since the ion channels restrict movement of ions on the basis of their size and charge properties, they can be modeled as electrical **resistors** (R_{ion}), as shown in Figures 11B through 11D. By measuring current carried across the membrane by particular ions, one can estimate the resistance value for ion channels (from Ohm's law). The reciprocal of resistance, **conductance** (g), is a measure of the ease of passage of ions through their channels. The greater the conductance, the more readily ions pass through available channels.

The value of the potential across C_m can be estimated from the Goldman equation (E_m).

Charge on the Membrane

The amount of charge needed to create the membrane potential can be calculated from the following equation:

$$Q \text{ (coulombs of charge)} = C_m E_m$$

Measured values for C_m are 1 $\mu F/cm^2$ of membrane, and for E_m, usually 90 to 100 mV.

Hence a charge of 10^{-7} coulomb/cm^2 is necessary to produce a membrane potential of 100 mV. This is equivalent to 10^{-12} mole of univalent cations (Q/F, where F is Faraday's constant, the number of coulombs per mole of ions, or about 10^5). Note that this amount is very small compared with the total number of available ions in the cell (see Fig. 7A).

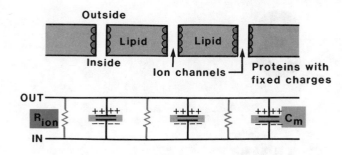

C_m = membrane capacitance (determined by lipid)

R_{ion} = electrical resistance of ion channel

A

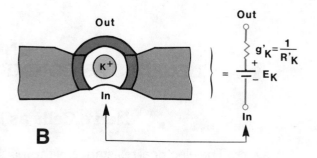

B

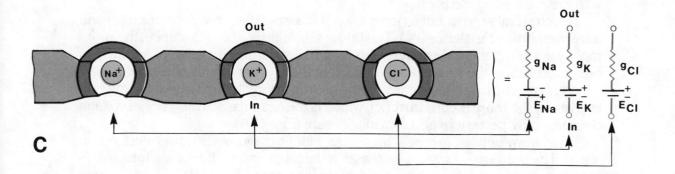

C

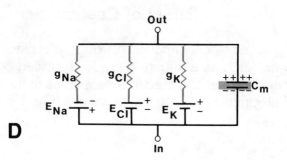

D

Figure 11 *A* to *D*, Ionic channels and their electrical equivalents. (*B* and *C*, Modified after Kandel ER, Schwartz JH. Principles of neural science. New York: Elsevier, 1985:61, 62.)

3

NERVE IMPULSE

UNIT 12
NEURONS AS CONDUCTORS OF ELECTRICITY

Nerve Cells as Electrical Cables

The electrical resistance of the inside of a nerve axon is much higher than that of a metal wire of similar size. A voltage change induced by a pulse of current dies out a few millimeters from the point of application, because the electrical resistance of the nerve cell impedes longitudinal flow of current, and membrane channels allow it to leak out of the core (Fig. 12A). Voltage declines exponentially with distance along the axon.

Each small segment of a nerve axon has associated core resistance (r_i) and transmembrane resistance (r_m). The larger the value of core resistance, the more rapidly applied current dissipates with length. The larger the value of transmembrane resistance, the less leakage of current there is per length of axon.

A measure of the effectiveness of the neuron in longitudinal signal conduction is given by the **length constant** (λ), which is the distance at which signal voltage declines to 37 percent (l/e)* of its initial value (Fig. 12A).

For unmyelinated axons, λ increases with fiber diameter (lower core resistance). The presence of myelin increases λ, because myelin increases total membrane resistance and less current leaks from the core (Fig. 12B).

Effect of Capacitance

Charging an electrical capacitor through a resistor takes time. An abruptly changing signal such as a square wave is "rounded off" in its time course by membrane capacitance. The electrical properties of the membrane limit the rate of change of electrical signals in the nerve cell (Fig. 12C).

---

* e is the base of natural logarithms, 2.7182. The mathematical description of voltage distribution along the axon is: $V_x = V_o e^{-x/\lambda}$, where: V_x is voltage at a distance x from point of current application and V_o is voltage at the point of current application.

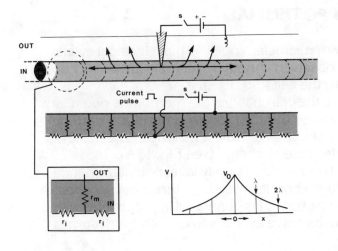

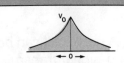

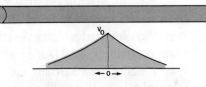

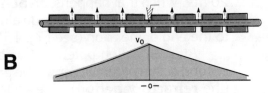

A

B

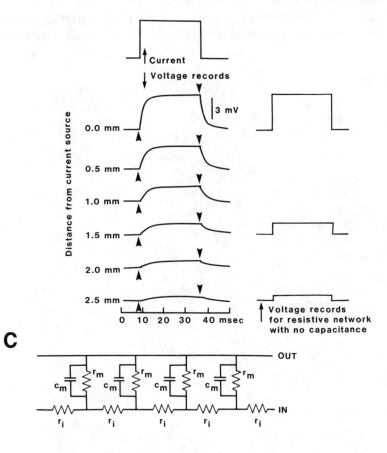

C

Figure 12 *A,* Resistive elements of the neuron. *B,* The effect of axon size and myelin on the spread of an electrical signal. *C,* The effect of capacitative properties of the neuron. (*A,* Modified after Kuffler SW, Nicholls JG, Martin AR. From neuron to brain. Sunderland, MA: Sinauer Associates Inc., 1984: 169. *C,* Modified after Hodgkin AL, Rushton WAH. The electrical constants of a crustacean nerve fibre. Proc R Soc Lond [Series B] 1946; 133:462.)

UNIT 13
ACTION POTENTIAL

A nerve cell can be penetrated with microelectrodes so that electrical events during signal transmission may be observed. Another microelectrode can be inserted to inject electrical current into the cell (Fig. 13A).

Passing extra negative current into the cell changes the membrane potential to a more negative level (**hyperpolarizes** the cell) locally around the current-passing electrode. However, the signal dies out within a few millimeters because of core resistance and transmembrane leakage of charge (see Fig. 13A).

Passing extra positive current also generates a purely local potential change (**depolarizes** the cell) unless the voltage change exceeds a "threshold" of about 20 mV. When that happens, an **action potential** is generated. It propagates with constant velocity and amplitude along the nerve axon and dies out when it comes to the end of the axon (see Fig. 13A).

After an action potential has been produced by stimulation of the axon, a second action potential cannot be produced for a period of 0.5 to 1 msec afterward (the **refractory period**). Thereafter, for about 0.5 to 2 msec a second action potential can occur, but it is smaller, and more current is needed to produce it (**relative refractory period**). Absolute and relative refractory periods are illustrated in Figure 13B. The refractory period limits the frequency response of the nerve axon to a value usually between 500 and 1,000 impulses per second.

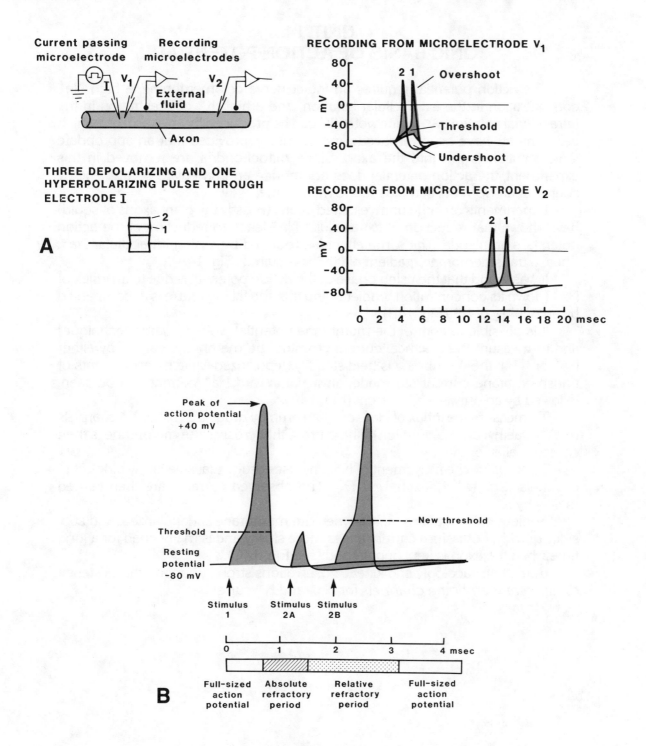

Figure 13 *A*, Subthreshold and suprathreshold stimuli. *B*, Threshold and refractory period. (*A*, Modified after Kuffler SW, Nicholls JG, Martin AR. From neuron to brain. Sunderland, MA: Sinauer Associates Inc., 1984:104.)

UNIT 14
IONIC BASIS OF ACTION POTENTIAL

The action potential requires an intact nerve cell membrane, a high Na^+ concentration in the extracellular solution, and a high K^+ concentration in the intracellular solution. An action potential can be produced by an axon from which cell contents have been removed experimentally, provided that an appropriate ionic solution is put into the axon. Since mitochondria are removed in this experiment, the action potential does not require an immediate cellular energy source apart from the stimulus to the membrane.

Experiments on large unmyelinated axons (mostly the giant axons of squid) have shown that reduction of extracellular Na^+ leads to reduction of the action potential's amplitude. The same effect is produced by raising intracellular Na^+. Thus, a transmembrane gradient of Na^+ is required (Fig. 14A).

It was found that the rising phase of the action potential is due to an influx of Na^+ (down its concentration gradient) and that the falling phase is accompanied by an outflow of K^+ (Fig. 14B).

It is possible to control the membrane potential (voltage clamp technique) and to measure the electrical current crossing the membrane carried by either Na^+ or K^+. If the membrane is held steadily depolarized while measurements of transmembrane current are made, an initial inward Na^+ current can be seen, followed by an outward K^+ current (Fig. 14C).

To measure the influx of Na^+, one can employ drugs that block K^+ channels (e.g., tetraethyl ammonium ion). The current that crosses the membrane is then carried mainly by Na^+.

To measure the movement of K^+, one uses drugs that selectively block Na^+ channels (e.g., tetrodotoxin, or TTX). The observed currents are then carried mainly by K^+.

Sodium current arises rapidly when the membrane is depolarized, and subsides quickly. Potassium current arises more slowly and is maintained for a long time when the axon is kept depolarized (see Fig. 14C).

Both pharmacologic and kinetic observations strongly support the existence of *different membrane channels* for Na^+ and K^+ currents.

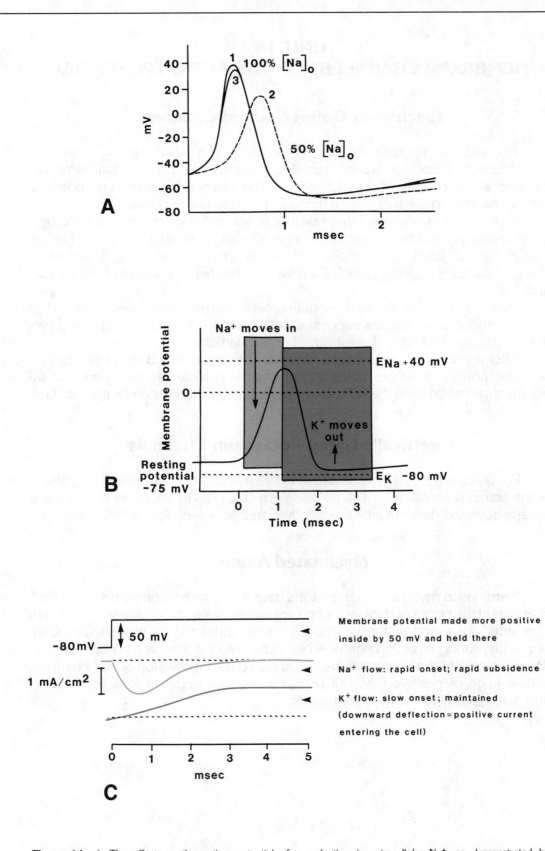

Figure 14 *A,* The effect on the action potential of a reduction in extracellular Na⁺, as demonstrated by experiments on large unmyelinated axons. *B,* Action potential in large unmyelinated axon. *C,* Current flow during depolarization of a large unmyelinated axon. (*A,* Adapted from Hodgkin AL, Katz B. The effect of sodium ions on the electrical activity of the giant axon of the squid. J Physiol 1949; 108:48. *C,* Modified after Hodgkin AL, Huxley AF. Currents carried by sodium and potassium ions through the membrane of the giant axon of *Loligo.* J Physiol 1952; 116:451.)

UNIT 15
MEMBRANE CHANNELS FOR THE ACTION POTENTIAL

Electrically Gated Sodium Channels

The stimulus for obtaining a nerve impulse is a positive-going change in membrane potential (which can be obtained by application of electrical current or by mechanical or chemical perturbation). The change in membrane potential opens channels in the membrane through which ions can move.

In particular, a relatively large number of sodium channels are opened by a positive-going membrane potential change, allowing inward movement of Na^+. A model for the opening of sodium channels involves microdisplacement of charged particles ("gating particles") near the channel as shown in Figures 15A and 15B.

Note that in the model, all three gating particles must be displaced for Na^+ to enter. Actual measurements suggest inward rotation of negatively charged particles or outward rotation of positively charged particles.

After a sodium channel opens, it rapidly becomes **inactivated** by another process, thought to involve movement of another particle into the opened channel. Inactivation explains the **refractory period** of the nerve membrane (see Unit 13).

Electrically Gated Potassium Channels

Potassium channels open to allow K^+ to leave the cell during the falling phase of the action potential (Fig. 15C). Potassium channels in the nerve axon have a voltage-activated gate but lack the inactivation that is seen for Na^+ channels.

Myelinated Axons

Mammalian myelinated nerve axons have a very heavy concentration of Na^+ channels at the nodes of Ranvier, but no voltage-activated K^+ channels (Fig. 15D). The latter are found in the internode region under the myelin sheath. Consequently, during an action potential Na^+ flows into the axon at the node, but the downstroke of the action potential is accompanied by inactivation of Na^+ channels and leakage of positive ions out of the axon, and negative ions in, through non-gated (passive) membrane channels.

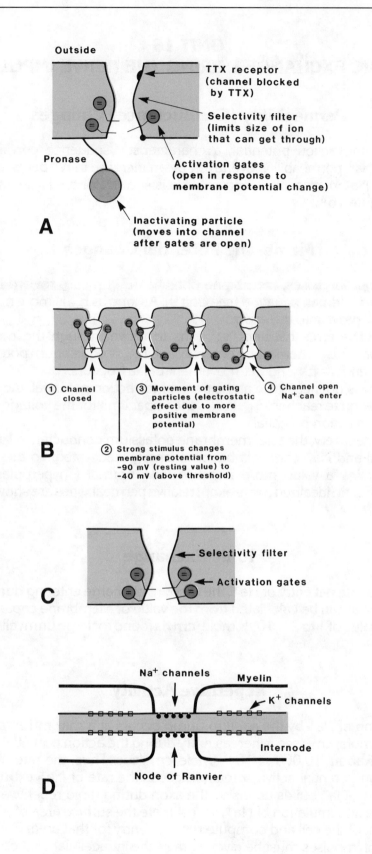

Figure 15 *A,* Sodium channel. *B,* Sequence of events in the opening of sodium channels. *C,* Voltage-gated potassium channel. *D,* Location of sodium and potassium channels in mammalian myelinated axons. (*B,* Modified after Armstrong CM. Sodium channels and gating currents. Physiol Rev 1981; 61:652.)

UNIT 16
IONIC EXCHANGE DURING THE NERVE IMPULSE

Permeability (Conductance) Changes

During the action potential, a characteristic sequence consisting of an increase in Na^+ permeability, overtaken by an increase in K^+ permeability and a decrease in Na^+ permeability, occurs. This is shown (for the large unmyelinated axon) in Figure 16A.

Membrane Potential Changes

When g_{Na} increases, membrane potential (E_m) moves toward E_{Na}, as predicted by the Goldman equation (see Unit 9). As long as E_m is more negative than E_{Na}, Na^+ will move into the axon.

The motive force causing Na^+ ions to move through the membrane is $(E - E_{Na})$, where E = membrane potential and E_{Na} = equilibrium potential for the Na^+ ion. When $E = E_{Na}$, no net movement of Na^+ occurs.

Since g_K is not negligible at the peak of the action potential, the membrane voltage never quite reaches E_{Na}. E_{Na} is the upper limit for the voltage that can be attained by an action potential.

During recovery, the total membrane potassium conductance (g_K) is higher than normal and Na^+ channels become largely inactivated, so the membrane potential attains a value more negative than normal ("hyperpolarizing after-potential"). For an idealized nerve axon, relative permeabilities are shown in Figure 16C.

Ionic Exchange

To calculate net entry of Na^+, the amount of charge entering during a single action potential can be calculated from the value of membrane capacitance (see Unit 11). A value of 1 to 2×10^{-12} mole/cm^2 is found for large unmyelinated fibers (Fig. 16B).

Repetitive Activity

Extrusion of Na^+ by the sodium pump occurs at a maximum rate of about 50×10^{-12} mole/cm^2/sec, whereas entry during the action potential occurs at a peak rate of about $10,000 \times 10^{-12}$ mole/cm^2/sec. Thus, the rate of Na^+ entry during action potential activity greatly exceeds the rate of Na^+ extrusion by the sodium pump. Na^+ builds up inside the axon during rapid repetitive activity. To calculate the accumulation of Na^+, we estimate the surface area of a representative segment of the cell and compute net Na^+ entry for that area. For large cells, thousands of impulses must be given to raise the intracellular Na^+ concentration by a few millimoles per liter. For small cells, relatively few impulses can make an appreciable difference in intracellular Na^+.

Ionic balance is restored more slowly by the Na^+-K^+ pump acting continuously during the "resting" period of the axon. Energy is used (ATP split) for this purpose, but not for the impulse itself. The impulse is a downhill reaction. Apart from the initiating stimulus itself, the energy source for the impulse is derived from ionic gradients created and maintained largely by the sodium pump.

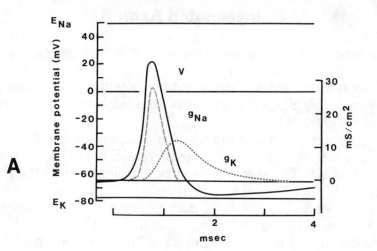

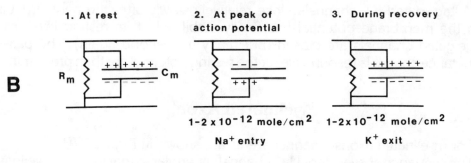

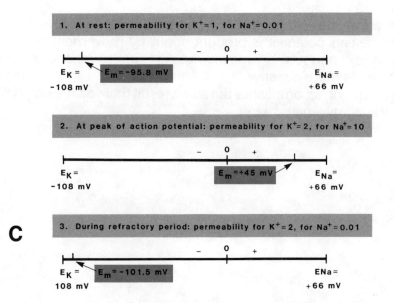

Figure 16 *A,* Conductance changes for a large unmyelinated axon. *B,* Charge movement in a large unmyelinated axon. *C,* Membrane potential and equilibrium potentials during the action potential. (*A,* Modified after Hodgkin AL, Huxley AF. A quantitative description of membrane current and its application to conduction and excitation in nerve. J Physiol 1952; 117:530.)

UNIT 17
SEQUENCE OF EVENTS FOR CHANNELS DURING THE NERVE IMPULSE

Unmyelinated Axon

For unmyelinated axons of standard type, channel events are shown in Figure 17A.

Depolarization to the threshold membrane potential opens many voltage-gated Na^+ channels. This allows Na^+ to flow into the cell; both diffusion and electrostatic attraction aid entry of Na^+.

As the membrane becomes progressively depolarized, voltage-gated K^+ channels start to open and Na^+ channels inactivate. Entry of Na^+ slows until it is overtaken by exit of K^+. Thereafter, K^+ exit predominates until the membrane potential is restored.

The refractory period is the time during which a large number of Na^+ channels are inactivated by the preceding depolarization.

Repolarization of the membrane reverses Na^+ channel inactivation; the channels are now closed, but ready to respond to another stimulus.

Voltage-gated K^+ channels close relatively slowly after the nerve impulse. When the membrane potential has finally stabilized at its resting level, most voltage-gated channels are closed (but ready to respond again). The passive conductance channels responsible for the resting potential are then predominant.

Myelinated Axon

For myelinated axons, channel events are shown in Figure 17B.

The sequence of events for Na^+ channels is similar to that in an unmyelinated axon.

Since there are no voltage-gated K^+ channels at the node of Ranvier, repolarization to the resting potential is brought about by movement of ions through passive (leakage) channels: K^+ moves out, Cl^- moves in, and the membrane potential becomes more negative.

Leakage current accomplishes the same result that voltage-gated K^+ current achieves in the unmyelinated axon.

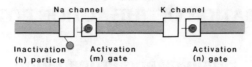

1. Membrane at rest

Na channel   K channel

Inactivation   Activation   Activation
(h) particle   (m) gate   (n) gate

2. Initial stimulus: sodium channel opens,
   Na+ enters axon

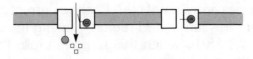

3. At peak of impulse: sodium channel inactivates,
   potassium channel opens, K+ leaves axon:
   refractory period

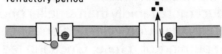

A   4. After refractory period: sodium channel inactivation
      removed, both channels closed

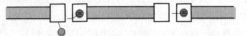

1. Membrane at rest

                  Leakage channels
Na channel   (K+)   (Cl−)

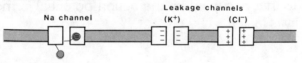

2. Initial stimulus: sodium channel opens, Na+ enters

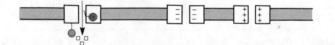

3. At peak of impulse: sodium channel inactivates, K+ and Cl−
   flow through leakage channels to repolarize membrane

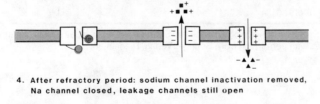

B   4. After refractory period: sodium channel inactivation removed,
      Na channel closed, leakage channels still open

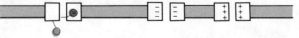

Figure 17   *A*, Sequence of events during the nerve impulse in a large unmyelinated axon. *B*, Sequence of events during the nerve impulse in a mammalian myelinated axon at the node of Ranvier.

UNIT 18
PROPAGATION OF THE ACTION POTENTIAL

Stimulus and Propagation

Depolarization of the axonal membrane to threshold (by electrical current or by natural means) causes an inflow of Na^+. Positive current spreads along the core of the axon away from the stimulated region, making the adjacent region more positive (Figs. 18A and 18B). When this region in turn reaches threshold, the regenerative increase in g_{Na} occurs there as well. Thus, the action potential is a self-propagating event; it serves as the stimulus for the adjacent region of the axon. Once the action potential has been initiated, it propagates with constant velocity.

Large axons conduct more rapidly than smaller ones; myelinated axons (Fig. 18C) conduct more rapidly than unmyelinated ones of equivalent size (Table 18).

An analogy is the burning of a fuse. Once ignited by a flame (stimulus), it burns with constant velocity along its length. However, unlike a fuse, the axonal membrane renews itself for another stimulus (recovery from the refractory period).

The length of axon occupied by an action potential at any one instant is related to conduction velocity. An impulse conducting at 100 m/sec and lasting 1 msec occupies 10 cm of axon; one conducting at 10 m/sec and lasting 1 msec occupies 1 cm of axon.

Since the longitudinal spread of current is more effective in axons of larger diameter and consequent longer length constant (see Unit 12), excitation of regions adjacent to that occupied by the action potential is more effective, and conduction velocity is faster.

TABLE 18   Conduction Velocity and Size of Afferent Myelinated Nerve Axons in the Cat

Function of Nerve Fiber	Mean Fiber Diameter (μm)	Mean Conduction Velocity (m/sec)
Primary muscle spindle afferents	13	75
Mechanoreceptors of the skin	9	55
Deep pressure sensitivity of the muscle	3	11
Unmyelinated pain fibers	1	1

Adapted from Dudel J. Excitation of nerve and muscle. In: Schmidt RF, ed. Fundamentals of neurophysiology. New York: Springer-Verlag, 1975:62. With permission from Springer-Verlag, Heidelberg.

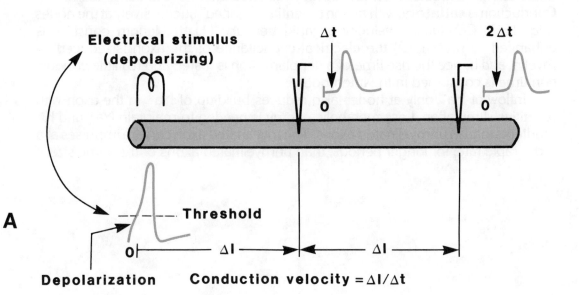

Electrical stimulus (depolarizing)

Δt

$2\Delta t$

0

0

Threshold

0

Δl

Δl

Depolarization

Conduction velocity $= \Delta l / \Delta t$

A

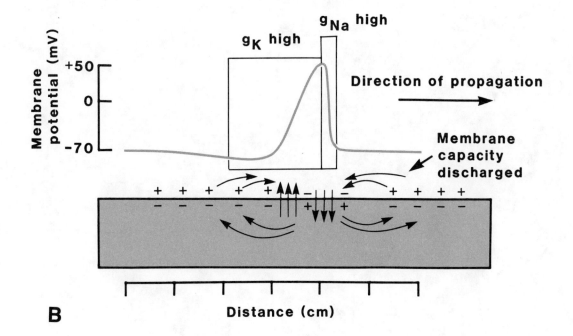

g_K **high**

g_{Na} **high**

Membrane potential (mV)

+50

0

−70

Direction of propagation

Membrane capacity discharged

+ + + + + − − + + + +
− − − − − + + − − − −

Distance (cm)

B

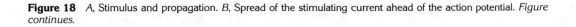

Figure 18 *A*, Stimulus and propagation. *B*, Spread of the stimulating current ahead of the action potential. *Figure continues.*

Myelinated Axons

Regenerative increase in g_{Na} occurs only at nodes. Passive spread of incoming positive charge at one node effectively depolarizes the next, since there is little loss through the myelin sheath of the internode. (Length constant of the myelinated axons is greater than for an unmyelinated axon of the same diameter.) Conduction is **saltatory**, with action potentials "ignited" successively at the nodes (Fig. 18C). Conduction velocity is rapid because (1) the length constant is enhanced by myelin; (2) the electrical capacitance of the axon is reduced by myelin, and hence the rise time of a depolarization is faster; and (3) little conduction time is consumed in the internodes.

Inflow of Na^+ only at nodes also reduces build-up of Na^+ in the axon with repetitive stimulation. Less metabolic energy is needed to maintain Na^+ and K^+ gradients than in unmyelinated axons. The myelinated axon can fire impulses at a more rapid rate, for longer periods, than unmyelinated axons of the same size.

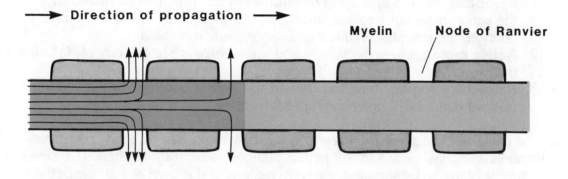

Direction of propagation →

Myelin Node of Ranvier

Nodes are depolarized by current from nearby action potential

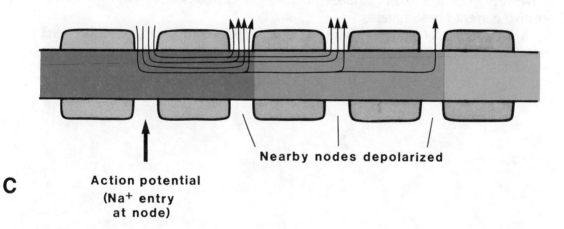

Nearby nodes depolarized

C

Action potential
(Na⁺ entry
at node)

Figure 18(*continued*)   *C,* Saltatory conduction in myelinated axons. (*B,* Modified after Kuffler SW, Nicholls JG, Martin AR. From neuron to brain. Sunderland, MA: Sinauer Associates Inc., 1984:178.)

UNIT 19
INTRACELLULAR AND EXTRACELLULAR ACTION POTENTIALS

Action potentials in the nervous system and in skeletal muscle fibers are often monitored by extracellular electrodes. These electrodes do not impale the cell, but record small voltage changes (often less than 1 mV) close to its surface which are set up by currents entering and leaving the cell during the action potential (Fig. 19A).

In simplifed form, three regions of the axonal membrane can be identified:

1. **Region of forward spread of depolarizing current**, traveling in advance of the action potential. Positive current passes along the core of the axon and changes the potential on the membrane toward threshold.
2. **Active region**, where g_{Na} is high and where there is a large entry of Na^+ into the axon.
3. **Refractory region**, traveling behind the action potential, where outward positive current (K^+ or leakage) predominates.

The extracellular recording reflects these three phases. At a single electrode location, a triphasic extracellular action potential is seen most often. The same picture is obtained by sampling different regions of the axon at a single point in time (Fig. 19B).

The large negative-going "peak" of voltage occurs with Na^+ entry into the active region of the axon. Smaller positive-going peaks occur where outward positive current predominates.

(For a more detailed treatment, consult the reference given for Figure 19B.)

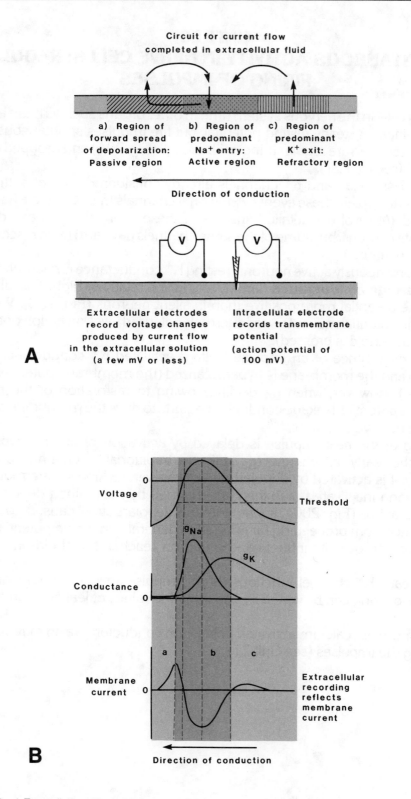

Figure 19 *A,* Extracellular and intracellular recording of action potentials. *B,* Membrane voltage and membrane current. (*B,* Modified after Dudel J. Excitation of nerve and muscle. In: Schmidt RF, ed. Fundamentals of neurophysiology. New York: Springer-Verlag, 1975:58.)

UNIT 20
SPONTANEOUS ACTIVITY IN NERVE CELLS: REGULAR FIRING OF IMPULSES

Many cells in the nervous system (and in other organs such as heart and gut) do not maintain a steady resting potential, but fire impulses spontaneously. Two patterns often seen are regular firing or "beating" (Fig. 20A) and grouped firing or "bursting" (see Unit 21).

The classic Na^+ and K^+ channels already considered are not sufficient in themselves to explain these events. Additional channels that play a role have been discovered. (Most of the detailed analysis of these channels has been done on invertebrate neurons, but some of the same channels have also been discovered in vertebrate neurons.)

In spontaneously active neurons, resting K^+ conductance is relatively low and resting **leakage conductance** (largely for Na^+) is relatively high. This dictates a membrane potential more positive than in silent neurons (Fig. 20B). When the membrane potential moves toward such a depolarized level, an action potential is fired (the threshold is crossed).

With occurrence of an impulse, voltage-activated K^+ conductance (g_K) is turned on and the membrane is hyperpolarized (the membrane potential moves toward E_K). However, when g_K declines owing to restoration of the negative membrane potential, leakage conductance starts to drive the membrane potential again in a positive direction.

Firing of the next impulse is delayed by activation of another type of K^+ channel, the "early" K^+ channel (g_A). Like the traditional K^+ channel considered previously, it is activated by depolarization; however, its kinetics are more rapid, and it is soon inactivated (like the Na^+ channel) by maintained depolarization. While it is active (Fig. 20C), it *prevents* the depolarization caused by leakage conductance from proceeding far enough to generate an action potential. When inactivation removes its influence, the neuron reaches threshold and fires an impulse.

The early K^+ channel functions as an "impulse spacer" for regularly firing cells. Rate of firing can be varied by changing the values of leakage conductance and g_A.

In some cells, calcium-activated potassium conductance also may play a role in spacing the impulses (see Unit 21).

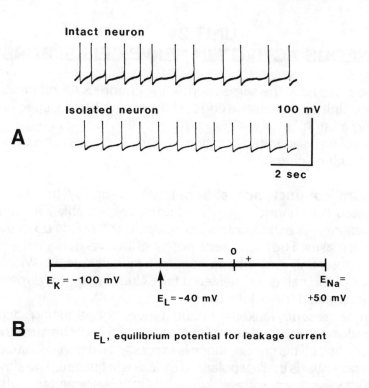

Intact neuron

Isolated neuron

A

100 mV

2 sec

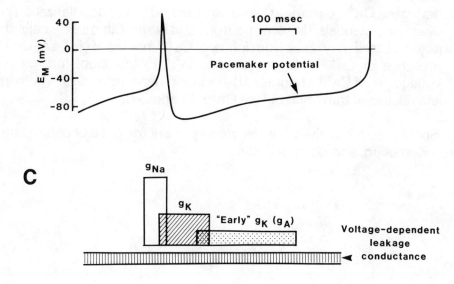

$E_K = -100$ mV
$E_L = -40$ mV

0

$E_{Na} = +50$ mV

B

E_L, equilibrium potential for leakage current

100 msec

Pacemaker potential

E_M (mV)

40
0
-40
-80

C

g_{Na}

g_K

"Early" g_K (g_A)

Voltage-dependent
leakage
conductance

Figure 20 *A*, Spontaneous regular firing of impulses. *B*, Leakage conductance is higher than in silent neurons. *C*, The role of "early" K+ current as a "brake" to space impulses. (*A*, Adapted from Alving BO. Spontaneous activity in isolated somata of *Aplysia* pacemaker neurons. J Gen Physiol 1968; 51:35. *C*, Modified after Connor JA, Stevens CF. Prediction of repetitive firing behaviour from voltage clamp data on an isolated neurone soma. J Physiol 1971; 213:47.)

UNIT 21
SPONTANEOUS ACTIVITY IN NERVE CELLS: BURSTING

Bursting neurons have the same membrane channels found in neurons that fire regularly (see Unit 20), and these conductances regulate the spacing of action potentials during a burst.

The pattern of well-separated bursts of action potentials is brought about by additional conductance channels.

1. A **potassium conductance channel** turned on by intracellular Ca^{++} (calcium-gated K^+ channel, $g_{K(Ca)}$) is largely responsible for the interburst hyperpolarization. As action potentials occur, Ca^{++} builds up in the neuron, and $g_{K(Ca)}$ increases. The membrane potential is driven toward the potassium equilibrium potential, and thus is kept at a negative level. When Ca^{++}_i is pumped out of the cell or sequestered (see Unit 34), $g_{K(Ca)}$ diminishes, and depolarizing conductances take over.

2. In addition to resting leakage conductance, the bursting neuron typically has a **slow, voltage-dependent conductance channel** that admits Na^+, Ca^{++}, or both. This conductance is expressed when $g_{K(Ca)}$ subsides. The membrane potential is then depolarized by leakage current. The slow depolarizing conductances predominate during the impulse-generating phase of the burst cycle (see "Depolarizing conductances" in Figure 21).

3. Entry of Ca^{++} into the neuron is brought about largely through **voltage-activated Ca^{++} channels**, which are opened by the depolarization produced by action potentials. (In some neurons and in smooth muscle cells, the action potential itself may result from inflow of Ca^{++} instead of Na^+; see Unit 56.) The presence of Ca^{++} channels allows Ca^{++} to build up, turning on $g_{K(Ca)}$. Voltage-gated Ca^{++} channels also occur in nerve terminals, where they regulate release of transmitters (see Units 33 and 34).

Spontaneously active neurons are important for circuits controlling respiration, locomotion, and other activities.

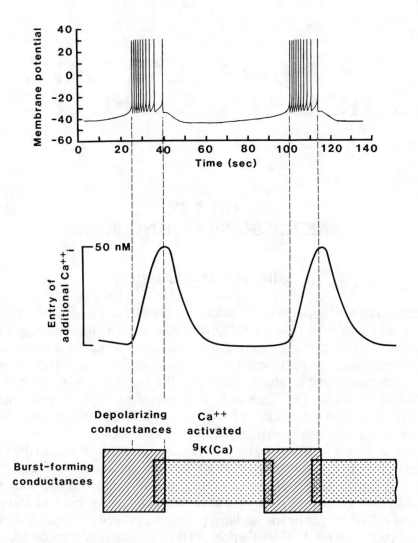

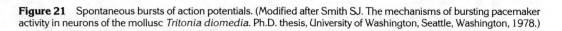

Figure 21 Spontaneous bursts of action potentials. (Modified after Smith SJ. The mechanisms of bursting pacemaker activity in neurons of the mollusc *Tritonia diomedia*. Ph.D. thesis, University of Washington, Seattle, Washington, 1978.)

4

MOLECULAR AND INTRACELLULAR PROCESSES

UNIT 22
ENERGY SUPPLY OF NEURONS

Glucose and Oxygen

Nervous tissue (especially the brain) is critically dependent on a continuous supply of glucose and oxygen for production of the high-energy phosphate compounds ATP and phosphocreatine. These compounds are the immediate source of energy for cellular reactions. There is little glycogen in mammalian nerve cells, and glucose must be transported into the central nervous system through the blood–brain barrier (see Unit 2) to maintain the supply of substrate for ATP production (Fig. 22A). Amounts of oxygen consumed and carbon dioxide produced show that glucose is almost fully oxidized to CO_2.

Neurons take up glucose by carrier-mediated transport. Within the cell, ATP is produced and subsequently used in metabolic reactions. A major consumer (accounting for up to 40 percent of energy consumption) is the sodium pump. ATP production in the brain is linked to neural activity: As more action potentials occur, more ATP is split by the sodium pump and more adenosine diphosphate (ADP) is produced. As ADP levels rise, ATP production is stimulated, and more glucose is required.

Regions of the brain that are more active have higher rates of glucose uptake and increased local blood circulation. New imaging techniques are available to monitor these changes in vivo.

ATP

Production of ATP in nervous tissue proceeds mainly through the aerobic pathways associated with mitochondria (Fig. 22B). Glycolytic metabolism is less productive and cannot sustain brain function for more than a few minutes. Oxygen deprivation leads to irreversible changes that result in cell death.

The sodium pump is one of many ATPases that draw energy from ATP and, secondarily, from the "energy buffer," phosphocreatine. ATPase activity leads to ADP production; ADP is used in enzymatic reactions that regenerate ATP (see Fig. 22B).

Under conditions of high energy demand, phosphocreatine is used to regenerate ATP, and the cellular levels of ATP remain nearly constant until the phosphocreatine supply is exhausted. This rarely occurs in nervous tissue. Total "energy charge" (ATP plus phosphocreatine) is generally regulated within a narrow range, even though the *rate of energy consumption* varies greatly with functional demand. Local blood flow increases in regions of the brain that are active.

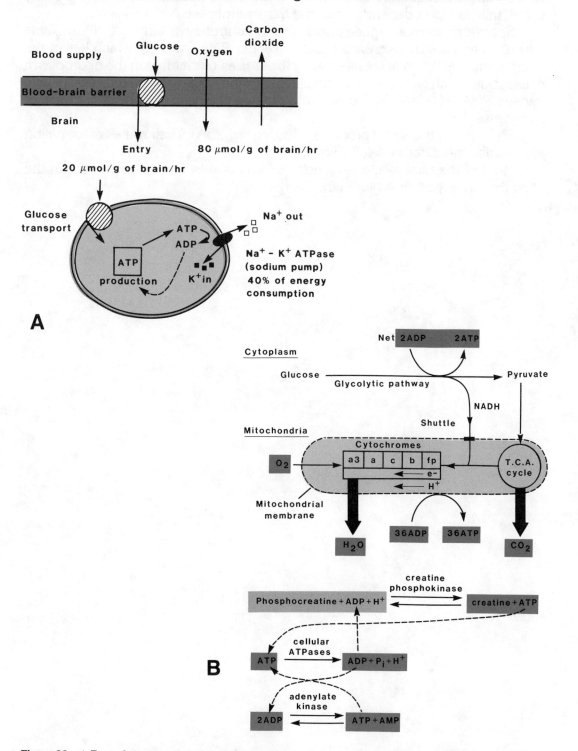

Figure 22 *A*, Entry of glucose into the brain and into neurons. *B*, Production of ATP from glucose. (*B*, Adapted from Carlson FD, Wilkie DR. Muscle physiology. Englewood Cliffs: Prentice-Hall, 1974:97.)

UNIT 23
NEURONAL PROTEINS

Protein synthesis requires substrate amino acids, which reach the central nervous system by specific transport mechanisms at the blood-brain barrier (see Unit 2) and subsequently enter nerve cells by membrane transport. (In many cases, this transport depends upon the transmembrane Na^+ gradient.)

Specific proteins are made under genetic control. Segments of DNA available for expression are **transcribed** into messenger RNA (mRNA), which leaves the nucleus and becomes associated with **ribosomes** (either free in the neuroplasm or associated with endoplasmic reticulum). Amino acids (associated with specific transfer RNA, or tRNA) are formed into peptide chains in the polyribosomes, or polysomes.

Three major classes of protein are found (Fig. 23A). Their routes of formation and distribution differ in detail (Fig. 23B).

More of the total available genetic information in DNA is expressed in the brain than in any other organ in the body.

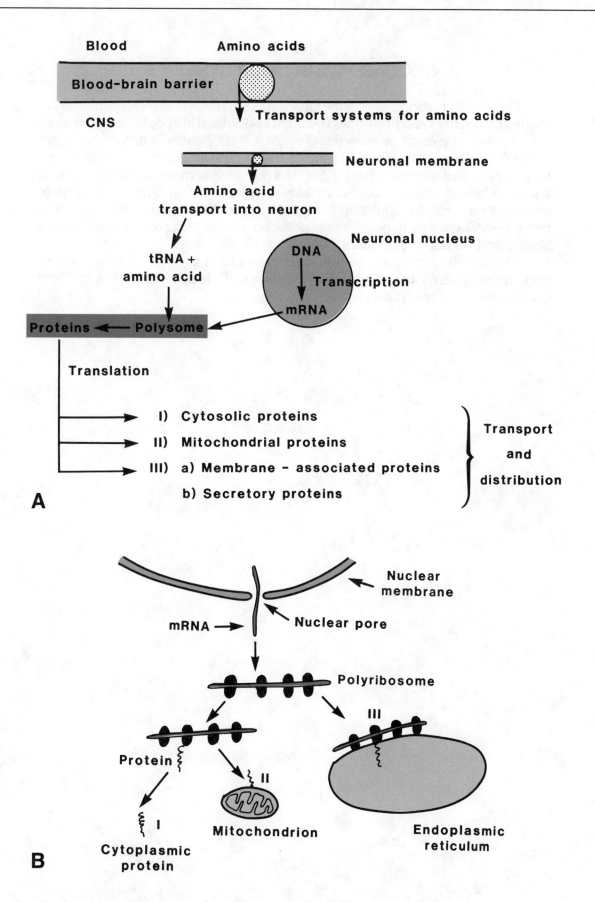

Figure 23 *A,* General path for protein synthesis. *B,* Details of protein synthesis.

UNIT 24
SECOND MESSENGER SYSTEMS

Nerve cells respond to changes in impulse activity or to extracellular signals (neurotransmitters and hormones) through specialized intracellular signaling systems known as second messengers (Fig. 24A, II). In general, extracellular signals or ion fluxes (especially of Ca^{++}) activate membrane-associated enzyme systems for production of a second messenger. The messenger molecule in turn activates a protein kinase, which phosphorylates a substrate protein. The phosphorylated protein plays a role in regulating a physiological or biochemical response of the nerve cell. Control of genetic expression can also be regulated by extracellular signals and second messengers.

Cyclic AMP provides a well-studied example of the way in which second messenger systems work (Fig. 24B). Physiological effects mediated by cAMP are considered later (see Unit 41).

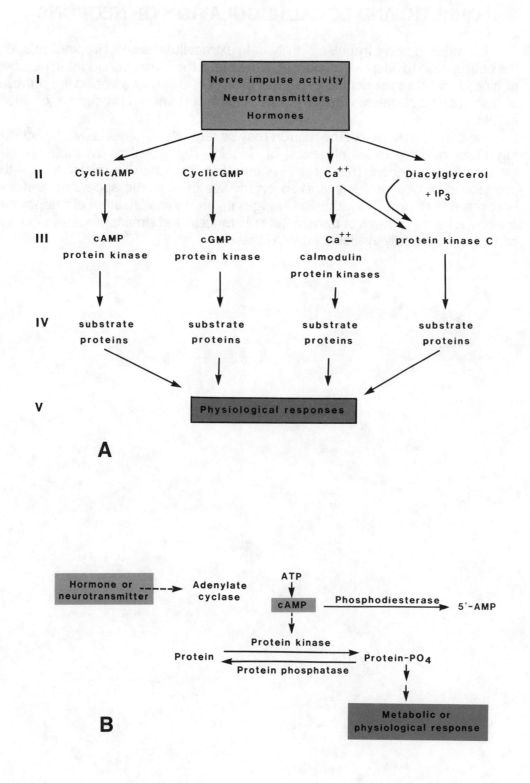

Figure 24 *A*, General overview of the role of second messenger systems. *B*, Cyclic AMP as a second messenger: protein phosphorylation. (*B*, Adapted from Greengard P. Phosphorylated proteins as physiological effectors. Science 1978; 199:147.)

UNIT 25
GENETIC AND LOCAL REGULATION OF NEURONS

Changes in nerve impulse activity or in extracellular signals impinging upon the neuron lead to adaptive responses. These take the form of changes in number or type of membrane channels, changes in level of enzymes involved in synthesis of transmitter substances, growth or retraction of neuronal processes, or other events.

Adaptive responses of the neuron may be regulated "genetically" (by activating a new or different set of genes) or "locally" (by activating available protein kinases through second messenger systems; Fig. 25). Changes related to growth, production of new proteins, and so on involve the genetic apparatus and the mechanisms of protein synthesis. Changes involving modification of membrane channels, local synthesis of transmitter substances, and similar processes can be carried out by locally available protein kinases.

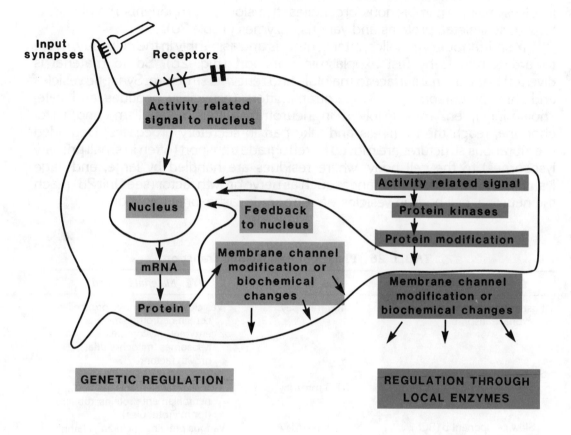

Figure 25 Genetic regulation versus local regulation of neuronal physiological properties. (Modified after Atwood HL. Modifiability of single identified neurons in crustaceans. In: Alkon DL, Woody CD, eds. Neural mechanisms of conditioning. New York: Plenum Press, 1985:332.)

UNIT 26
AXONAL TRANSPORT: PROCESSES AND MATERIALS

Proteins synthesized in the neuronal cell body are moved to axon terminals by **axonal transport**. In motoneurons that have long axons, distances of centimeters to meters are involved.

Axonal transport has **fast** and **slow** components. The fast component involves mainly membranous organelles, the slower components mainly structural (cytoskeletal) proteins and various enzymes (Table 26).

Membranous organelles, after synthesis and assembly in the cell body, move toward terminals by fast axoplasmic transport (Fig. 26). Some material is diverted to the axonal surface to maintain and renew its structure. Synaptic vesicles and their precursors, some neurotransmitters (especially peptides and catecholamines), enzymes involved in neurotransmitter metabolism, and mitochondria, reach the terminals and take part in secretory processes. Degraded membranous structures are moved by retrograde transport (often in small primary lysosomes) to the cell body, where residues are handled by large, end-stage lysosomes. In addition, substances such as nerve growth factor (see Unit 28) reach the neuronal cell body in vesicles via retrograde fast axonal transport.

TABLE 26   Phases of Axoplasmic Transport

Phase	Rate of Transport	Materials Moved
Fast anterograde or retrograde axonal transport	400 mm/day	Vesicles, membranous organelles, certain neurotransmitters, enzymes, glycoproteins, lysosomes, mitochondria, growth factors
Slow axoplasmic flow		
Slow component a (SCa)	0.5-3 mm/day	Cytoskeletal elements, particularly: neurofilament proteins; tubulins (for microtubules)
Slow component b (SCb)	5-10 mm/day	Various proteins, including clathrin, actin, metabolic enzymes

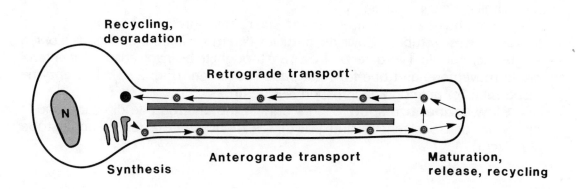

Figure 26   Fast axoplasmic transport. (Modified after Kandell ER, Schwartz JH. Principles of neural science. New York: Elsevier, 1985:42.)

UNIT 27
AXONAL TRANSPORT: MECHANISMS

Fast axonal transport involves microtubules and an ATP-splitting enzyme (ATPase), referred to as a force-generating enzyme (FGE). The FGE is normally present as a soluble protein in axoplasm, but can attach to both microtubules and vesicles.

The neuronal cell body is not required for fast axonal transport. Particles can be moved by microtubules in axoplasm extracted from an axon, provided that ATP is available.

Recent evidence suggests that the FGE attaches preferentially to the microtubule and to membrane-bound vesicles. Splitting of ATP leads to a relative force between the microtubule and the vesicle (Fig. 27A). The force is probably generated by a conformational change of the FGE induced by ATP splitting (see Unit 55 for a similar case in muscle).

Microtubules are "polarized" so that the relative force is exerted in one direction along a microtubule. However, particles can move in both directions along a single microtubule. Two different FGEs are thought to be involved: one for anterograde movement, and one for retrograde movement (Fig. 27B). The enzyme responsible for anterograde transport is **kinesin**.

Slow axonal transport occurs only in the anterograde direction and is necessary for axonal renewal and growth. The motive force is not well understood at present.

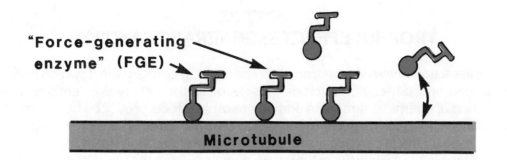

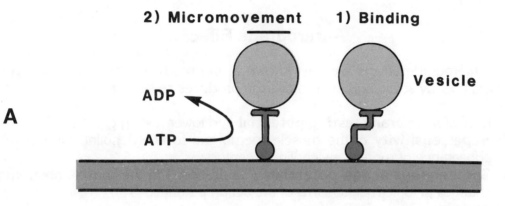

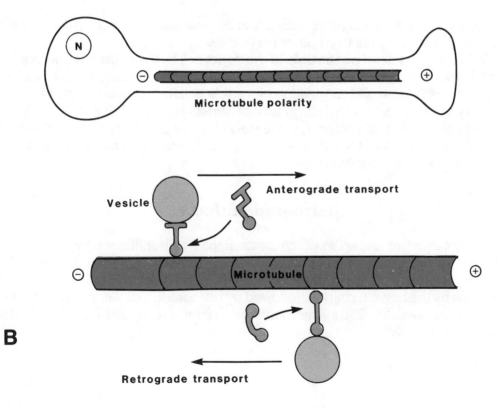

Figure 27 *A,* Force-generating enzyme and microtubule. *B,* Anterograde and retrograde fast axonal transport. (*B,* Modified after Schnapp BJ, Reese TS. New developments in understanding rapid axonal transport. Trends Neurosci 1986; 9(4):161.)

UNIT 28
TROPHIC EFFECTS: GENERAL FEATURES

Interaction between a neuron and other cells in contact with it (which may be other neurons, target cells such as muscle, or glial cells) involves emission and reception of chemical signals. In addition to rapid effects produced by transmitter substances, long-term effects (often called **trophic effects**) are produced.

Trophic effects can occur in the **anterograde** direction (from the neuron to the target; Fig. 28A) or in the **retrograde** direction (from the postsynaptic target to the neuron; Fig. 28B).

Anterograde Effects

Anterograde effects are best known in the motor system. Denervating a muscle fiber by sectioning the motor axon produces several effects:

1. Loss of **membrane resting potential** and lower resting g_K;
2. **Supersensitivity** of the muscle membrane to acetylcholine, due to the appearance of more acetylcholine receptors;
3. **Spontaneous action potentials** ("fibrillation") in the muscle fiber, and changes in ionic mechanisms of the action potential;
4. **Atrophy** of the muscle fiber; and
5. **Loss of acetylcholinesterase activity** at the motor end-plate.

Some of these effects (especially 2 and 3) have also been seen in nerve cells that have lost their inputs from other nerve cells.

Induction of **action potentials** in the target cell by the neuron is one trophic effect. Thus, treating motor axons with a local anesthetic, with consequent block of synaptic transmission and elimination of muscle action potentials, leads to supersensitivity of the target, even though axonal transport can still occur.

It is also likely that molecules released in small amounts from the axonal terminals are important for some of the trophic effects (such as maintenance of the resting membrane potential).

Retrograde Effects

Many cases are known in which postsynaptic cells influence the neuron. In particular, **nerve growth factor** taken up by neurons causes them to elongate.

The general mechanism for retrograde effects is pinocytotic uptake of trophic molecules by the nerve terminals, followed by retrograde axoplasmic transport to the cell body (see Fig. 28B). Presynaptic membrane receptors for trophic substances may be involved in some cases.

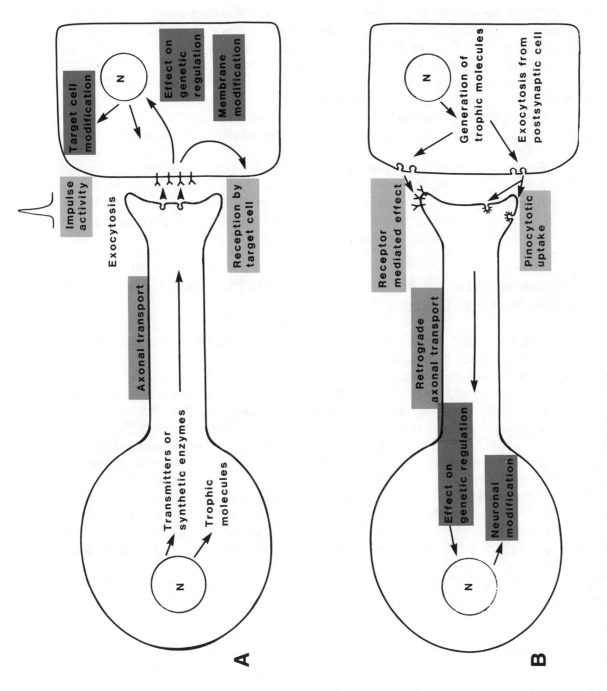

Figure 28 *A,* Trophic effects of neuron on target. *B,* Trophic effects of target on neuron.

UNIT 29
TROPHIC EFFECTS: NERVE GROWTH, SPECIFICITY

Nerve growth factor. Nerve growth factor (NGF) is extracted from various tissues. It promotes growth of axons in culture. Antibodies against NGF inhibit development of the sympathetic nervous system.

Cellular adhesion molecule. A cellular adhesion molecule (CAM) is a membrane glycoprotein that promotes interaction of axons to form nerve bundles. Antibodies against CAM inhibit the formation of axon bundles.

Glial cells. Schwann cells from peripheral nerves promote growth of central axons; growth is not promoted by glial cells from the central nervous system (Fig. 29).

Embryonic brain cell transplants. Regeneration of axons in the central nervous system is promoted by transplantation of embryonic brain cells.

Specificity in regeneration. In lower vertebrates, axons of retinal ganglion cells grow back after transection to connect specific parts of the retina to the correct parts of the central nervous system (optic tectum).

Mechanisms for Establishing Specificity and Final Connections in the Nervous System

1. **Cell lineage.** During development, groups of cells are genetically predestined to form parts of the nervous system.
2. **Growth and guidance.** Axons are guided by trophic factors and cell-to-cell surface interactions to form specific connections. "Instruction molecules" are important in this process; probably there is a large number of them.
3. **Cell death.** Cells that are less active, or less able to form specific connections, die during development. In some parts of the central nervous system and in peripheral ganglia, there is a considerable loss of neurons during development.
4. **Competition.** Terminals of surviving and developing cells compete for available connection sites of target cells. Overall activity and functional demand shape and remodel the pathways in the central nervous system. During adult life, synapse elimination and terminal growth can still occur.

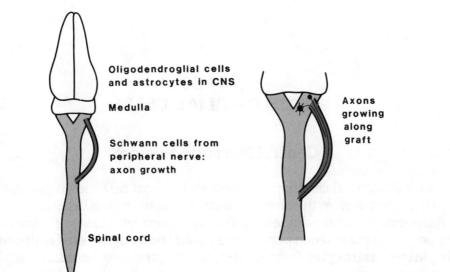

Oligodendroglial cells
and astrocytes in CNS

Medulla

Schwann cells from
peripheral nerve:
axon growth

Spinal cord

Axons
growing
along
graft

Figure 29   Growth of central neurons along Schwann cell bridge. (Modified after David S, Aguayo AJ. Axonal elongation into peripheral nervous system injury in adult rats. Science 1981; 214:931.)

5

GLIAL CELLS

UNIT 30
TYPES OF GLIAL CELLS

Central Nervous System

Glial cells are smaller than neurons and at least 50 times more numerous. The major types seen in the central nervous system (Fig. 30A) are:

Astrocytes. "Star-shaped" cells with many processes. **Fibrous astrocytes** are found in axon-rich parts of the central nervous system (**white matter**). **Protoplasmic astrocytes** (with shorter, stouter processes) predominate in parts of the central nervous system containing neuronal cell bodies and synapses (**gray matter**). Astrocytes often come into contact with both neurons and capillaries.

Oligodendrocytes. Small glial cells with few processes. They are responsible for forming the myelin sheath around myelinated axons. One oligodendrocyte forms the myelin for several central axons (Fig. 30B).

Other types of glial cells in the central nervous system are **ependymal cells**, which occur in the lining of the central canal system of the brain and spinal cord, and **microglia**, which are mobilized in response to injury or disease and become phagocytic (removing debris or damaged tissue).

Peripheral Nervous System

Schwann cell. The counterpart of the oligodendrocyte in peripheral nerves. Each Schwann cell is associated with one axon and forms a single myelin segment over approximately 1 mm of axon.

Unmyelinated axons are enclosed singly or in groups within ensheathing glial cells that do not form tight wrappings of myelin.

Myelin sheath is composed of Schwann cell wrappings from which the cytoplasm has largely disappeared. It is 80 percent lipid and 20 percent protein.

At the gaps between adjacent myelin wrappings, the axon is partly or completely exposed (the **node of Ranvier**). The myelinated section of axon between two nodes of Ranvier is an **internode**.

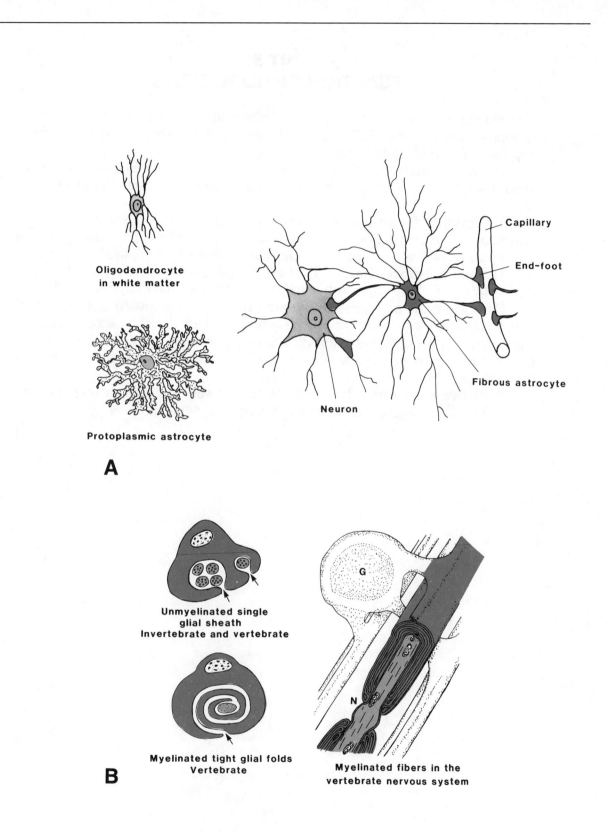

Figure 30 *A*, Types of glial cells. *B*, Relationships between axons and glial cells. (*A*, Modified after Kandel ER, Schwartz JH. Principles of neural science. New York: Elsevier, 1985:18. *B*, From Shepherd GM. Neurobiology. New York: Oxford University Press, 1988:62 and adapted from Bunge MB, Bunge RP, Ris H. Ultrastructural study of remyelination in an experimental lesion in adult cat spinal cord. J Biophys Biochem Cytol 1961; 10:79.)

UNIT 31
FUNCTION OF GLIAL CELLS

Structural. Astrocytes provide support for neurons and separation for groups of neurons, or individual parts of neurons. Astrocyte processes also cover capillaries in the central nervous system.

Nerve conduction. Oligodendrocytes and Schwann cells form the myelin sheath around myelinated axons, enabling them to conduct impulses more rapidly (see Unit 18).

Buffering of extracellular ionic concentrations. Some of the K^+ released by nerve cells during activity is taken up by glial cells. Astrocytes may convey some of this liberated K^+ to capillaries, where it enters the bloodstream.

Uptake of transmitters. Transmitters released by neurons are taken up rapidly by glial cells through high-affinity transport systems (Fig. 31)(see Unit 38).

Development and growth. Some glial cells are involved in growth of neurons to specific locations during development. Nerve regeneration is aided or prevented by glial cells (see Unit 29). Schwann cells promote regeneration of peripheral neurons; glial cell proliferation in the central nervous system after injury prevents regeneration of central neurons.

Nutritive functions. It is possible, but not well established except in a few cases, that glial cells provide metabolic support for neurons.

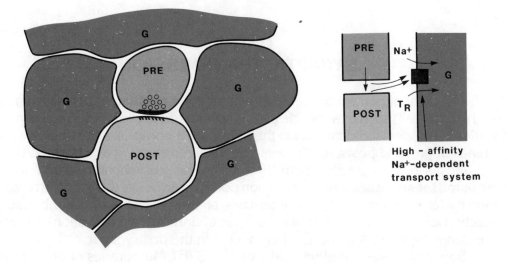

Figure 31 Inactivation of transmitter substance (T_R) by glial cell (G) uptake.

6

SYNAPSES

UNIT 32
SYNAPTIC TRANSMISSION

The point of contact between one neuron and another, or between a neuron and a target cell (such as a muscle cell), is specialized to allow cell-to-cell communication. The specialized contact is the **synapse**; it comprises the adjacent membranes of pre- and postsynaptic cells and the intervening space (Fig. 32A).

Most synapses are **chemical** (Fig. 32B). The presynaptic neuron releases a **transmitter substance** when an action potential arrives at the axon terminal. The transmitter substance acts on **receptors** of the postsynaptic membrane. The reaction leads to opening or closing of ionic channels, *or* to activation of a second messenger system. A response then occurs in the postsynaptic cell.

Some synapses are **electrical** (see Fig. 32B). Membranes of pre- and postsynaptic cells are joined by connecting channels that bridge a narrow separation (**gap junction**). Electrical current can flow directly into the postsynaptic cell from the presynaptic cell.

Electrical synapses are found in pathways involved in rapid stereotyped responses and also among brain cells in which near-synchronous electrical activity occurs.

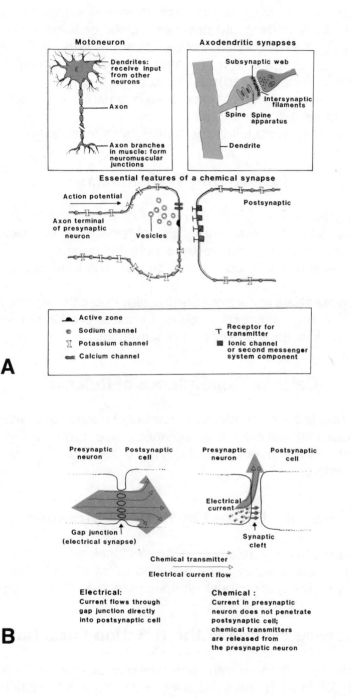

Figure 32 *A*, Synapses. *B*, Chemical and electrical transmission.

UNIT 33
RELEASE OF TRANSMITTER SUBSTANCES

Action potentials arriving at the nerve terminal stop there because they cannot drive electrical current into the postsynaptic cell and they cannot return along the presynaptic axon (because of the refractory period).

The major role of the action potential in releasing transmitter is to open **calcium channels** (voltage-gated). Ca^{++} enters the presynaptic nerve terminal. A calcium-catalyzed reaction leads to exocytosis of synaptic vesicles. (The nature of the reaction is not yet fully worked out.)

A summary of the events leading to transmitter release is given in Figure 33A.

Fast-Acting Transmitters

Each exocytotic event (probably release of the contents of one synaptic vesicle) results in a few thousand molecules of transmitter substance hitting the postsynaptic membrane. A small electrical potential appears in the postsynaptic cell. The potential is relatively constant in size, so it is termed a quantal unit of transmission.

Synaptic potentials result from one to many quantal units acting **synchronously** (Fig. 33B). Asynchronous release does not produce a large synaptic potential, because individual events do not summate.

Calcium Dependence of Release

The amount of transmitter released (number of quantal units) depends on the amount of calcium that enters the presynaptic nerve terminal (Fig. 33C). Thus, reducing calcium in the extracellular solution, or blocking Ca^{++} channels, reduces transmitter secretion.

Release Evoked by Action Potentials

An action potential is a relatively large electrical event, and it opens many voltage-gated calcium channels. The resulting influx of Ca^{++} favors release of many synaptic vesicles; a large, brief synaptic potential often occurs.

Release Evoked Without Action Potentials

In many neurons the membrane potential may be changed without evoking an action potential. In such cases, relatively few voltage-gated calcium channels are opened (or closed), and a small change in presynaptic Ca^{++} results. The resulting postsynaptic potential is usually smaller and slower than it would be if an action potential were to occur in the same presynaptic neuron (see Fig. 33C). However, many cells in the retina (and elsewhere) transmit without action potentials.

Recently, some cells in the retina have been found to transmit in the absence of calcium, so there may be more than one mechanism for transmitter release.

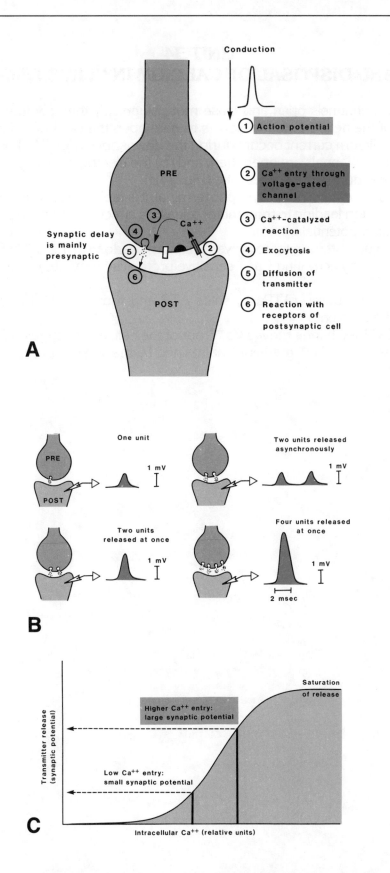

Figure 33 *A*, Action potential triggers release of transmitter. *B*, Each unit of release has a small postsynaptic effect. *C*, Dependence of transmitter release on intracellular calcium. (*C*, Adapted from Atwood HL, Wojtowicz JM. Short-term and long-term plasticity and physiological differentiation of crustacean motor synapses. Int Rev Neurobiol 1986; 28:306.)

UNIT 34
ENTRY AND DISPOSAL OF CALCIUM IN NERVE TERMINALS

Calcium channels open and close more sluggishly than sodium channels. The peak of the action potential serves to gate open the calcium channels, but maximum calcium current occurs during the downstroke (Fig. 34A) because (a) more calcium channels are open then, and (b) the electrical driving force ($E_m - E_{Ca}$) is greater during the downstroke (Fig. 34B).

Once Ca^{++} enters the presynaptic terminal, it is rapidly inactivated (Fig. 34C). Thus the reaction leading to transmitter release is effective for only 0.5 to 2 msec after the action potential.

Two major systems exist to prevent calcium overload in the cell (which could destroy the cell by activating Ca^{++}-sensitive proteolytic enzymes):

1. The calcium pump (ATPase) splits ATP and moves Ca^{++} out of the cell against a gradient.
2. Na^+-Ca^{++} exchange moves Ca^{++} out of the cell in exchange for Na^+ entry; requires a steep Na^+ gradient (maintained by the sodium pump).

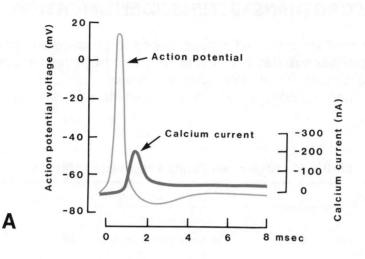

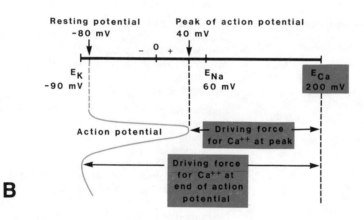

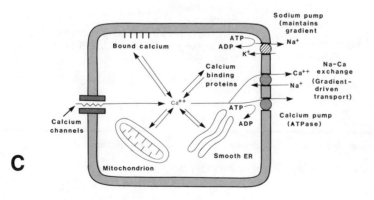

Figure 34 *A*, Calcium current (giant synapse). *B*, Electrical force acting on calcium. *C*, Fate of intracellular calcium. (*A*, Modified after Llinas R. Calcium in synaptic transmission. Sci Am 1982; 247:64-65.)

UNIT 35
NEUROTRANSMITTERS: IDENTIFICATION

Individual neurons are genetically regulated to produce one or more substances (**transmitter substances**) that are released from the nerve terminals to affect postsynaptic cells (most often other neurons).

The major known and suspected neurotransmitters are listed in Table 35.

TABLE 35   Known and Putative Neurotransmitters

System	Compound
Cholinergic	Acetylcholine (Ach)
Amino acidergic (amino acid transmitters)	Gamma-aminobutyric acid (GABA) Aspartate Glutamate Glycine Histamine Taurine
Monoaminergic (biogenic amine transmitters)	Adrenaline (epinephrine)† Dopamine† Noradrenaline (norepinephrine)† Serotonin (5-hydroxytryptamine, or 5-HT) Tryptamine Octopamine
Peptidergic*	Angiotensin Bombesin Carnosine Cholecystokinin Endorphins, Dynorphin Luteinizing hormone releasing hormone (LHRH) Methionine and leucine enkephalins Motilin Neuromedins (A to C) Neuropeptide Y Neurotensin Oxytocin Somatostatin Substance P Thyroid hormone releasing hormone (TRH) Vasoactive intestinal peptide (VIP) Vasopressin
Purinergic	Adenosine ADP AMP ATP

* Other peptides are suspected to be neurotransmitters, but are less well established.
† Catecholamines.
Adapted from Bradford HF. Chemical neurobiology. New York: WH Freeman, 1986:157.

Criteria for Identifying a Transmitter Substance

To be classified as a neurotransmitter a substance must meet the following criteria:

1. It produces the physiological effects of normal synaptic transmission.
2. It is present in the presynaptic nerve terminals.
3. The presynaptic neuron has the enzymes to make the transmitter.
4. The substance is released in sufficient quantity by nerve impulses to produce the known physiological effects.

Not all the substances listed in Table 35 have met these criteria, but they have met at least some of them.

Neuromodulators and Co-Transmitters

Substances that modify the action or release of a neurotransmitter, but do not have a strong effect by themselves, are termed **neuromodulators**. (Examples include several peptides and 5-hydroxytryptamine.)

Two (or possibly more) substances may be released from the same terminal and cause different effects. Usually one substance is a peptide, which may act as a neuromodulator.

General Classification

As shown in Table 35, several classes of molecule are used as transmitters.

Peptides must be made in the cell body and transported to the terminals for release. Most of the other compounds can be made in the terminals, by enzymes transported from the cell body, from precursors taken up by the neuron (Fig. 35).

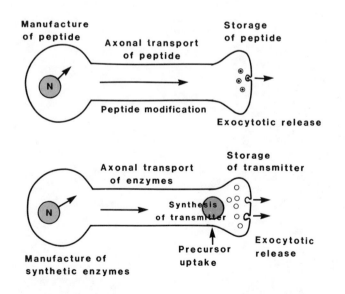

Figure 35 Peptide and nonpeptide traffic in the neuron.

UNIT 36
ACETYLCHOLINE

Acetylcholine is generated within the nerve terminal by reaction of the precursors **choline** and **acetyl coenzyme A**, catalyzed by **choline acetyltransferase**.

Choline acetyltransferase is synthesized in the neuron and delivered by axonal transport. **Acetyl coenzyme A** is derived from glucose metabolism (via pyruvate) by mitochondrial enzymes. **Choline** is taken into the nerve terminal by specific transport molecules. Availability of substrates becomes rate-limiting during activity.

After it is released from synaptic vesicles (some claim it is released directly from the cytoplasm and not from vesicles), acetylcholine is hydrolyzed and some of the choline is recycled into the nerve terminal.

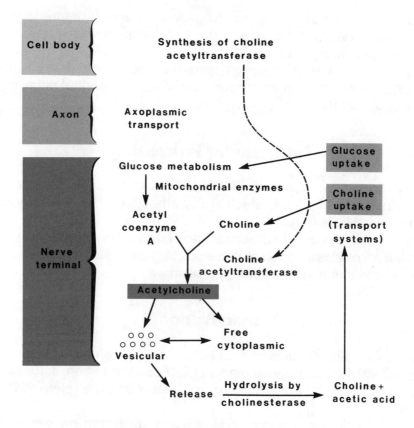

Figure 36 Steps in the synthesis and breakdown of acetylcholine.

UNIT 37
MONOAMINES

Synthesis

The precursor **tyrosine** gives rise to catecholamines (noradrenaline, adrenaline, dopamine). Tyrosine is derived from cellular metabolism and also arrives through the blood-brain barrier (Fig. 37A).

The precursor **tryptophan** gives rise to the indolamine serotonin (Fig. 37B). Tryptophan is derived from dietary sources and reaches central neurons through the blood-brain barrier.

Intracellular Processing

Amines are produced in the cell body, axon, and terminals. They are incorporated into dense-cored vesicles, which are synthesized in the cell body and transported to the terminals (Fig. 37C).

Dense-cored vesicles of noradrenergic neurons contain the enzyme **dopamine beta-hydroxylase**, which makes noradrenaline from dopamine. They also contain ATP and a transmitter-binding protein.

Inactivation

Monoamines are inactivated after release by high-affinity transport systems (Na^+-dependent) in neurons and adjacent glial cells. In addition, diffusion from the synapse, and low-affinity transport systems, remove some released transmitter (Fig. 37D).

Within the cell, the mitochondrial enzyme **monoamine oxidase** (MAO) breaks down some of the free transmitter. Inhibition of this enzyme elevates levels of monoamine transmitters in the neuron.

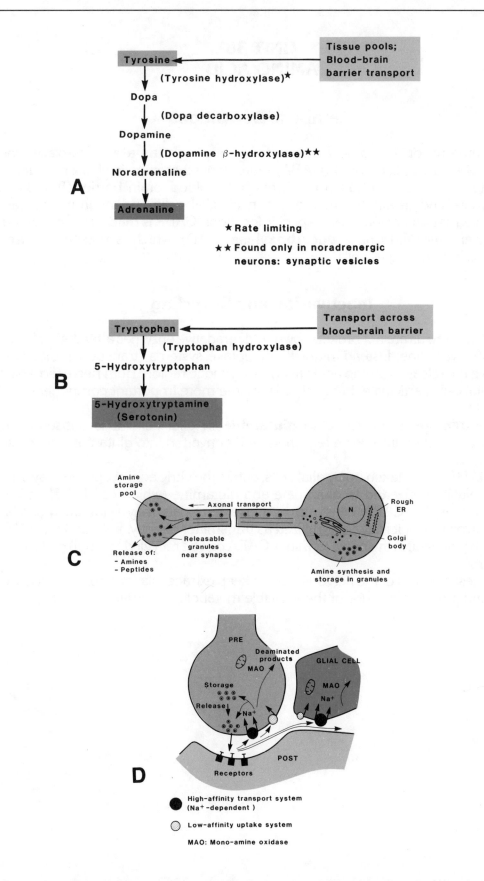

Figure 37   *A*, Synthesis of catecholamines. *B*, Synthesis of serotonin. *C*, Transport and storage of biogenic amines. *D*, Inactivation of monoamines (MAO). (*C*, Modified after Bradford HF. Chemical neurobiology. New York: WH Freeman, 1986:268.)

UNIT 38
AMINO ACID

Metabolic Derivations

Three major amino acid neurotransmitters — **glutamate**, **aspartate**, and **gamma-aminobutyric acid** (GABA) — are derived metabolically from glucose and do not have to be taken up through the blood-brain barrier (Fig. 38A). Glutamate and aspartate are present in all glial cells and neurons, but are employed as transmitters only in specific locations. GABA is made from glutamate by the enzyme **glutamate decarboxylase** (GAD), which is present in some neurons but not in glial cells.

Inactivation and Recycling

Amino acids are not broken down by degradative enzymes after their release, as is acetylcholine. Instead, high-affinity uptake systems (transport molecules) remove the released amino acids from the synaptic region. Both nerve terminals and glial cells participate, but glial cells are the more important component (see Unit 31).

Glutamate is converted to **glutamine** in glial cells. It is subsequently released, taken up into nerve terminals, and converted into glutamate for re-use (Fig. 38B).

GABA, when taken up by glial cells, enters the citric acid cycle and may then eventually be converted to glutamate and glutamine (which can be relayed to nerve terminals). GABA taken up by nerve terminals may undergo a similar transformation, or it may be re-utilized as transmitter directly. Provided that GAD enzyme is present in the nerve terminal, GABA can be recycled through glutamate (Fig. 38C).

These features of the nervous system keep extracellular amino acids at a low level and provide for re-use of the available metabolic substrates.

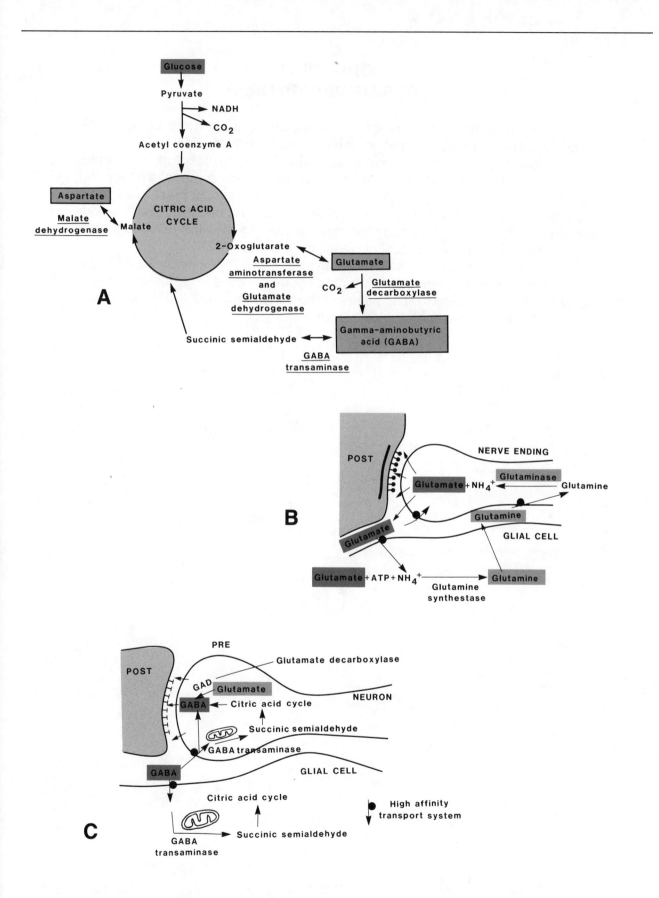

Figure 38 *A*, Simplified scheme showing the derivation of amino acid neurotransmitters. *B*, Recycling of glutamate. *C*, Recycling of gamma-aminobutyric acid (GABA). (Modified after Bradford HF. Chemical neurobiology. New York: WH Freeman, 1986:121, 143, 218.)

UNIT 39
TYPES OF RECEPTORS

For each of the "small-molecule" neurotransmitters, there are generally several types of receptor mediating different physiological effects. Some of the better-known receptors are summarized in Table 39. Many receptors are coupled to second messenger systems, and hence act on cellular metabolism (see Unit 41). The complexities of receptor distribution and effect must be studied separately for each region of the central nervous system and for each effector. The wide range of available receptors and their modulation provides the nervous system and its effectors with a great deal of plasticity.

In general, responses evoked by a transmitter are governed by the nature of the receptors and the elements to which they are coupled (e.g., ionic channels, second messenger system). The nature of the transmitter itself is not the primary factor determining the physiological response.

TABLE 39   Types of Receptor

Transmitter System	Receptor Type	Pharmacologic Agents	Examples of Mechanism and Location
Acetylcholine	Nicotinic	Blocked by curare; activated by nicotine	Neuromuscular junction (ionic channels)
	Muscarinic	Blocked by atropine; activated by muscarine	Smooth muscle; cardiac muscle, central brain regions (involves second messenger)
Monoamines	Alpha-adrenoreceptor (for norepinephrine)	Blocked by phentolamine	Glands; smooth muscle (Ca^{++} influx and other ionic events)
	Beta-adrenoreceptor (for norepinephrine)	Blocked by propranolol	Heart; smooth muscle (coupled to adenylate cyclase; protein phosphorylation)
	Dopamine receptors D1 type	Bind dopamine preferentially	Central nervous system; sympathetic ganglia coupled to adenylate cyclase)
	D2 type	Preferentially blocked by haloperidol and other neuroleptic drugs	Central nervous system; pituitary gland (may activate second messengers or ionic channels)
	Serotonin receptors S1 type	Preferentially activated by serotonin	Central nervous system (inhibitory effect; linked to adenylate cyclase)
	S2 type	Preferentially binds spiroperidol	Central nervous system (excitatory effect)
Amino Acids	$GABA_A$ receptors	Blocked by bicuculline and picrotoxin; activated by muscimol	Central nervous system; both pre- and postsynaptic (activate Cl^- channels to cause inhibition)
	$GABA_B$ receptors	Activated by baclofen	Central nervous system; often presynaptic (Ca^{++} channels; inhibits adenylate cyclase activity)
	Glycine receptors	Blocked by strychnine	Spinal cord (inhibition)
	Glutamate receptors Q type	Activated by quisqualate	Central nervous system (ionic channels for monovalent cations)
	K type	Activated by kainate	Central nervous system (ionic channels for monovalent cations)
	NMDA type	Activated by N-Methyl-D-aspartate	Central nervous system (normally blocked by Mg^{++}; unblocked by depolarization; admit Ca^{++} with secondary intracellular effects)
Peptides	Opiate and peptide receptors	Blocked by naloxone and other opiate antagonists	Central nervous system and smooth muscle

UNIT 40
PERMEABILITY CHANGES DUE TO RECEPTORS

Classes of Receptor

Two general classes of receptor mediate signal transmission at synapses:

1. Receptors that open (or close) a conductance channel in the membrane. Their action is very *fast*.
2. Receptors that mediate a change in cellular metabolism, with resulting physiological effects. Their action is relatively *slow* (see Unit 41).

Receptor-Ionophore Complex

Receptors that cause rapid conductance changes are coupled to a membrane channel (ionophore) that is selective for certain species of ions (Fig. 40A). When the transmitter reacts with the receptor, a conformational change in the channel's protein subunits takes place and the channel is available for passage of ions across the membrane (Fig. 40B).

Selectivity

The selectivity of the channel for ionic species determines whether the synapse has an *excitatory* or *inhibitory* effect on the target cell. Generally, **excitatory** synapses have channels that allow cations (usually Na^+ and K^+) to cross the membrane (see Fig. 40B). This leads to membrane depolarization. **Inhibitory** synapses have channels that allow Cl^- (or K^+) to cross the membrane. This leads to membrane hyperpolarization or to counteraction of depolarizing changes (see Units 43 and 44).

Desensitization

Continuous exposure of receptors to their transmitter leads to **desensitization**; that is, the receptor-transmitter reaction no longer leads to a permeability change. Normally, transmitter released by the presynaptic ending is removed rapidly and desensitization does not occur.

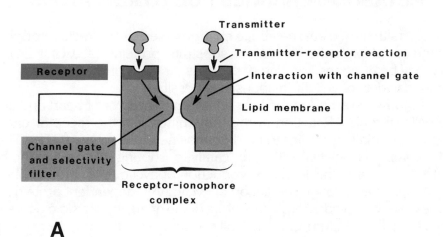

A

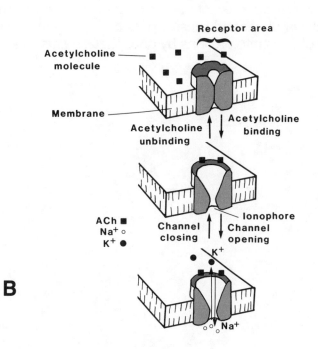

B

Figure 40 *A*, General organization of receptors coupled to ionic channels (ionophores). *B*, Acetylcholine receptor and permeability change. (*B*, Modified after Stevens CF. The neuron. Sci Am 1979; 241:65.)

UNIT 41
METABOLIC CHANGES DUE TO RECEPTORS

Receptors that mediate metabolic changes exert their effects through phosphorylation (or dephosphorylation) of substrate proteins (see Unit 24). Such proteins may be enzymes, regulatory proteins, or parts of membrane channels. Thus, a wide variety of cellular responses is possible.

A well-studied example is the beta-adrenergic receptor of heart and smooth muscle cells (Fig. 41). Reaction of the transmitter with the receptor enables a transducing protein (G-protein) to bind guanosine triphosphate (GTP). The activated G-protein associates with the catalytic subunit of membrane-bound adenylate cyclase, and this leads to production of cyclic AMP. Protein phosphorylation then ensues through mediation of cyclic AMP-dependent protein kinase.

In the case of beta-adrenergic receptors of the heart, the physiological effect is an increase in the calcium current: Voltage-sensitive calcium channels in the membrane become phosphorylated, and this causes them to change from an inactive to an active (responsive) form. The cardiac action potential is increased in amplitude as a result (see Unit 60).

Termination of metabolic events set in motion by the transmitter occurs through (a) breakdown of second messengers by hydrolytic enzymes, and (b) dephosphorylation of substrate proteins by phosphatase enzymes.

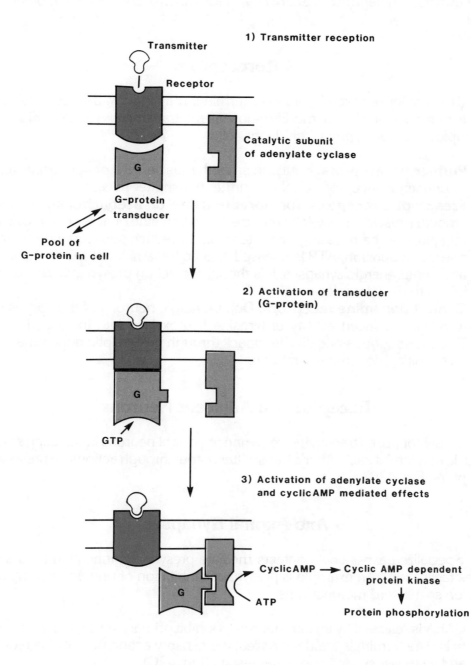

1) Transmitter reception

Transmitter

Receptor

Catalytic subunit
of adenylate cyclase

G

G-protein
transducer

Pool of
G-protein in cell

2) Activation of transducer
(G-protein)

G

GTP

3) Activation of adenylate cyclase
and cyclic AMP mediated effects

G

CyclicAMP → Cyclic AMP dependent
protein kinase

ATP

Protein phosphorylation

Figure 41 Coupling of transmitter action to metabolism.

UNIT 42
PRESYNAPTIC RECEPTORS

Many transmitter-releasing nerve terminals are endowed with receptors for their own transmitters (**autoreceptors**) or for transmitters released by other nerve cells.

Autoreceptors

Transmitter released by a nerve terminal may react with receptors on the same nerve terminal and modify subsequent transmitter release (Fig. 42A). Examples of autoreceptors include the following:

1. **Purinergic receptors.** Found in smooth muscle. ATP or adenosine acts on P_1 purinergic receptors to inhibit further transmitter release.
2. **Presynaptic receptors for noradrenaline or acetylcholine.** Found in smooth muscle and skeletal muscle. Noradrenaline or acetylcholine acts on receptors of the releasing nerve terminal to reduce subsequent transmitter release. In addition, ATP is released as a co-transmitter at many cholinergic and noradrenergic synapses; it is thought to act on presynaptic receptors to inhibit transmitter release.
3. **Central dopamine receptors.** Dopaminergic neurons of the corpus striatum show reduced activity of tyrosine hydroxylase with increased activity. Evidence suggests negative feedback through presynaptic dopamine receptors, limiting dopamine synthesis.

Receptors on Adjacent Neurons

Closely opposed transmitter-releasing regions of neurons innervating smooth muscle may inhibit each other's transmitter output through actions on presynaptic receptors (Fig. 42B).

Axo-Axonal Synapses

Specialized axo-axonal contacts mediate presynaptic inhibition (and sometimes facilitation). An example is presynaptic inhibition of primary sensory afferents on spinal cord motoneurons.

1. GABA is released by an interneuron to inhibit primary sensory afferent terminals. The terminals are depolarized, the sensory action potential is reduced, and a smaller synaptic potential results (Fig. 42C).
2. Pain fiber terminals (releasing substance P) are inhibited by enkephalin-releasing neurons (see Unit 47).

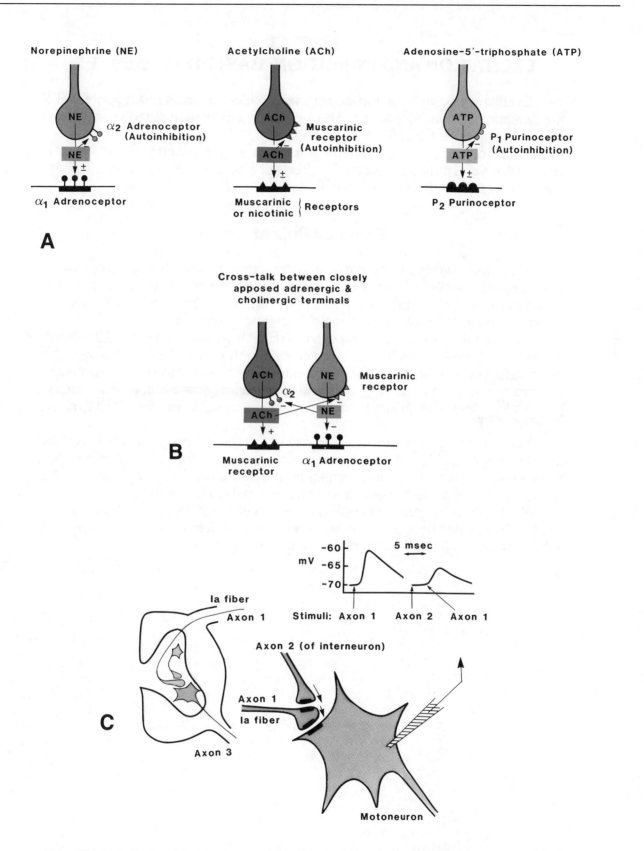

Figure 42 *A,* Feedback to releasing nerve terminal. *B,* Feedback to adjacent nerve terminal. *C,* An axo-axonal synapse. (*A* and *B,* Modified after Burnstock G. Recent concepts of chemical communication between excitable cells. In: Osborne NN, ed. Dale's principle and communication between neurons. New York: Pergamon Press, 1983:14. *C,* Modified after Bradford HF. Chemical neurobiology. New York: WH Freeman, 1986:239.)

UNIT 43
EXCITATION AND INHIBITION: BASIC DIFFERENCES

Excitatory synaptic action **depolarizes** the cell from its resting potential. If the synaptic potential is large enough, threshold for the action potential is attained and an action potential is fired (Fig. 43A)

Inhibitory synaptic action **hyperpolarizes** the cell *when the membrane is depolarized*, and thus counteracts the effects of excitatory transmission. Inhibition can prevent the cell from firing an action potential (Fig. 43B).

Reversal Potentials

When the membrane potential is systematically varied by injecting current into the postsynaptic cell (see Fig. 43A), a membrane potential can be found at which the synaptic potential reverses its polarity (i.e., current flows in the reverse direction across the membrane through synaptic channels).

For *excitatory* synapses, this potential (E_{rev}) is usually between -20 mV and $+30$ mV (Fig. 43A and 43C). This indicates a high permeability of the synaptic channel for Na^+ (or Ca^{++}), and *some* permeability for K^+ (so the reversal potential is more negative than E_{Na} or E_{Ca}). During synaptic transmission, the membrane potential is directed toward E_{rev}; this normally causes the membrane to be depolarized.

For *inhibitory* synapses, E_{rev} is close to the resting potential and is usually equal to E_{Cl} (see Fig. 43C). (In some cases, it is equal to E_K.) During synaptic transmission, the membrane potential is directed toward E_{rev}; this causes the membrane potential to remain close to the normal resting potential.

Most cells in the nervous system receive both excitatory and inhibitory synapses. The balance between excitation and inhibition determines whether the cell will fire an action potential or remain silent (see Fig. 43B).

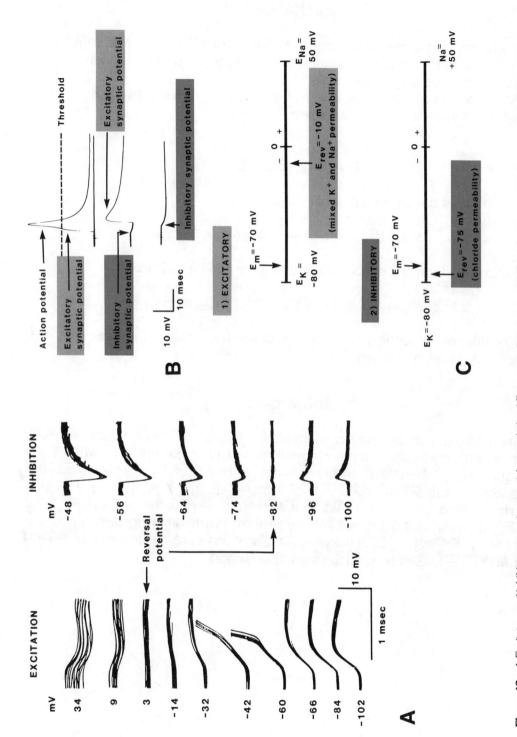

Figure 43 *A*, Excitatory and inhibitory synaptic potentials recorded at different membrane potentials. *B*, Inhibition counters excitation. *C*, Reversal potentials. (*A*, *Left*, adapted from Coombs JS, Eccles JC, Fatt P. Excitatory synaptic action in motoneurones. J Physiol 1955; 130:377. *Right*, adapted from Coombs JS, Eccles JC, Fatt P. The specific ionic conductances and the ionic movements across the motoneuronal membrane that produce the inhibitory post-synaptic potential. J Physiol 1955; 130:329.)

UNIT 44
EXCITATION AND INHIBITION: ELECTRICAL MODELS

Excitation

Excitatory transmitter opens channels for cations (Na^+, K^+, and sometimes Ca^{++}). The transmitter-gated channels are separate from the channels responsible for resting and action potentials.

At the **reversal potential**, inward Na^+ current equals outward K^+ current through the channels. From Ohm's law:

$$I_{Na} = \Delta g_{Na} (E_m - E_{Na})$$
$$I_K = \Delta g_K (E_m - E_K)$$

Since $I_{Na} = I_K$, at the reversal potential, E_{rev}

$$\Delta g_{Na} (E_{rev} - E_{Na}) = - \Delta g_K (E_{rev} - E_K)$$

Ratio of sodium to potassium conductance can be estimated:

$$\Delta g_{Na} / \Delta g_K = -(E_{rev} - E_K) / E_{rev} - E_{Na})$$

For the acetylcholine-gated channel of the motor end-plate (see Unit 45), $\Delta g_{Na} / \Delta g_K$ is approximately 1.3.

Inhibition

Inhibitory transmitter opens channels for chloride (Cl^-) or potassium (K^+). When the inhibitory conductance channel is open, ionic current flows when E_m is not equal to E_{Cl}. When the membrane is depolarized from E_m, Cl^- flows *into* the cell and makes the membrane potential more negative (i.e., there is a **hyperpolarizing** synaptic potential). When the membrane potential is more negative than E_{Cl}, Cl^- flows *out of* the cell and a **depolarization** inhibitory synaptic potential is seen. No matter which of these occurs, inhibitory synaptic action opposes the ion currents generated by excitatory synaptic action.

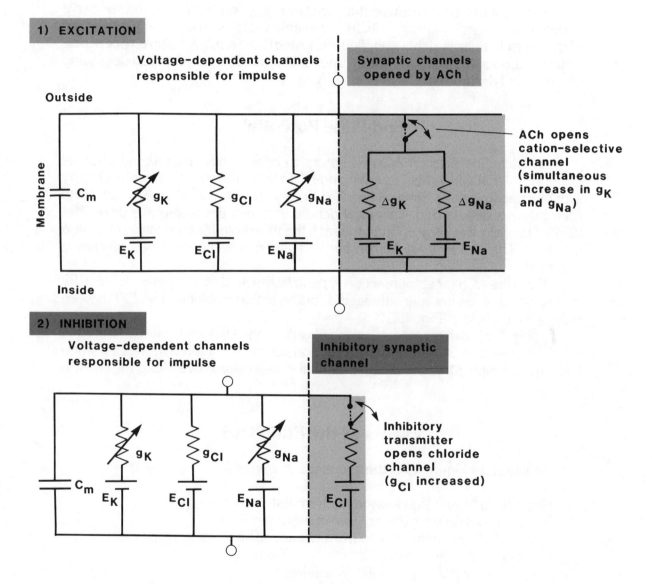

Figure 44 Electrical models of excitation and inhibition. (Adapted from Kuffler SW, Nicholls JG, Martin AR. From neuron to brain. Sunderland, MA: Sinauer Associates Inc., 1984:226, 230.)

UNIT 45
NEUROMUSCULAR JUNCTION

Neuromuscular Junction or End-Plate

This is the best-studied excitatory synapse. Most mammalian striated muscle fibers are innervated by a single branch of a motor axon which forms a large excitatory synapse (**neuromuscular junction** or **end-plate**). The motor nerve ending contains acetylcholine (ACh) in synaptic vesicles. The underlying surface of the muscle fiber is richly supplied with **nicotinic acetylcholine receptors**, while the associated basal lamina in junctional folds contains the ACh-degrading enzyme **acetylcholinesterase** (Fig. 45A).

End-Plate Potential

Acetylcholine acts on ACh receptors to open a transmembrane channel (ionophore) that allows Na^+ to enter and K^+ to leave the muscle fiber (excitatory synaptic transmission). Since at first Na^+ enters more rapidly than K^+ leaves, the membrane is depolarized. This local depolarization is the **end-plate potential** (EPP). Normally it is large enough to reach the threshold for generating an action potential. The action potential propagates along the muscle fiber, triggering contraction.

When the ACh-receptor reaction is partially blocked by curare, a smaller EPP is seen which does not reach threshold for the action potential. The EPP is seen only at the end-plate (Fig. 45B)

Note: Two different electrical events are seen at the end-plate: (a) the EPP, caused by reaction of ACh, and (b) the action potential triggered by the EPP when it is large enough. Only the action potential is seen elsewhere along the muscle fiber.

Events at the End-Plate

As shown in Figure 45C, the sequence of events is:

1. Entry of Ca^{++} into the presynaptic terminal.
2. Reaction leading to release of transmitter.
3. Diffusion of transmitter (ACh) from release site across synaptic cleft.
4. Reaction of ACh with receptor.
5. Breakdown of ACh by acetylcholinesterase.
6. Uptake of choline (active transport).
7. Resynthesis of ACh and creation of ACh-filled synaptic vesicles.

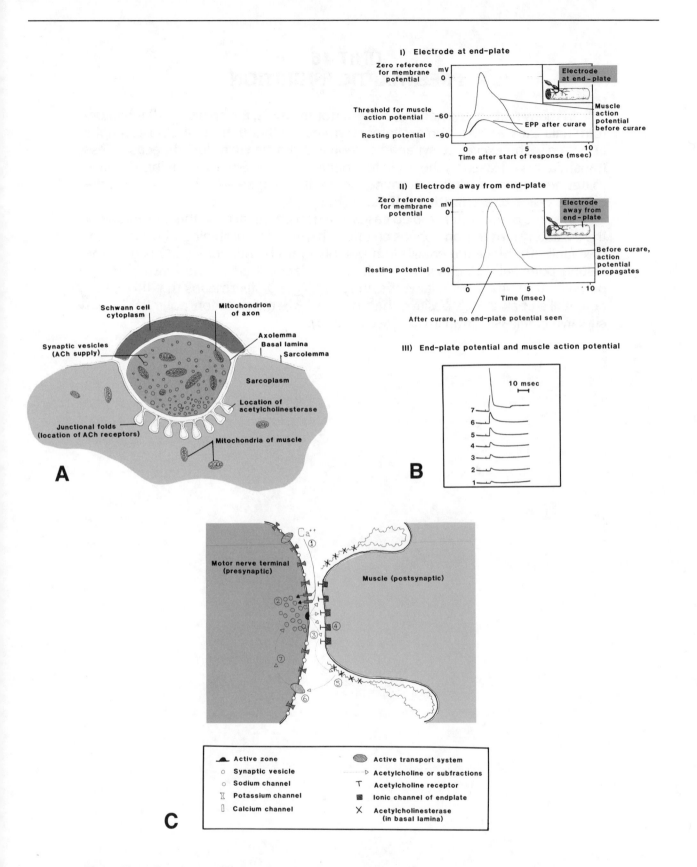

I) Electrode at end-plate

Zero reference for membrane potential

Threshold for muscle action potential

Resting potential

Electrode at end-plate

Muscle action potential before curare

EPP after curare

Time after start of response (msec)

II) Electrode away from end-plate

Zero reference for membrane potential

Resting potential

Electrode away from end-plate

Before curare, action potential propagates

After curare, no end-plate potential seen

Time (msec)

III) End-plate potential and muscle action potential

10 msec

Schwann cell cytoplasm

Mitochondrion of axon

Synaptic vesicles (ACh supply)

Axolemma
Basal lamina
Sarcolemma

Sarcoplasm

Location of acetylcholinesterase

Junctional folds (location of ACh receptors)

Mitochondria of muscle

A

B

Ca++

Motor nerve terminal (presynaptic)

Muscle (postsynaptic)

Active zone
Synaptic vesicle
Sodium channel
Potassium channel
Calcium channel

Active transport system
Acetylcholine or subfractions
Acetylcholine receptor
Ionic channel of endplate
Acetylcholinesterase (in basal lamina)

C

Figure 45 *A*, Cross section of motor nerve ending at end-plate. *B*, Excitation of muscle fiber by motor axon. *C*, Summary of events at the end-plate following arrival of the nerve action potential. (*A*, Adapted from Copenhaver WM, Kelly DE, Wood RL. Bailey's textbook of histology. Baltimore: Williams & Wilkins, 1978:336. *B*, III, Adapted from Nastuk WL. Neuromuscular transmission. Am J Med 1955; 19:665.)

UNIT 46
PRESYNAPTIC INHIBITION

In many parts of the nervous system (for example, the spinal cord) inhibitory terminals exert an effect on excitatory terminals rather than on the postsynaptic target cell. The excitatory synaptic potential is drastically reduced because less transmitter is released by the excitatory nerve terminal. Since the inhibitory transmitter acts on the excitatory terminal before its synapse with the target cell, the effect is called **presynaptic inhibition** (Fig. 46A).

In some of the better-studied cases, the transmitter acts on the membrane of the excitatory terminal and opens chloride channels by combining with a receptor (see Unit 40). Since the equilibrium potential for chloride ions (Cl^-) is near the resting potential, Cl^- enters the cell as it is depolarized by the arriving action potential (Fig. 46B). Simultaneous entry of Cl^- and Na^+ means that the action potential's peak is less positive than normal. A smaller action potential is less effective in releasing transmitter (see Unit 33).

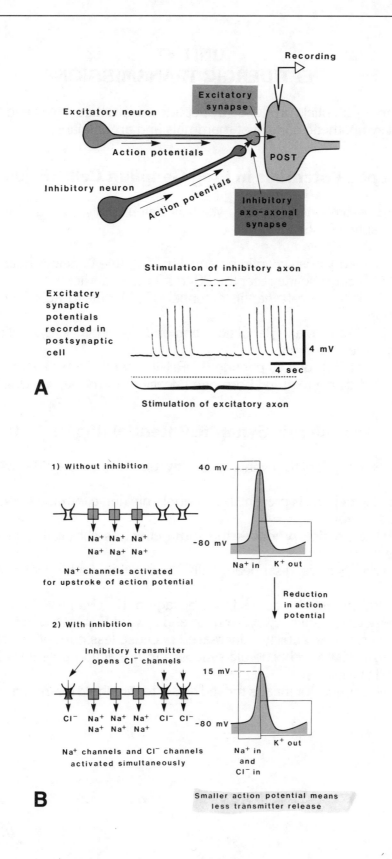

Recording

Excitatory neuron

Excitatory synapse

Action potentials

POST

Inhibitory neuron

Action potentials

Inhibitory axo-axonal synapse

Stimulation of inhibitory axon

Excitatory synaptic potentials recorded in postsynaptic cell

4 mV

4 sec

Stimulation of excitatory axon

A

1) Without inhibition

40 mV

Na⁺ Na⁺ Na⁺
Na⁺ Na⁺ Na⁺

-80 mV

Na⁺ in   K⁺ out

Na⁺ channels activated
for upstroke of action potential

Reduction in action potential

2) With inhibition

Inhibitory transmitter
opens Cl⁻ channels

15 mV

Cl⁻   Na⁺ Na⁺ Na⁺   Cl⁻ Cl⁻
      Na⁺ Na⁺ Na⁺

-80 mV

Na⁺ channels and Cl⁻ channels
activated simultaneously

Na⁺ in
and
Cl⁻ in   K⁺ out

B

Smaller action potential means
less transmitter release

Figure 46 *A*, Presynaptic inhibition. *B*, Ionic mechanism in the excitatory presynaptic terminal. (*A*, Adapted from Wiens TJ, Atwood HL. Dual inhibitory control in crab leg muscles. J Comp Physiol 1975; 99:221.)

UNIT 47
PEPTIDERGIC TRANSMISSION

Synaptic potentials produced by peptide transmitters have been well studied in several sympathetic ganglia of mammals and amphibians.

Synaptic Potentials in Frog Ganglion Cells (Figure 47A)

In this respresentative case, which is better analyzed than for mammals, several synaptic events occur:

1. Fast excitatory postsynaptic potential (EPSP) due to acetylcholine acting on nicotinic acetylcholine receptor: 30 to 50 msec duration.
2. Slow inhibitory postsynaptic potential (IPSP) due to acetylcholine: 2 sec duration.
3. Slow EPSP due to acetylcholine acting on muscarinic acetylcholine receptor: 30 to 60 sec duration.
4. Late slow EPSP due to peptide (LHRH-like peptide): 5 to 10 min duration. (Note: LHRH = luteinizing hormone releasing hormone; see Unit 94.)

Peptidergic Synaptic Potential (Figure 47B)

Further analysis of the events caused by release of the peptide has shown that

1. LHRH-like peptide is present in preganglionic nerve terminals and is released by stimulation.
2. LHRH-like peptide produces the same effect as stimulation of peptidergic nerve fibers.
3. LHRH-like peptide disappears with denervation (cutting of preganglionic axons).
4. Late slow potential is caused by blockage of K^+ channels; hence the membrane potential shifts away from E_K and toward E_{Na} (see Unit 9).
5. The neuron's excitability is increased because less current has to be generated by excitatory cholinergic synapses to fire action potentials in the postsynaptic cell.
6. The membrane potential is moved closer to threshold for the action potential.

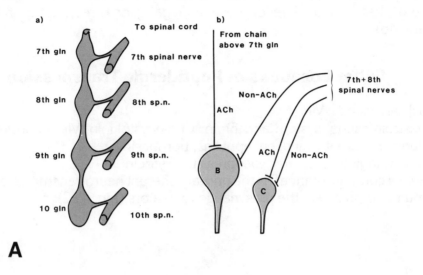

A

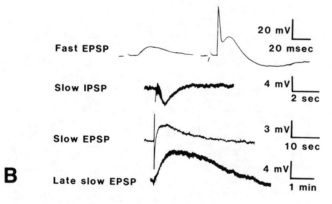

B

Figure 47 *A*, Sympathetic ganglion cell innervation. *B*, Cholinergic and peptidergic synaptic potentials. *Figure continues.*

Other Cases of Peptidergic Transmission in Sympathetic Ganglia

1. Mammalian inferior mesenteric ganglion: Slow peptidergic EPSP and fast cholinergic EPSP. Substance P is the peptide transmitter.
2. Presynaptic effects of enkephalin: Depression of both cholinergic and peptidergic EPSPs in the inferior mesenteric ganglion (presynaptic inhibition; see Unit 46).

Other Locations of Peptidergic Transmission

1. Salivary glands: VIP.
2. Gastrointestinal system and brain: Cholecystokinin, VIP, neurotensin, substance P, somatostatin, enkephalins, bombesin.
3. Brain: Angiotensin, TRH, vasopressin, oxytocin.
4. Spinal cord: Substance P is the primary afferent neurotransmitter; enkephalin and endorphins are the presynaptic regulators (Fig. 47C).

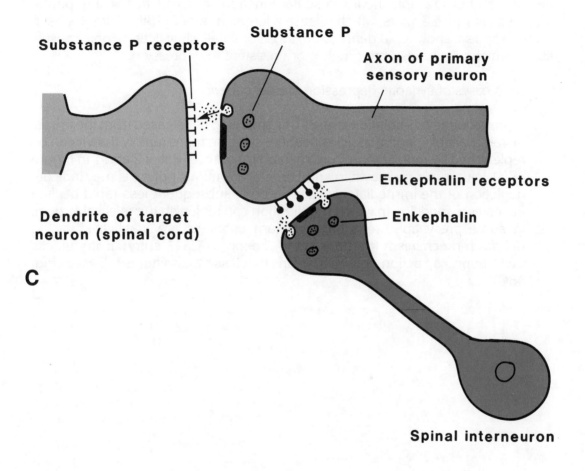

Substance P receptors

Substance P

Axon of primary sensory neuron

Enkephalin receptors

Enkephalin

Dendrite of target neuron (spinal cord)

C

Spinal interneuron

Figure 47 *(continued)* C, Peptide transmitters in the spinal cord. (*A* and *B*, From Jan YN, Jan LY, Kuffler SW. A peptide as a possible transmitter in sympathetic ganglia of the frog. Proc Natl Acad Sci USA 1979; 76:1502. With permission from Dr. Y.N. Jan. *C*, Modified after Iversen LL. The chemistry of the brain. Sci Am 1979; 241(3):146.)

UNIT 48
SYNAPTIC DEPRESSION

Synapses activated by many impulses commonly show **depression** (or fatigue) — a decline in amplitude of the synaptic potential (Fig. 48A). This is almost always attributable to release of a lesser amount of transmitter from the pre-synaptic nerve terminal (*not* to desensitization of postsynaptic receptors). A few cases are known in which rapid desensitization plays a role.

In general, synapses that release a lot of transmitter for each impulse depress more rapidly with repeated use than those which release a small amount of transmitter. For example, neuromuscular junctions of large, fast-acting, phasic mammalian muscle fibers, which release a large amount of transmitter for each motor impulse, show rapid depression; those of small, slow-acting, tonic muscle fibers, which release less, are much more resistant to depression.

Two cases of synaptic depression are described:

1. High-frequency stimulation causes transmitter to be released from the immediately available pool of vesicles near the synapse more rapidly than it can be replenished by mobilization from metabolic sources (Rates 2 and 1 in Figure 48B). Initial rapid run-down in amplitude of a synaptic potential may indicate depletion of the immediately available pool; subsequent less rapid decline indicates a condition in which mobilization can replenish the releasable pool.
2. In some presynaptic terminals, calcium channels are inactivated by an unknown mechanism (perhaps set in motion by Ca^{++} entry). Entry of less Ca^{++} during an action potential means that less transmitter is released (Fig. 48C).

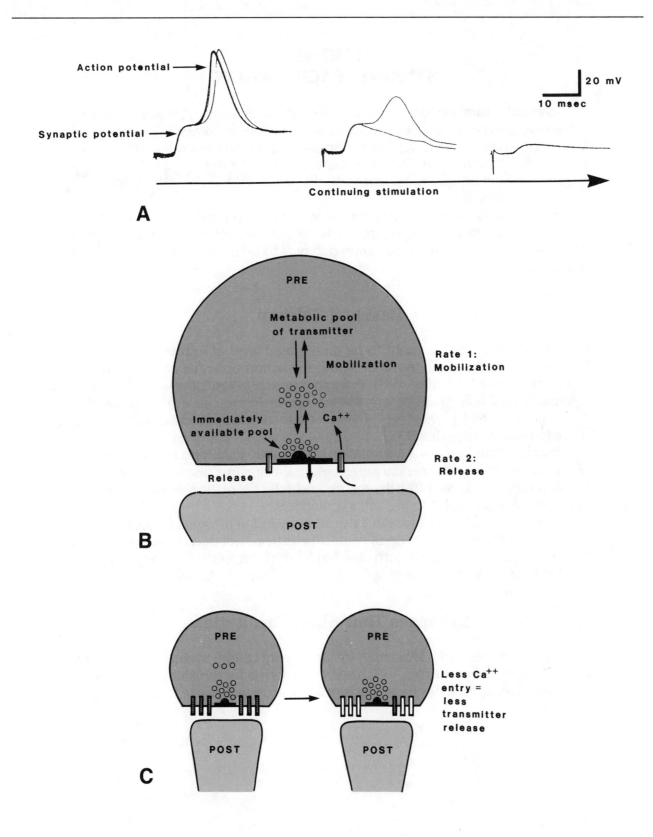

Figure 48 *A*, Stages of synaptic depression. *B*, Mobilization and release of transmitter. *C*, Depression due to inactivation of calcium channels. (*A*, Adapted from Atwood HL, Jahromi SS. Fast-axon synapses of a crab leg muscle. J Neurobiol 1978; 9:3.)

UNIT 49
SYNAPTIC FACILITATION

Synaptic facilitation occurs at many synapses when impulses follow each other closely in time. Synaptic potentials after the first are larger; in Figure 49A, 1, V_2 is larger than V_1. When a train of impulses occurs in the presynaptic neuron, progressive growth of synaptic potentials is seen. The postsynaptic cell can be made to fire action potentials when a high-frequency train of stimulation is delivered (Fig. 49A, 2).

Facilitation is due to a progressive increase in release of transmitter substance from the presynaptic neuron. The presynaptic action potential leaves an after-effect that causes the next action potential to be more effective in releasing transmitter.

Residual Calcium

The after-effect is thought to be an elevated level of intracellular calcium. Calcium enters the nerve terminal during the action potential and remains elevated for a short time (Fig. 49B). If another action potential arrives when extra calcium from the first is still there, the sum of "entering calcium" and "residual calcium" provides a higher level of intracellular calcium. This leads to release of more transmitter (see Unit 33).

Summation (temporal summation) of synaptic potentials (see Fig. 49A, 2) occurs when a second potential arises before the first has decayed. Both facilitation and summation can bring the membrane potential of the postsynaptic cell up to threshold and cause it to fire action potentials.

Summation also occurs with calcium entry in the presynaptic terminal (see Fig. 49B). However, *facilitation of calcium entry* has not been observed in nerve terminals; the amount of calcium entering for each impulse (Ca_e) stays constant (or decreases in some cases of synaptic depression; see Unit 48).

Synapses That Show Facilitation

Synapses that show facilitation include many central synapses; motor synapses of crustacean muscles, which serve as models for the study of facilitation; and some vertebrate neuromuscular junctions, especially those found in smooth muscle.

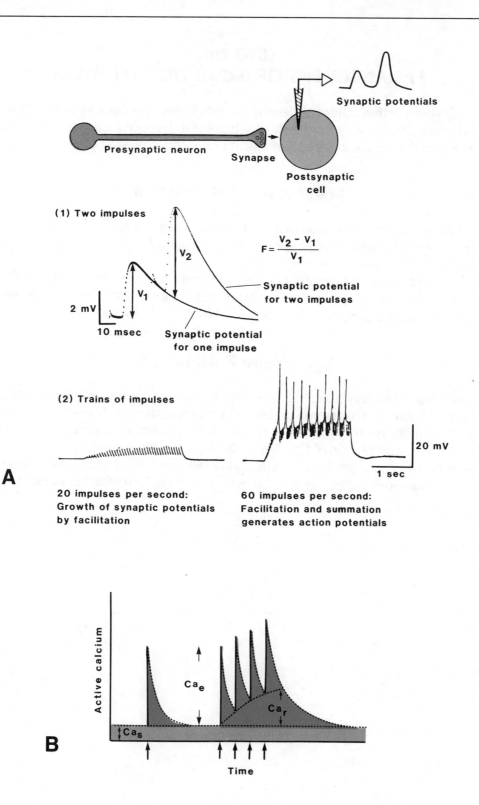

Figure 49 *A*, Synaptic facilitation. *B*, The residual calcium hypothesis. (*A1*, Adapted from Stephens PJ, Atwood HL. Thermal acclimation in a crustacean neuromuscular system. J Exp Biol 1982; 98:41. *A2*, Adapted from Atwood HL, Bittner GD. Matching of excitatory and inhibitory inputs to crustacean muscle fibers. J Neurophysiol 1971; 34:159. *B*, From Zucker RS, Lara-Estrella LO. Post-tetanic decay of evoked and spontaneous transmitter release and a residual-calcium model of synaptic facilitation of crayfish neuromuscular junctions. J Gen Physiol 1983; 81:366. With permission from Rockefeller University Press.)

UNIT 50
ENHANCEMENT OF SYNAPTIC PATHWAYS

Repetitive action potentials lead to several types of enhancement of synaptic transmission, some very long-lasting. These mechanisms may enhance active pathways in the nervous system, allowing better transmission of information.

Post-tetanic Potentiation

High-frequency activation of a motor axon or other nerve cell yields a much larger synaptic potential after the burst of activity (Fig. 50A). The enhanced response may persist for several minutes.

The mechanism of post-tetanic potentiation involves accumulation of Ca^{++} and Na^{+} in the nerve terminals. Increased intracellular Ca^{++} leads to release of more transmitter during an action potential (see Units 33 and 34).

Long-Term Facilitation

Maintained activity in a single neuron leads to growth of synaptic potentials and enhancement of transmission lasting for hours after the burst of activity (Fig. 50B). The increase in synaptic potential during repetitive stimulation involves progressive accumulation of Ca^{++} and Na^{+} in the nerve terminals, which leads to release of more transmitter. The long-lasting after-effect probably involves a second messenger system associated with the nerve terminal membrane.

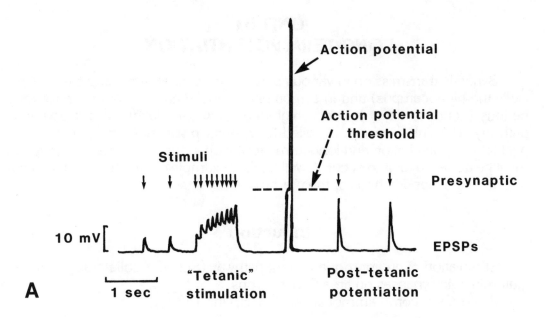

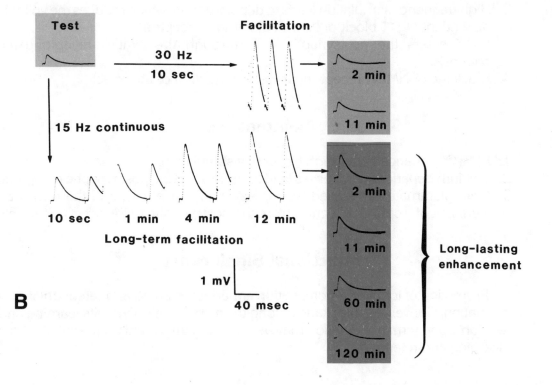

Figure 50 *A*, Post-tetanic potentiation. *B*, Long-term facilitation. (*B*, Adapted from Swenarchuk L. Long-term facilitation of transmission at a crayfish neuromuscular synapse. Ph.D. thesis, University of Toronto, 1975.)

UNIT 51
LONG-TERM POTENTIATION

Synaptic transmission in various parts of the central nervous system (especially the hippocampus) and in sympathetic ganglia can be enhanced for long periods (hours to days) by brief, high-frequency stimulation of a presynaptic pathway. The enhancement is called **long-term potentiation**. It differs from post-tetanic potentiation and long-term facilitation in that postsynaptic receptors must be activated for it to occur. A well-studied example of long-term potentiation occurs in the hippocampus of the mammalian brain.

Induction

Stimulation of an appropriate input pathway (Schaffer collaterals) activates glutaminergic synapses on area CA1 neurons.

(Note: CA = cornu ammonis; see Fig. E, Unit 143.)

1. Glutamate (GLU) generates an EPSP via the K and/or Q types of glutamate receptors (see Unit 39).
2. High-frequency stimulation leads to depolarization, which reduces the voltage-dependent Mg^{++} block of NMDA glutamate receptors.
3. Ca^{++} enters the postsynaptic cells through the NMDA receptor-gated channels.
4. Blockage of NMDA receptors prevents induction of the effect.

Maintenance

1. EPSP is enhanced after high-frequency stimulation.
2. Calcium-dependent processes lead to more available postsynaptic receptors.
3. More glutamate is released from presynaptic terminals, and there may be feedback of trophic molecules from the postsynaptic to the presynaptic cell.

Functional Significance

Promotion of long-term potentiation enhances learning and retention of new information. Conversely, blockage of long-term potentiation inhibits learning and retention. Long-term potentiation may be especially important for the initial stages of learning and retention.

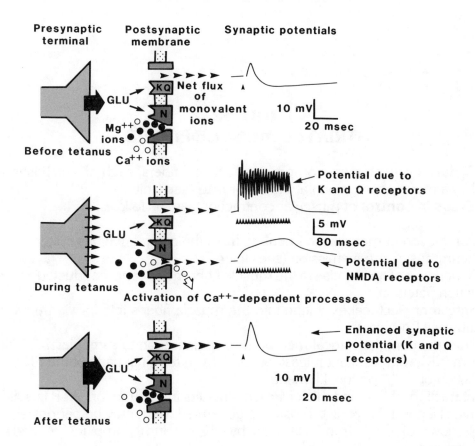

Figure 51 Hypothesis for long-term potentiation. (Adapted from Collingridge GL, Bliss TVP. NMDA receptors — their role in long-term potentiation. Trends Neurosci 1987; 10:292.)

7

EFFECTORS

UNIT 52
STRIATED MUSCLE FIBERS

Striated muscles are composed of muscle fibers, each of which is innervated by a motor axon branch at the **end-plate** (see Unit 45).
Steps in control of muscular contractions are as follows:

1. Conduction of motor axon impulses from the central nervous system.
2. Neuromuscular transmission (see Unit 45).
3. Generation of an impulse in the muscle fiber membrane; conducted muscle action potential.
4. Spread of electrical excitation into the muscle fiber's interior via transverse tubules (T-tubules).
5. Transduction of electrical membrane depolarization to sarcoplasmic reticulum (SR), with resultant release of Ca^{++} from terminal parts of the SR.
6. Action of Ca^{++} on thin filaments.
7. Interaction of thin and thick filaments results in contraction. ATP is split by thick filaments (myosin). Tension is generated; work may be performed.
8. Removal of Ca^{++} from filaments by the calcium pump in SR leads to relaxation.

The path of electrical events is outlined in Figure 52A.

Calcium-controlled chemical events lead to interaction of thick (myosin) and thin (actin-troponin-tropomyosin) filaments (Fig. 52B). Calcium removes the inhibitory effect of troponin so that actin and myosin can react. The ATPase activity of actomyosin is high; ATP is split and contraction ensues.

Contraction of muscle is caused by rotation of myosin cross-bridges attached to the thin filament; this rotation causes relative movement of the thick and thin filaments (see Fig. 52B). ATP must be present for the cross-bridge cycle to be completed. Lack of ATP results in arrest of the cross-bridge cycle in a "locked" position ("rigor mortis").

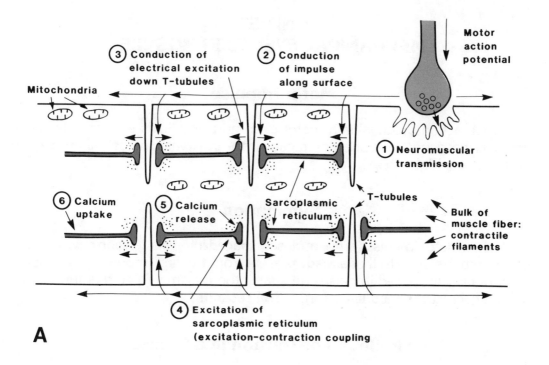

③ Conduction of electrical excitation down T-tubules

② Conduction of impulse along surface

Motor action potential

Mitochondria

① Neuromuscular transmission

⑥ Calcium uptake

⑤ Calcium release

Sarcoplasmic reticulum

T-tubules

Bulk of muscle fiber: contractile filaments

④ Excitation of sarcoplasmic reticulum (excitation-contraction coupling)

A

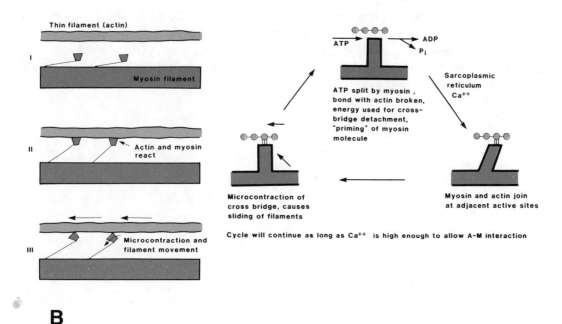

Thin filament (actin)

I

Myosin filament

ATP → ADP, Pi

ATP split by myosin, bond with actin broken, energy used for cross-bridge detachment, "priming" of myosin molecule

Sarcoplasmic reticulum Ca++

II

Actin and myosin react

Myosin and actin join at adjacent active sites

Microcontraction of cross bridge, causes sliding of filaments

III

Microcontraction and filament movement

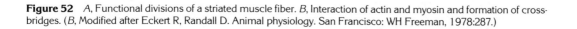

Cycle will continue as long as Ca++ is high enough to allow A-M interaction

B

Figure 52 *A*, Functional divisions of a striated muscle fiber. *B*, Interaction of actin and myosin and formation of cross-bridges. (*B*, Modified after Eckert R, Randall D. Animal physiology. San Francisco: WH Freeman, 1978:287.)

UNIT 53
MECHANICAL EVENTS IN MUSCLE

Motor Impulse

Each action potential in a motor axon normally leads to a muscle action potential that generates a brief contraction in the innervated muscle fibers (**twitch contraction**; Figure 53A).

Summation

When motor impulses arrive at closely spaced intervals, tension developed by a later impulse adds to that already present from the first impulse (Fig. 53B). A burst of closely spaced impulses generates the maximal force possible for the muscle fiber (**tetanic contraction**, or **full tetanus**).

Gradation of Tension in a Muscle

Each muscle fiber can develop any degree of tension between the twitch and full tetanus, depending on the temporal sequence of nerve impulses. Each motor axon innervates a group of muscle fibers (**motor unit**). An impulse in the motor axon recruits all fibers in the motor unit. Tension developed by the muscle as a whole reflects the *number of motor units* active at that time (Fig. 53C).

The number of muscle fibers in a motor unit varies greatly from one muscle to another. Large limb muscles have many muscle fibers in a motor unit, while small eye and finger muscles have relatively few.

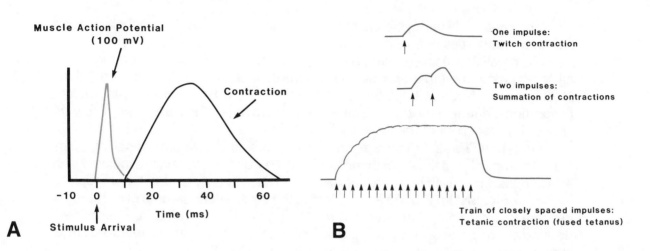

A, Muscle Action Potential (100 mV), Contraction, Time (ms), Stimulus Arrival

B, One impulse: Twitch contraction. Two impulses: Summation of contractions. Train of closely spaced impulses: Tetanic contraction (fused tetanus)

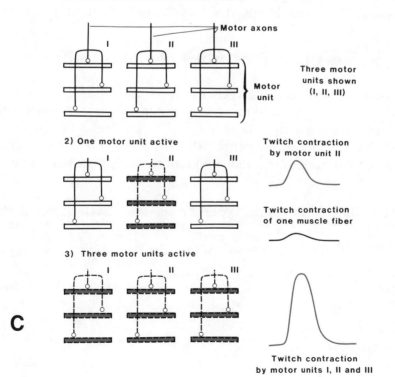

C

1) Muscle at rest: no motor units active

Motor axons

I II III

Motor unit

Three motor units shown (I, II, III)

2) One motor unit active

I II III

Twitch contraction by motor unit II

Twitch contraction of one muscle fiber

3) Three motor units active

I II III

Twitch contraction by motor units I, II and III

Figure 53 *A*, Action potential and contraction. *B*, Twitch contraction and tetanic contraction. *C*, Motor unit recruitment.

UNIT 54
TYPES OF MUSCLE FIBER

Mammalian Muscle Fibers

The contractile performance of a motor unit is limited by the biochemical and structural properties of the muscle fibers.

Mammalian muscles usually have three main types of muscle fiber (Fig. 54A), all of which contract in response to action potentials produced at the end-plate. Most muscles have at least two and often all three types of fiber, in varying proportions. Within a motor unit, all muscle fibers are of the same type. Table 54 shows the properties of the three major types.

Myosin ATPase.   The rate at which ATP is split by myosin is determined by specific properties of the myosin molecule and regulatory proteins associated with it. In general, fibers with high rates of myosin ATPase activity contract more rapidly.

Fast glycolytic (FG) fibers.   Most of the cross-sectional area of FG fibers is devoted to contractile filaments, and relatively little to mitochondria. These fibers develop a large force but fatigue rapidly. Motor units containing FG fibers are large, are used for maximal exertions, and are silent most of the time.

Slow oxidative (SO) fibers.   SO fibers contain numerous mitochondria and contract relatively slowly. Motor units containing them are active much of the time in postural activities.

Fast oxidative and glycolytic (FOG) fibers.   These are fast-acting fatigue-resistance fibers, used in normal locomotory activities.

Functional Properties of Motor Units

Slow motor units are recruited most easily for use in postural activities. When extra effort is required, more and more fast motor units are recruited (Fig. 54C). Recruitment mechanisms are "built into" the nervous system. This orderly recruitment is known as the **size principle** of motor unit activation, since motor neurons of slow motor units are smaller and more easily depolarized by excitatory

TABLE 54   Differences Among Types of Mammalian Skeletal Muscle Fiber

	Fast Glycolytic (FG) or Fast-Twitch White Fibers	Slow Oxidative (SO) or Slow-Twitch Intermediate Fibers	Fast Oxidative and Glycolytic (FOG) or Fast-Twitch Red Fibers
Fiber diameter	Large	Intermediate	Small
Myoglobin content	Low	High	High
Myosin ATPase activity (relative rate at normal pH)	High	Low	High
Contraction speed (relative)	Fast	Slow	Fast
Glycolytic enzymes	High	Low	Intermediate
Resistance to fatigue	Low	High	Intermediate to high
Mitochondrial content and oxidative enzymes	Low	High	High

Trophic effects: (1) *Increased activity* converts FG fibers to FOG fibers. (2) *Cross-reinnervation* of a muscle by a nerve from another muscle can convert the contraction speed and many other properties of slow fibers to fast, and vice versa. SO fibers are sometimes termed "type I" fibers while FG and FOG fibers are sometimes termed "type II" fibers.

synaptic input, and hence more likely to produce action potentials, than those of fast motor units.

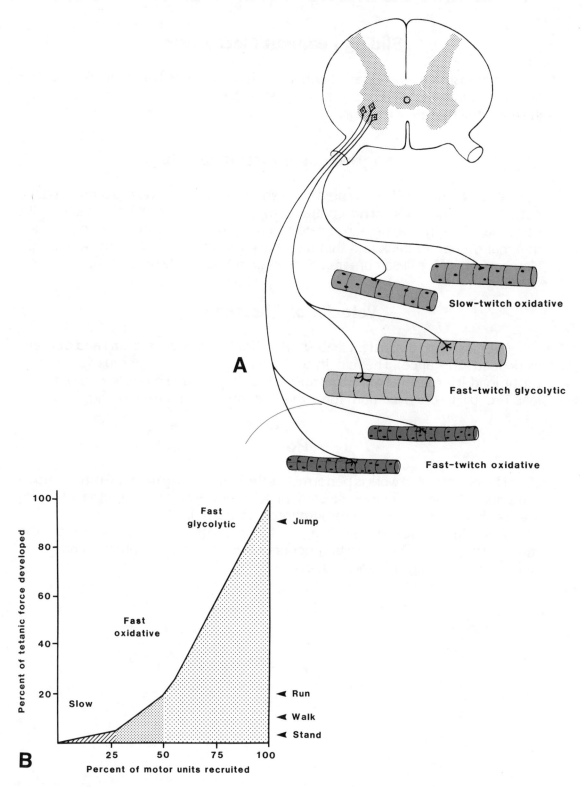

Figure 54 *A*, Mammalian muscle fibers. *B*, Mammalian muscle function. (*B*, Modified from Walmsley B, Hodgson JA, Burke RE. Forces produced by medial gastrocnemius and soleus muscles during locomotion in freely moving cats. J Neurophysiol 1978; 41:1213.)

UNIT 55
MECHANICAL EVENTS AND INFLUENCE OF LOAD

Sliding Filament Mechanism

As myosin cross-bridges attached to thin filaments rotate, thick and thin filaments within each sarcomere move past each other. As all sarcomeres shorten in series, the muscle fiber shortens.

Length-Tension Relationship

When the muscle is prevented from shortening, it develops tension but does not move a load (**isometric** contraction). The amount of tension varies with sarcomere length. It approaches zero when the muscle is stretched to produce minimal overlap of thick and thin filaments. It is maximal when thick and thin filaments of each half-sarcomere are overlapped optimally (Fig. 55A).

Velocity of Shortening

Muscles lifting a constant load shorten (**isotonic contraction**) and perform work (load × distance). The velocity of shortening for a particular muscle depends on the load. It is maximal when the muscle is unloaded, and drops to zero when the load is equal to the maximum force that the muscle can develop (Fig. 55B).

Power

The rate at which work is performed is the **power output** of the muscle (load × distance × time^{-1}). For most striated muscles, power output is maximal when the load is about one-third the maximum force (Fig. 55C).

When the muscle contracts against a force greater than it develops, the muscle lengthens. This condition occurs often in the body when antagonistic muscles contract against each other.

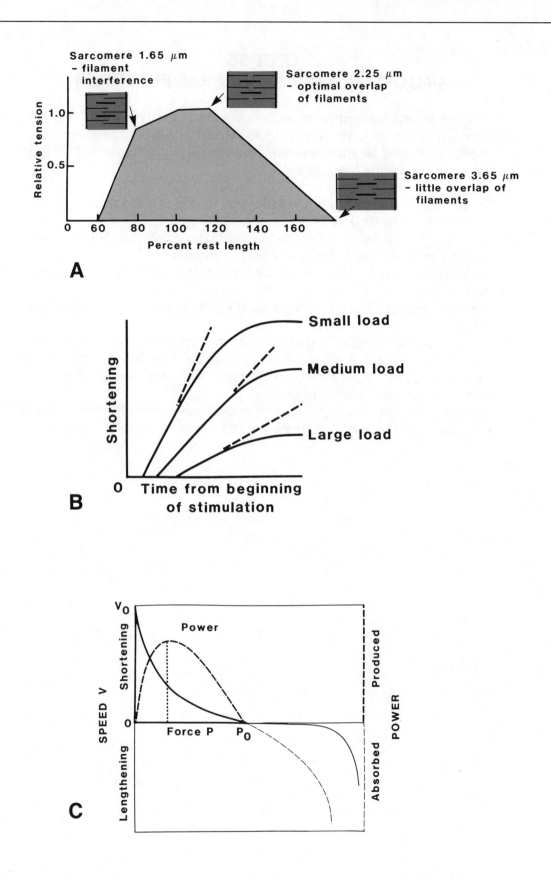

Figure 55 *A,* Length-tension relationship. *B,* Load-velocity relationship. *C,* Power output. (*A,* Modified from Eckert R, Randall D. Animal Physiology. San Francisco: WH Freeman, 1978:285. *B* and *C,* From Carlson FD, Wilkie DR. Muscle physiology. Englewood Cliffs, NJ: Prentice-Hall, 1974:39. With permission from Appleton & Lange.)

UNIT 56
SMOOTH MUSCLES: GENERAL FEATURES

Smooth muscles are important components of many organs controlled by the autonomic nervous system (e.g., blood vessels, gastrointestinal system, uterus). Features shared by most smooth muscles, and distinguishing them from skeletal muscles, are the following:

1. Small muscle fibers (2 to 5 μm wide, 100 to 200 μm long); spindle-shaped, associated in sheets (Fig. 56A).
2. Lack of regular array of contractile filaments (no striations). Actin and myosin are present, but do not form ordered sarcomeres.
3. Lack of transverse tubular system. Calcium enters the cell through the suface membrane.
4. Calcium-dependent action potentials (Fig. 56B) and frequent spontaneous activity.
5. Regulation of contractile filament activity by calcium-calmodulin activation of myosin kinase, which phosphorylates myosin (Fig. 56C). Phosphorylated myosin can form detachable cross-bridges with actin and produce relative movement of thick and thin filaments.
6. Presence of membrane receptors for acetylcholine, noradrenaline, and often peptides; these receptors regulate the cell's activity.

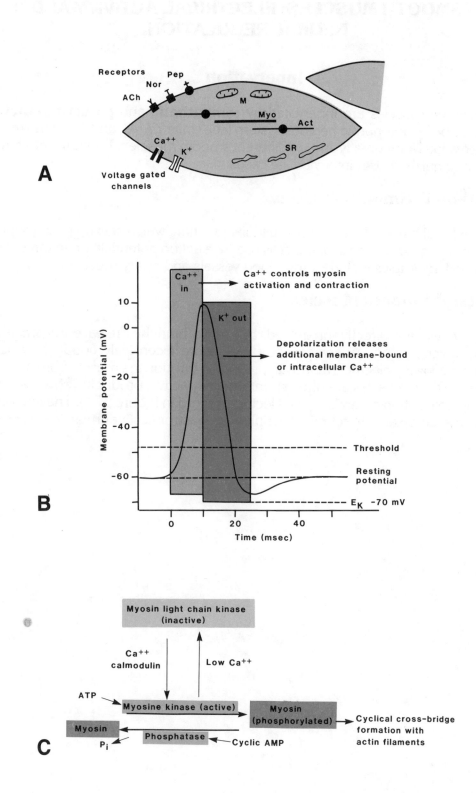

Figure 56 *A,* Smooth muscle cells. *B,* Calcium-dependent action potential. *C,* Control of myosin activation by calcium.

UNIT 57
SMOOTH MUSCLES: ELECTRICAL ACTIVITY AND NEURAL REGULATION

Innervation

Smooth muscles are innervated by **sympathetic** and **parasympathetic** branches of the autonomic nervous system (see Units 77, 78, and 89). The mode of innervation varies greatly among different smooth muscles. Two extremes have been distinguished, with intermediate cases:

"Multi-unit" Smooth Muscles

Each cell has a "close" neuromuscular junction, which sets up postsynaptic potentials (Fig. 57A). Some of the cells produce action potentials when threshold is reached. Examples include large blood vessels and ciliary muscle.

"Unitary" Smooth Muscles

Few cells are directly innervated, but nerve branches release transmitters nearby which act on surface receptors. Cells are extensively coupled by gap junctions, allowing electrical activity to propagate through the muscle from a point of origin. These muscles are often spontaneously active, producing **slow waves** that generate action potentials (see electrical record in Figure 57A). Their activity varies when they are stretched. Examples are gastrointestinal muscles and the uterus.

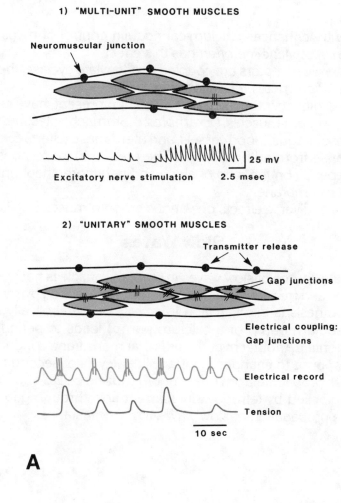

Figure 57 *A*, Two styles of innervation. *Figure continues.*

Effects of Neurotransmitters

Two classes of effect arise from the action of transmitters:

Electrical Effects

Ionic conductances are altered and the muscle cells depolarized toward threshold (more action potentials and more contraction produced) or hyperpolarized away from threshold (fewer action potentials produced).

Second Messenger Effects

1. Calcium entry enhances calcium-calmodulin control of myosin, promoting contraction. Acetylcholine *often* has this effect.
2. Beta-adrenergic receptors are coupled to adenylate cyclase; the resulting rise in cyclic AMP promotes relaxation (Fig. 57B).
3. Beta-adrenergic receptors (see Unit 39), when present, have different effects in different smooth muscles. (*Examples:* Stomach, intestine, and colon are inhibited; esophagus, blood vessels, and uterus are excited.) Excitatory effects probably arise from entry of Ca^{++}. The predominant response to norepinephrine depends on the ratio of alpha and beta norepinephrine receptors in the muscle membrane.
4. Peptides have diverse effects on various smooth muscles.

Slow Waves

The ultimate source of slow waves in smooth muscle is not well understood. The occurrence and frequency of these events is influenced by metabolic conditions. One hypothesis is that variation in activity of metabolically driven pumps (perhaps the sodium pump or a calcium pump) leads to periodic changes in membrane potential. Another hypothesis is that membrane conductance for Na^+ oscillates in response to changes in intracellular levels of second messengers.

Slow waves propagate from one smooth muscle cell to another when nerve cell activity is blocked by tetrodotoxin. Current flow through gap junctions can account for the propagation of slow waves in many instances.

1) ELECTRICAL EFFECTS

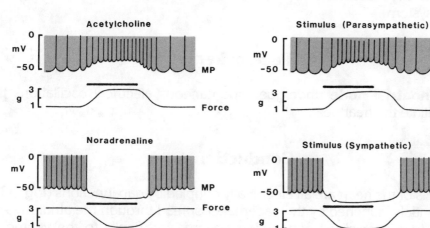

2) SECOND MESSENGER EFFECTS

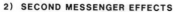
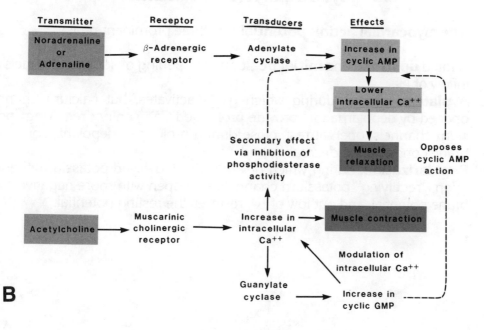

Figure 57 *(continued)* *B*, Effects of neurotransmitters. (*B1*, from Janig W. The autonomic nervous system. In: Schmidt RF, ed. Fundamentals of neurophysiology. New York: Springer-Verlag, 1975:245, 252. With permission from Springer-Verlag, Heidelberg.)

UNIT 58
HEART: ELECTRICAL ACTIVITY

The heart is functionally organized (Fig. 58A) into **pacemaker, conducting system,** and **myocardium** (contractile tissue that moves blood through the circulatory system).

Pacemaker

The **sinoatrial node** undergoes spontaneous electrical oscillations that normally initiate the heartbeat.

Conduction

The cells of the heart are all electrically coupled by gap junctions (Fig. 58A). Action potentials launched by the pacemaker spread through the atrial myocardium, then to a specialized conducting system, and finally to the ventricular myocardium.

Myocardial Action Potential

The **myocardial action potential** has three prominent phases:

1. A rapid **upstroke** and **initial peak** due to opening of sodium channels and inflow of Na^+;
2. A **plateau phase**, during which g_{Na} inactivates, but calcium channels, opened by depolarization, provide prolonged Ca^{++} entry; "rectifying" potassium channels, open at rest, close during prolonged depolarization (membrane conductance *decrease*); and
3. **Repolarization**, during which g_{Ca} subsides, delayed potassium channels open, "rectifying" potassium channels also open with more negative membrane potential, and outflow of K^+ restores the resting potential.

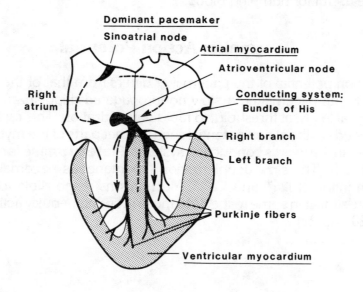

Dominant pacemaker
Sinoatrial node
Atrial myocardium
Atrioventricular node
Right atrium
Conducting system:
Bundle of His
Right branch
Left branch
Purkinje fibers
Ventricular myocardium

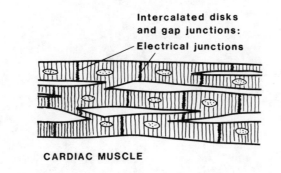

Intercalated disks
and gap junctions:
Electrical junctions

A   CARDIAC MUSCLE

Figure 58   *A*, Organization of the heart. *Figure continues.*

Refractory Period

Cardiac tissue has a prolonged refractory period after the action potential (Fig. 58B), due largely to inactivation of sodium channels. Functionally, this feature prevents rapid re-excitation of the heart and limits its frequency of response to the range useful for pumping blood.

Pacemaker Action Potential

The action potential of the pacemaker differs from that of the myocardium (Fig. 58C). In the pacemaker, a slow nonpropagated depolarization after each action potential leads, at threshold, to rapid depolarization. This rapid depolarization corresponds to the action potential seen in other parts of the myocardium and is propagated in the heart's conducting systems. **Plateau phase** is reduced in the pacemaker cells. The slow depolarization (spontaneous pacemaker potential) results from influx of Na^+ and Ca^{++}. Mechanisms responsible for pacemaker potentials are similar in some respects to those in spontaneously active nerve cells (see Units 20 and 21).

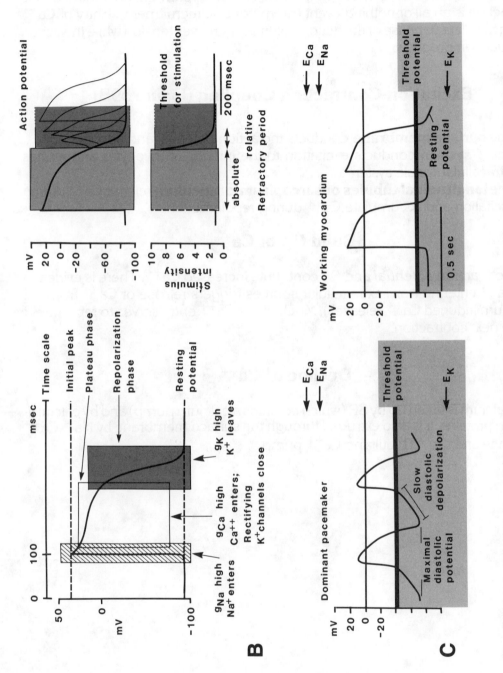

Figure 58 (continued)   B, Cardiac action potential and refractory period. C, Pacemaker and myocardial action potentials. (A, From Antoni H. Function of the heart. In: Schmidt RF, Thews G, eds. Human physiology. Heidelberg: Springer-Verlag, 1983:360. With permission from Springer-Verlag. Modified from Eckert R, Randall D. Animal physiology. San Francisco: WH Freeman, 1978:310. B and C, Adapted from Antoni H. Function of the heart. In: Schmidt RF, Thews G, eds. Human physiology. Heidelberg: Springer-Verlag, 1983: 361-363.)

UNIT 59
HEART: CONTRACTION

Unlike skeletal muscle, the heart cannot be tetanized, owing to its long action potential and refractory period (Fig. 59A). The syncytium ensures that cardiac contraction is an all-or-nothing event (no motor unit recruitment). Entry of Ca^{++} during the plateau phase of the action potential increases tension while the action potential is in progress.

Excitation-Contraction Coupling (Figure 59B)

1. The **surface membrane** conducts the action potential and admits Ca^{++}.
2. The **T-system** conducts excitation to the interior of myocytes and excites intracellular tubule systems.
3. The **longitudinal tubules or sarcoplasmic reticulum** release Ca^{++} during excitation and accumulate Ca^{++} during repolarization.

Build-Up of Ca^{++}

Both *action potential* and *SR* contribute increased Ca^{++}. There is evidence that Ca^{++} entering from extracellular sources triggers release of Ca^{++} from SR ("calcium-induced Ca^{++} release"). Much of the Ca^{++} entry serves to reprime SR for the next contraction.

Decline of Ca^{++}

Calcium is taken up by SR (which contains a calcium pump) and by calcium-binding proteins. It is also extruded through the surface membrane by Na^+-Ca^{++} exchange and the ATP-utilizing Ca^{++} pump.

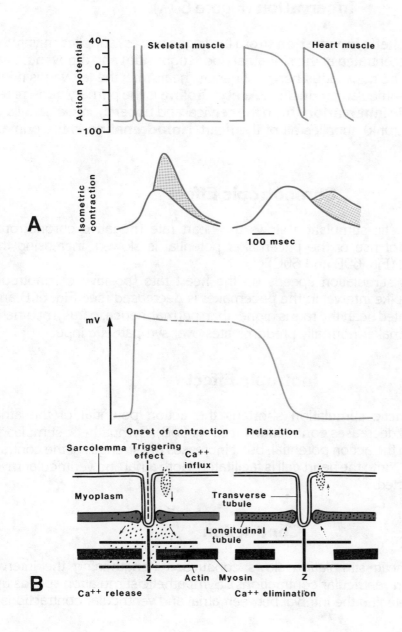

Figure 59 *A,* Relation of contraction to the action potential. *B,* Ionic events in contraction. (From Antoni H. Function of the heart. In: Schmidt RF, Thews G. Human physiology. Heidelberg: Springer-Verlag, 1983:364. With permission from Springer-Verlag, Heidelberg.)

UNIT 60
HEART: ACTION OF TRANSMITTERS

Innervation (Figure 60A)

Parasympathetic innervation (from the vagus nerves) supplies mainly the atrium and is concentrated at the sinoatrial node (right side) and atrioventricular node (left side). The right vagus nerve influences heart rate; the left vagus nerve influences atrioventricular conduction. **Acetylcholine** is the primary transmitter.

Sympathetic innervation (from the cervical and upper thoracic ganglia of the sympathetic trunk) supplies all of the heart. **Noradrenaline** is the primary transmitter.

Chronotropic Effect

Parasympathetic stimulation slows the heart rate (negative chronotropic effect). The rate of rise of the pacemaker potential is slowed, increasing the interspike interval (Fig. 60B and 60C).

Sympathetic stimulation speeds up the heart rate (positive chronotropic effect. The interspike interval in the pacemaker is decreased (see Fig. 60B and 60C). In a denervated heart the rate is higher than normal; hence, parasympathetic input to the pacemaker normally predominates over sympathetic input.

Inotropic Effect

Parasympathetic stimulation shortens the action potential of the atrial myocardium and decreases contraction (see Fig. 60B). Sympathetic stimulation has little effect on the action potential, but it increases the strength of the contraction. Entry of Ca^{++} into the heart cell is facilitated. Both atrial and ventricular myocardium are effected.

Conduction

Parasympathetic stimulation slows conduction (lengthening the interval between atrial and ventricular contractions). Sympathetic stimulation speeds up conduction (shortening the interval between atrial and ventricular contractions).

Transmitter Actions

The inhibitory effects of acetylcholine are largely due to an *increase in K^+ conductance*. Membrane potential is pulled toward E_K during transmission; outflow of K^+ generates a counter-current to Na^+ and Ca^{++} inflow during the time that the membrane is depolarized (see Unit 17).

Noradrenaline acts on beta-adrenergic receptors. In the myocardium, enhanced Ca^{++} entry through a larger number of calcium channels (see Unit 41) leads to more intense excitation-contraction coupling.

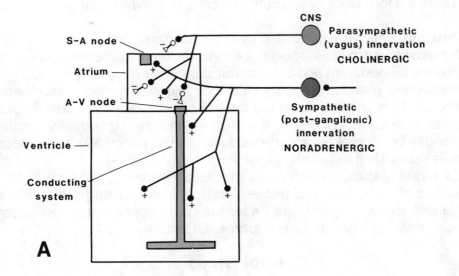

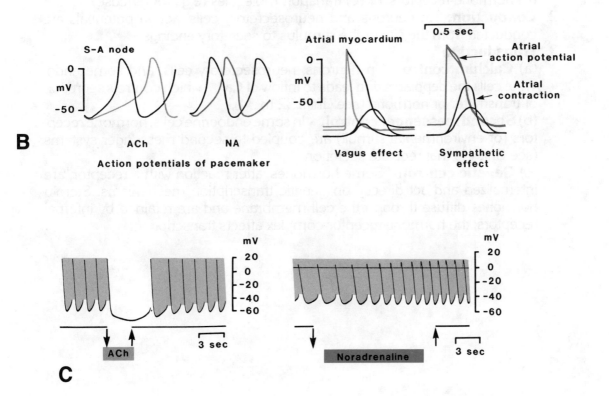

Figure 60 *A,* Distribution of innervation. *B,* Changes in action potentials and contraction in atrial myocardium and the pacemaker. *C,* Pacemaker frequency and transmitter action. (*B,* Adapted from Antoni H. Function of the heart. In: Schmidt RF, Thews G, eds. Human physiology. Heidelberg: Springer-Verlag, 1983:366. *C,* Adapted from Hutter OF, Trautwein W. Vagal and sympathetic effects on the pacemaker fibers in the sinus venosus of the heart. J Gen Physiol 1956; 39:720, 728.)

UNIT 61
SECRETORY EFFECTORS: GENERAL OVERVIEW

There are four types of secretory effectors (Fig. 61A):

1. **Neurons**, which are controlled by other neurons.
2. **Neurosecretory cells**, specialized neurons that release secretory products into the bloodstream and are controlled by other neurons (Fig. 61B)
3. **Endocrine glands**, secretory cells that release hormones into the blood-stream. They may be under the control of neurons (e.g., adrenal medulla), other endocrine cells (e.g., the thyroid and the reproductive endocrine glands), or internal environmental factors (e.g., pancreatic insulin-secreting cells responding to blood glucose levels).
4. **Exocrine glands**, secretory cells that release secretory products at the outer surface of the body (e.g., digestive glands, mucus-secreting goblet cells, sweat glands). Exocrine glands are under the control of neurons, neurosecretory cells, endocrine glands, or environmental factors.

Control Steps

1. **Stimulus.** The stimulus is usually receptor-mediated by (a) synapses, (b) hormone receptors, or (c) transport molecules (e.g., for glucose).
2. **Conduction.** In neurons and neurosecretory cells, action potentials are conducted from the site of the stimulus to secretory endings.
3. **Transduction**
   (a) **Calcium control.** In neurons, neurosecretory cells, and some endo-crine cells the depolarization leads to inflow of Ca^{++}, which controls secretion of transmitter or hormone (see Units 32 to 34).
   (b) **Second messenger control.** In some endocrine cells, hormone recep-tors (or environmental stimuli) are coupled to second messenger systems (see Unit 41) that regulate secretion.
   (c) **Genetic control.** Some hormones, after reaction with a receptor, are internalized and act directly on genetic transcription mechanisms. Steroid hormones diffuse through the cell membrane and are retained by internal receptors; the hormone-receptor complex affects transcription.

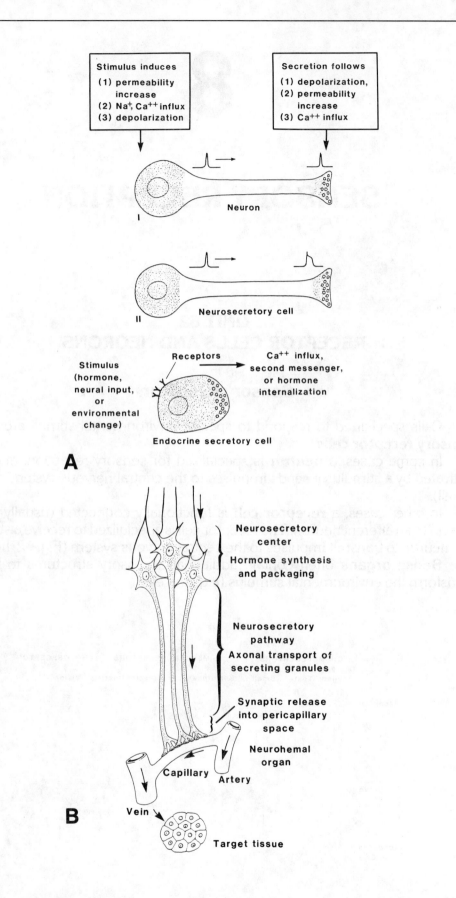

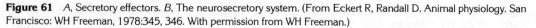

Figure 61 *A*, Secretory effectors. *B*, The neurosecretory system. (From Eckert R, Randall D. Animal physiology. San Francisco: WH Freeman, 1978:345, 346. With permission from WH Freeman.)

8

SENSORY RECEPTION

UNIT 62
RECEPTOR CELLS AND NEURONS

Sensory Receptors

Cells specialized to respond to specific environmental stimuli are termed **sensory receptor cells**.

In some cases, a **neuron** is specialized for sensory reception, and when activated by a stimulus it sends impulses to the central nervous system (Fig. 62, smell).

In other cases, a **receptor cell** is functionally connected (usually by synapses) to an afferent neuron. The receptor cell is specialized to receive a stimulus, the neuron to transmit impulses to the central nervous system (Fig. 62, hearing).

Sense organs often contain additional accessory structures to filter or transform the environmental stimulus (e.g., the eye).

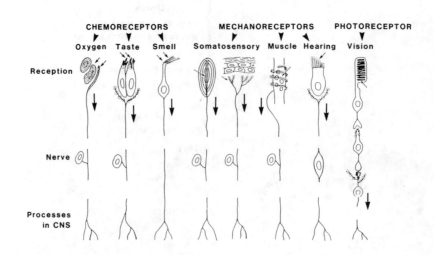

Figure 62   Types of sensory receptor cells. (Adapted from Shepherd GM. Neurobiology. New York: Oxford University Press, 1982:208.)

134

Sensory Modalities

Receptor cells respond specifically to certain stimuli (**receptor specificity**). The four major groups of receptors in mammals are mechanoreceptors, thermoreceptors, chemoreceptors, and photoreceptors. Examples are given in Table 62 and Figure 62.

TABLE 62   Sensory Modalities

Sensory Modality	Form of Energy	Receptor Organ	Receptor Cell	Type of Receptor
Chemical				
Common chemical	Molecules	Various	Free nerve endings	C
Arterial oxygen	O_2 tension	Carotid body	Cell and nerve endings	C
Toxins (vomiting)	Molecular	Medulla	Chemoreceptor cells	C
Osmotic pressure	Osmotic pressure	Hypothalamus	Osmoreceptors	C
Glucose	Glucose	Hypothalamus	Glucoreceptors	C
pH (cerebrospinal fluid)	Ions	Medulla	Ventricle cells	C
Taste	Ions and molecules	Tongue, pharynx	Taste bud cells	C
Smell	Molecules	Nose	Olfactory receptors	C
Somatosensory				
Touch	Mechanical	Skin	Encapsulated nerve terminals	M
Pressure	Mechanical	Skin, deep tissue	Encapsulated nerve endings	M
Temperature	Temperature	Skin, hypothalamus	Nerve terminals, central neurons	T
Pain	Various	Skin, various organs	Nerve terminals	M
Muscle				
Vascular pressure	Mechanical	Blood vessels	Nerve terminals	M
Muscle stretch	Mechanical	Muscle spindle	Nerve terminals	M
Muscle tension	Mechanical	Tendon organs	Nerve terminals	M
Joint pressure	Mechanical	Joint capsule, ligaments	Nerve terminals	M
Balance				
Linear acceleration (gravity)	Mechanical	Vestibular (otolith) organs	Hair cells	M
Angular acceleration	Mechanical	Vestibular organs (semicircular canals)	Hair cells	M
Hearing	Mechanical	Inner ear (cochlea)	Hair cells	M
Vision	Electromagnetic (photons)	Eye (retina)	Photoreceptors	P

C = chemoreceptor, T = thermoreceptor, M = mechanoreceptor, P = photoreceptor.

From Shepherd GM. Neurobiology. New York: Oxford University Press, 1983:188. Reprinted with permission from Oxford University Press.

UNIT 63
RECEPTION OF STIMULI: RESPONSE

Receptor Sequence

The steps in reception of a stimulus are outlined in Figure 63A for (i) a receptor neuron and for (ii) a receptor cell coupled synaptically to a neuron.

The key step in transduction is **change in membrane conductance** in the stimulated receptor cell. This leads to a **receptor potential**. Often this is caused by net flow of cations into the cell, leading to depolarization (most mechanoreceptors). If the receptor potential in a receptor neuron exceeds threshold of the adjacent excitable membrane, action potentials result. If the stimulus is weak, a subthreshold receptor potential results, seen only in the receptive endings of the neuron (Fig. 63B).

When synaptic transmission from a receptor cell to a second-order neuron is involved, the nonspiking receptor cell experiences a receptor potential, as above, which increases (or decreases) transmitter secretion at the synapse. A synaptic potential appears in the neuron. Impulses are generated by a depolarizing synaptic potential and inhibited if the synaptic potential is hyperpolarizing.

Transducer Systems

Membranes of receptor cells are endowed with channels that are gated open or shut in the resting condition (Fig. 63C). The stimulus alters the gate, changing membrane conductance. Ions flow to generate the receptor potential (see Unit 64).

Photoreceptors respond to light by generating a second messenger molecule, which acts internally to alter membrane conductance (see Unit 76).

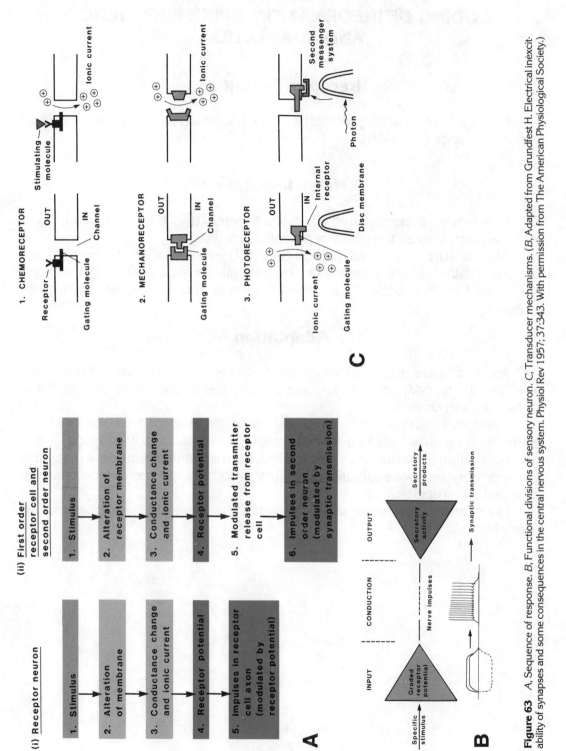

Figure 63 *A*, Sequence of response. *B*, Functional divisions of sensory neuron. *C*, Transducer mechanisms. (*B*, Adapted from Grundfest H. Electrical inexcitability of synapses and some consequences in the central nervous system. Physiol Rev 1957; 37:343. With permission from The American Physiological Society.)

UNIT 64
CODING OF INFORMATION: SPIKE FREQUENCY
AND ADAPTATION

Receptor Potential

Magnitude of receptor potential is graded: stronger stimuli produce a larger potential change (Fig. 64A).

Nerve Impulses

Impulses are generated by the receptor potential (Fig. 64B). The frequency of impulses increases as the receptor potential increases.

After each impulse, repolarization occurs. The rate at which the membrane is depolarized after recovery from an action potential increases with larger receptor potentials (see Fig. 64B). Thus, strength of stimulus is "coded" by impulse frequency.

Adaptation

A maintained stimulus usually produces a receptor potential that decreases with time (Figs. 64A and 64C). Consequently, the frequency of impulses also decreases with time.

Different sensory receptors show different rates of adaptation (see Fig. 64C). Some receptors are "rapidly adapting," while others are "slowly adapting."

Adaptation is produced by several different mechanisms. In some receptors, the accessory sensory structures play a role; in others, the membrane channels change their properties.

Functionally, adaptation allows for better detection of *changes* in environmental stimuli.

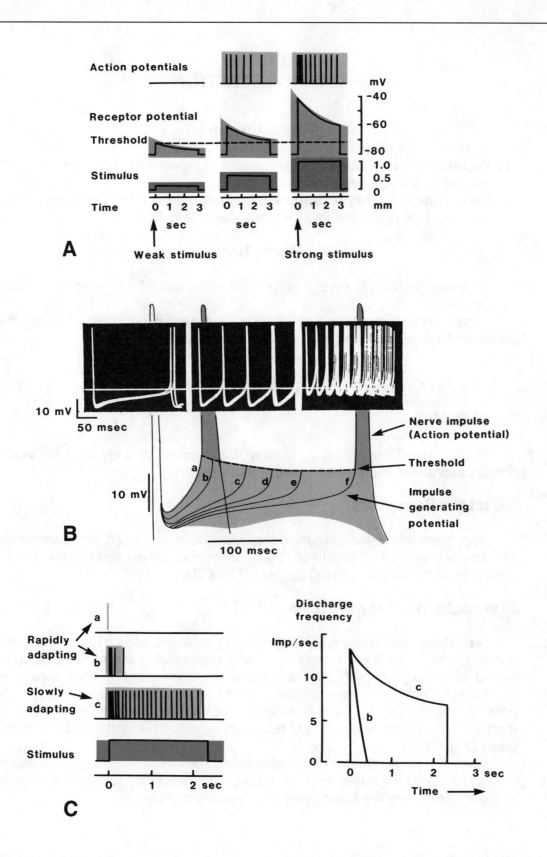

Figure 64 *A*, Coding of stimulus intensity into impulse frequency. *B*, The rate of rise of the impulse-generating potential determines the spike interval. *C*, Slow and rapid adaptation. (*A* and *C*, Adapted from Zimmerman M. Sensory system. In: Schmidt RF, ed. Fundamentals of neurophysiology. New York: Springer-Verlag, 1975:196, 197. *B*, Adapted from Eyzaguirre C, Kuffler SW. Processes of excitation in the dendrites and in the soma of single isolated sensory nerve cells of the lobster and crayfish. J Gen Physiol 1955; 39:102.)

UNIT 65
CHEMORECEPTION

Sense Organs

1. **Vertebrate taste buds** contain special receptor cells that synapse onto secondary afferent nerve axons.
2. **Vertebrate olfactory receptors** are primary afferent nerve cells with receptor processes projecting into the nasal cavity (Fig. 65A).

Reception

Receptor proteins of several types react with stimulating molecules to gate ionic channels.

Flow of ionic current produces a receptor potential that modulates impulse production in the primary or secondary nerve cell (see Unit 64).

Discrimination

Taste Buds

Four primary taste stimuli are known (sweet, sour, salt, and bitter). Individual sensory axons are differentially sensitive to these stimuli.

Olfactory Receptors

Approximately seven primary odors have been proposed for mammalian olfactory sensation. Individual sensory neurons may be excited or inhibited by particular odors, and to differing degrees (Fig. 65B).

Stereochemical Hypothesis

Size, shape, and charge of the stimulating molecule allow it to combine with one or more of the basic types of receptor molecule to produce a response. Individual sensory receptors may have more than one type of receptor molecule.

Discrimination of many different odors (several hundred for humans) is possible through (a) excitation or inhibition of impulse production in individual receptors, and (b) *combinations* of receptors recruited (or inhibited) by different odors (Fig. 65B3).

Given the large number of possible combinations of different active receptors, and the variation in impulse production, many different odors can be discriminated with relatively few basic types of receptor molecules.

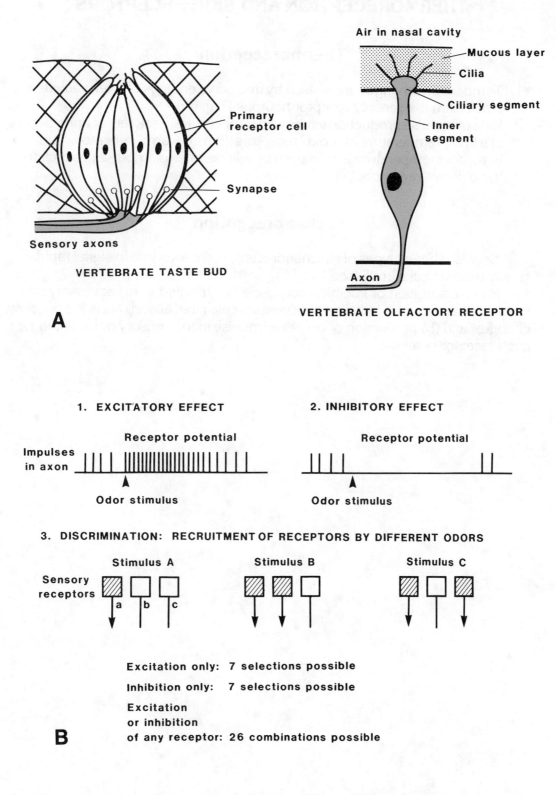

A

Primary
receptor cell

Synapse

Sensory axons

VERTEBRATE TASTE BUD

Air in nasal cavity

Mucous layer

Cilia

Ciliary segment

Inner
segment

Axon

VERTEBRATE OLFACTORY RECEPTOR

1. EXCITATORY EFFECT

Receptor potential

Impulses
in axon

Odor stimulus

2. INHIBITORY EFFECT

Receptor potential

Odor stimulus

3. DISCRIMINATION: RECRUITMENT OF RECEPTORS BY DIFFERENT ODORS

Sensory
receptors

Stimulus A

a b c

Stimulus B

Stimulus C

Excitation only: 7 selections possible

Inhibition only: 7 selections possible

Excitation
or inhibition
of any receptor: 26 combinations possible

B

Figure 65 *A*, Chemoreceptor organs: taste and smell. *B*, Electrical response: impulses. (*A*, Modified from Eckert R, Randall D. Animal physiology. San Francisco: WH Freeman, 1978:203.)

UNIT 66
THERMORECEPTION AND SKIN RECEPTORS

Thermoreception

1. Temperature changes are sensed by free nerve endings of intermediate- and small-diameter sensory receptor neurons (Fig. 66).
2. Rate of impulse production varies with temperature. Peak rate of firing occurs at a lower temperature in "cold" receptors than in "warm" receptors. Information about temperature is conveyed by relative rates of impulse production in the different receptors.

Mechanoreception

Several different types of mechanoreceptors are available to signal rapid and steady mechanical stimuli (see Fig. 66).

Rapid adaptation of Pacinian corpuscle is attributed to (a) accessory structures (concentric outer lamellae of accessory cells) that absorb and filter out slow changes, and (b) production of only one impulse in the sensory nerve ending for each receptor potential.

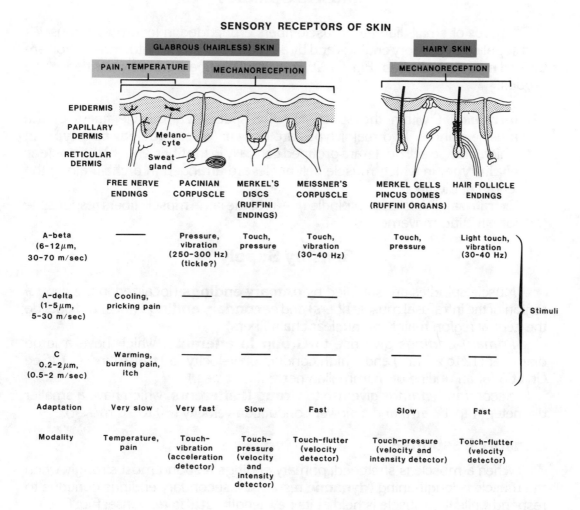

Figure 66 Sensory receptors of skin. (Adapted from Shepherd GM. Neurobiology. New York: Oxford University Press, 1983:232, 233.)

UNIT 67
MECHANORECEPTION IN MUSCLE

Muscle Spindles

Groups of small-diameter muscle fibers embedded in locomotory muscles and supplied by sensory endings and by a separate efferent motor innervation are termed **muscle spindles** (Fig. 67A). Thus, muscle fibers can be classified in two groups:

1. **Intrafusal** ("within the spindle") — the specialized muscle fibers of the muscle spindle. Two major types are known: (a) the **nuclear bag type**, in which muscle cell nuclei are grouped centrally in the fiber, and (b) the **nuclear chain type**, in which muscle cell nuclei are arranged in a chain along the length of the fiber.
2. **Extrafusal** ("outside the spindle") — all of the large muscle fibers responsible for effecting movement.

Sensory Supply

Muscle spindles are supplied by **primary endings** (localized in the central region of the intrafusal muscle fibers) and **secondary endings** (localized outside the central region mainly on nuclear chain fibers).

Primary endings give rise to **Group Ia afferents**, which have a large diameter (12 to 20 μm) and a high conduction velocity (80 to 120 m/sec). (See Unit 68 for an outline of mammalian nerve fiber types.)

Secondary endings give rise to **Group II afferents**, which have a smaller diameter (4 to 12 μm) and a slower conduction velocity (30 to 70 m/sec).

Sensory Response

When a muscle is stretched, primary endings respond most strongly when the muscle is lengthening (**dynamic** response); secondary endings continue to respond while the muscle is held at its new length (**static** response; Fig. 67B).

Golgi Tendon Organs

Endings of afferent nerve fibers embedded in tendons at the ends of muscles form **Golgi tendon organs** (see Fig. 67A). Their afferent axons are **Group Ib afferents**. The sensory stimulus is active **muscle tension** exerted in the tendon (*not* muscle lengthening or shortening).

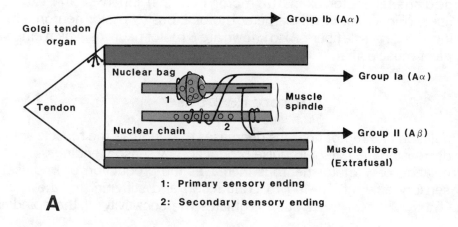

1: Primary sensory ending
2: Secondary sensory ending

A

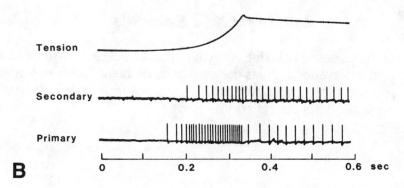

B

Figure 67 *A,* Sensory innervation of muscle. *B,* Impulses in primary and secondary sensory processes of muscle spindles. (*B,* Adapted from Matthews PBC. Mammalian muscle receptors and their central actions. London: Edward Arnold, 1972:148.)

UNIT 68
EFFERENT CONTROL OF MUSCLE SENSORY RECEPTORS AND AXON CLASSIFICATION

Efferent Innervation

Large-diameter motor axons (α motor neurons) innervate the extrafusal muscle fibers (Fig. 68A). Small-diameter motor axons (γ motor neurons) innervate the intrafusal muscle fibers. Also known are β motor neurons, which innervate both types of muscle fiber.

Sensory Response

Stimulation of α motor neurons decreases the length of the muscle spindle, thereby decreasing the rate of impulse production by sensory endings.

Stimulation of γ motor neurons increases the production of impulses in spindle sensory afferents, owing to contraction and stiffening of the muscle spindle. Thus, γ motor innervation regulates the sensitivity of the spindle to stretch.

Differences in response of Group I afferents to stretch during stimulation of *dynamic* γ innervation and *static* γ innervation are shown in Figure 68B. Dynamic innervation affects nuclear bag fibers. Static innervation affects nuclear chain fibers as well as some nuclear bag fibers.

Role of Muscle Spindles

Muscle spindles sense **relative length** of the muscle and **rate of change of length**. Efferent innervation adjusts the sensitivity of the spindles so that they can continue to provide information over a wide range of muscle length (particularly when the muscle shortens during contraction).

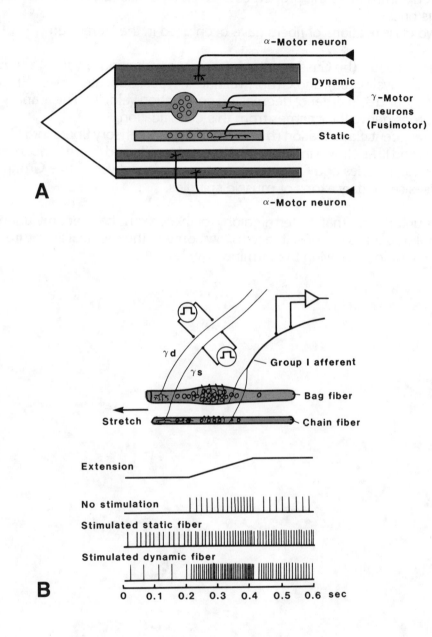

Figure 68 *A,* Efferent innvervation of muscle. *B,* Responses of Group I sensory endings to γ motor stimulation. (*B, Top,* From Kuffler SW, Nicholls JG, Martin AR. From neuron to brain. Sunderland, MA: Sinauer Associates, 1984:394. With permission from Sinauer Associates. *Bottom,* Adapted from Crowe A, Matthews PBC. The effects of stimulation of static and dynamic fusimotor fibres on the response of stretching of the primary endings of muscle spindles. J Physiol 1964; 174:112.)

Fiber Types

The classification of axons in mammalian peripheral nerve is shown in Table 68, which summarizes the properties of axon types discussed in this unit and in previous ones.

Two classifications of fibers have been used in the literature:

1. Classification (by Gasser) into A (rapidly conducting myelinated), B (autonomic myelinated), and C (unmyelinated) types. Subcategories of Type A are α, β, γ, and δ, in order of decreasing conduction velocity. The α and γ motorneurons derive their names from this classification.
2. More recent classification (by Lloyd) of Type A sensory fibers into Groups Ia, Ib, II, and III as shown in Table 68. Here, Groups Ia and Ib are sensory axons of muscle spindles and Golgi tendon organs, respectively, while Group II comprises secondary axons of muscle spindles.

It is unfortunate that the terminology for these axons has become unnecessarily complex, but it is not possible to follow some of the medical literature or even textbooks without knowing the terminology.

TABLE 68   Categories of Axon in Mammalian Peripheral Nerve

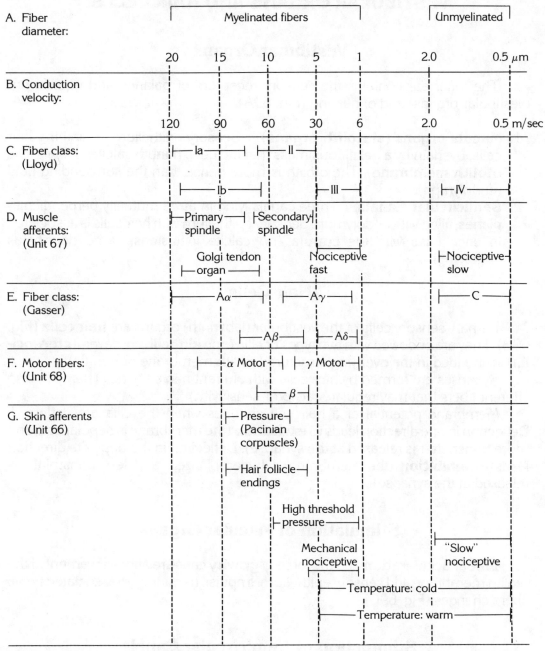

A. Fiber diameter:

| Myelinated fibers | Unmyelinated |

20   15   10   5   1   2.0   0.5 μm

B. Conduction velocity:

120   90   60   30   6   2.0   0.5 m/sec

C. Fiber class: (Lloyd)

Ia   II
Ib   III   IV

D. Muscle afferents: (Unit 67)

Primary spindle   Secondary spindle
Golgi tendon organ   Nociceptive fast   Nociceptive slow

E. Fiber class: (Gasser)

Aα   Aγ   C
Aβ   Aδ

F. Motor fibers: (Unit 68)

α Motor   γ Motor
β

G. Skin afferents (Unit 66)

Pressure (Pacinian corpuscles)
Hair follicle endings
High threshold pressure
Mechanical nociceptive   "Slow" nociceptive
Temperature: cold
Temperature: warm

Adapted from Somjen G. Sensory coding in the mammalian nervous system. New York: Meredith Corp., 1972:163.

149

UNIT 69
VESTIBULAR ORGANS AND HAIR CELLS

Vestibular Organs

The inner ear contains the sensory receptors of balance and equilibrium (vestibular organs) and of hearing (Fig. 69A).

1. **Macula organs (statolith organs).** Sensory epithelium containing hair cells, overlain by a gelatinous mass that includes minute calcite crystals (the **otolith membrane**). The otolith is more dense than the surrounding fluid (endolymph).
2. **Semicircular Canals.** Three canals lying in three mutually perpendicular planes, filled with endolymph. Sensory epithelium with hair cells is associated in each case with the **cupula** (no calcite inclusions, same density as endolymph).

Hair Cells

Primary sensory cells of the vestibular (labyrinth) organs are **hair cells** (Fig. 69B). They are endowed with two types of cilia (one **kinocilium**, several **stereocilia**) embedded in the overlying structure (otolith membrane or cupula).

Synapses are formed by hair cells with afferent nerve fibers. (There are also efferent fibers that may regulate receptor sensitivity.)

Membrane potential of a hair cell changes when the cilia are deflected. Deflection in one direction leads to **excitation** (the membrane is depolarized, and more transmitter is released at the synapse). Deflection in the opposite direction leads to **inhibition** (the membrane is hyperpolarized, and less transmitter is released at the synapse).

Stimulation of Macular Organs

Linear acceleration and the force of **gravity** cause relative movement of the otolith membrane and sensory epithelium. Impulse frequency in associated nerve fibers changes (Fig. 69C).

Stimulation of Semicircular Canals

Angular acceleration (head rotation) displaces the cupula relative to underlying hair cells. Inertia of the endolymph in the canal causes deflection of the cupula in the direction opposite head rotation. Impulse frequency in the sensory fiber changes with acceleration, but not with maintained position (see Fig. 69C).

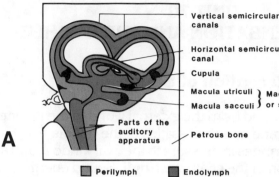

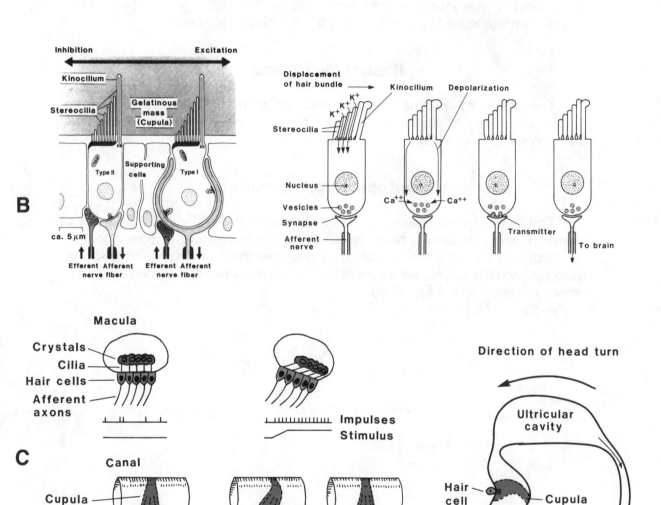

Figure 69 *A*, Vestibular organs. *B*, Vestibular hair cells. *C*, Stimuli for vestibular organs. (*A*, Adapted from Klinke R. Physiology of the sense of equilibrium, hearing and speech. In: Schmidt RF, Thews G, eds. Human physiology. Heidelberg: Springer-Verlag, 1983:274. *B, Left*, From Klinke R. Physiology of the sense of equilibrium, hearing and speech. In: Schmidt RF, Thews G, eds. Human physiology. Heidelberg: Springer-Verlag, 1983:275. With permission from Springer-Verlag, Heidelberg. *Right*, From Hudspeth AJ. The hair cells of the inner ear. Sci Am 1983; 248:64. With permission from WH Freeman. Copyright 1983 by Scientific American Inc. *C, Left,* Adapted from Shepherd GM. Neurobiology. New York: Oxford University Press, 1988:287. *Right*, From Somjen G. Neurophysiology—the essentials. Baltimore: Williams & Wilkins, 1983:342. Reproduced with permission from Williams & Wilkins.)

UNIT 70
AUDITORY SENSATION AND THE COCHLEA

Reception of Sound

Sound waves are transmitted from the external world to the inner ear (cochlea) via the tympanic membrane and the ossicles of the middle ear (Fig. 70A).

The ossicles transmit changes in pressure to the oval window, and a pressure wave appears in the perilymph of the **scala vestibuli**. Sound energy is dissipated in the **basilar membrane** and at the round window. Energy absorbed by the basilar membrane leads to excitation of the **cochlear hair cells**.

Basilar Membrane

The basilar membrane is elastic and has inertia; pressure waves in the perilymph cause it to vibrate. Vibrations ("ripples") move from base to apex as traveling waves (Fig. 70B).

Tonotopic Representation

The basilar membrane is narrower and stiffer at its base than at its apex. Vibrations of high frequency have their maximal amplitude near the base; those of low frequency have their maximal amplitude near the apex. Hair cells respond maximally to different sound frequencies (tones) at different locations along the basilar membrane (see Fig. 70B).

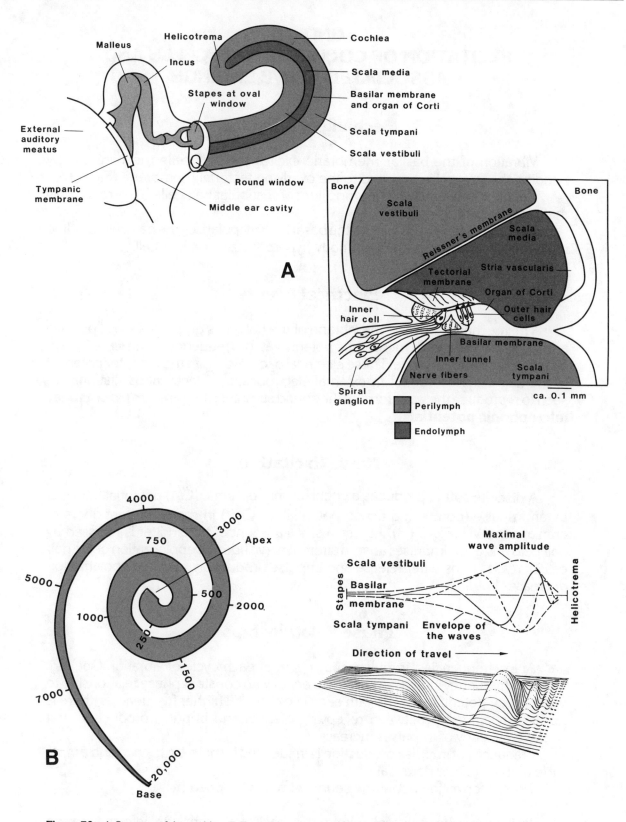

Figure 70 *A*, Structure of the cochlea. *B*, Tonotopic representation. (*A, Top,* Modified from Kandel ER, Schwartz JH. Principles of neural science. New York: Elsevier, 1985:398. *Bottom*, From Klinke R. Physiology of the sense of equilibrium, hearing and speech. In: Schmidt RF, Thews G, eds. Human physiology. Heidelberg: Springer-Verlag, 1983:281. With permission from Springer-Verlag, Heidelberg. *B*, Modified from Stuhlman O Jr. An introduction to biophysics. New York: John Wiley & Sons, 1943:286 and from Klinke R. Physiology of the sense of equilibrium, hearing and speech. In: Schmidt RF, Thews G, eds. Human physiology. Heidelberg: Springer-Verlag, 1983:285. With permission from Springer-Verlag, Heidelberg.)

UNIT 71
EXCITATION OF COCHLEAR HAIR CELLS AND ASSOCIATED NERVE ENDINGS

Mechanical Stimulus

Vibration of the basilar membrane excites the hair cells mechanically by bending the stereocilia attached to the overlying tectorial membrane (Fig. 71A).

Cochlear hair cells lack the kinocilium of vestibular hair cells. They retain only the basal body of this cilium.

Bending of stereocilia toward the basal body depolarizes the hair cell; bending of stereocilia away from the basal body hyperpolarizes the hair cell.

Electrical Events

The mechanoreceptive membrane of the hair cells generates small positive and negative changes in membrane potential at the frequency of the vibration set up in the basilar membrane. These electrical oscillations are the receptor potential of the hair cell. Recorded with external electrodes, the electrical oscillations are seen to reproduce the wave form of the sound stimulus; they are termed **cochlear microphonic potentials**.

Nerve Excitation

A discrete sound produces a cochlear microphonic (CM) potential followed by an impulse (compound action potential, or CAP) in many afferent fibers of cranial nerve VIII (Fig. 71B). At rest, a small amount of transmitter is released by hair cells and a few impulses arise in afferent nerve fibers. Depolarization of the hair cell increases transmitter release and impulse production, and hyperpolarization decreases both.

Phase Relationships

At low frequencies, impulses may occur at each cycle of vibration (see Fig. 71B). As frequency increases, impulses occur with constant phase relationship to the receptor potential, but not with each cycle. At still higher frequencies, there is no fixed relationship between receptor potential and impulse production, but overall frequency of impulses increases.

Frequency of impulse production is influenced by both *frequency* and *amplitude* of the receptor potential.

Thus, information about the sound stimulus is coded by:

1. Position of the hair cell along the basilar membrane: information on frequency.
2. Frequency of impulses in individual afferent nerve fibers: information on frequency.
3. Number of afferent nerve fibers recruited: information on intensity.

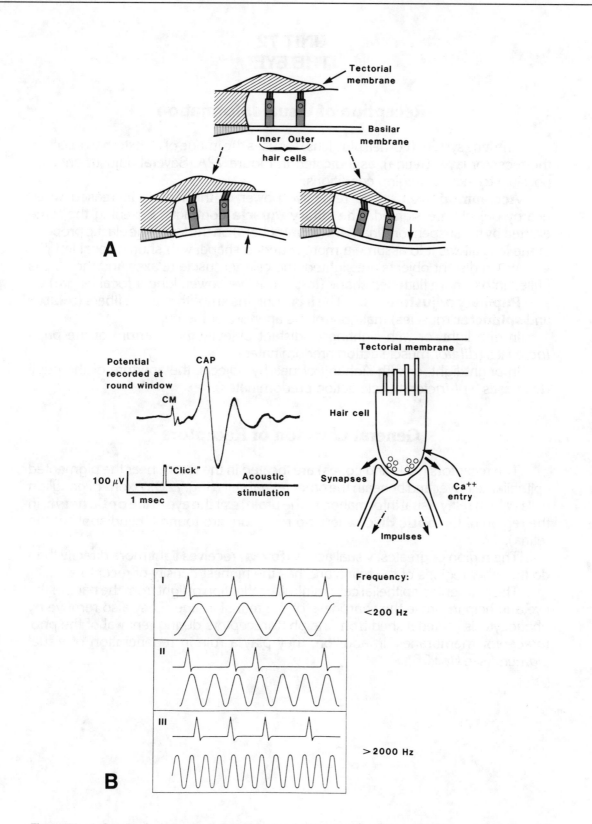

Figure 71 *A*, Stimulus for hair cells. *B*, Cochlear microphonic potentials and nerve impulse production. (*A* and *B, Bottom*, Adapted by Somjen G. Neurophysiology — the essentials. Baltimore: Williams & Wilkins, 1983:315, 320. *B, Top*, Adapted from Klinke R. Physiology of the sense of equilibrium, hearing and speech. In: Schmidt RF, Thews G, eds. Human physiology. Heidelberg: Springer-Verlag, 1983:286.)

UNIT 72
THE EYE

Reception of Visual Information

The lens system (cornea plus lens) focuses the image of an external object on the receptor layer (retina), as indicated in Figure 72A. Several adjustments are possible to meet changing conditions.

Accommodation. The refractive power of the lens is increased when nearby objects are sighted. The **ciliary muscle** contracts, lessening the force exerted by the suspensory ligament (zonule fibers) on the lens. The elastic property of the lens allows it to assume a more rounded shape, with shorter focal length.

When distant objects are sighted, the ciliary muscle relaxes and the lens is pulled into a more flattened shape (less refractive power, longer focal length).

Pupillary adjustments. The **iris** contains smooth muscle fibers (**dilator** and **sphincter** muscles) that control the aperture of the pupil.

In dim light, or with sighting of distant objects, the aperture of the pupil *increases* (*dilator* muscle action predominates).

In bright light, or with sighting of nearby objects, the aperture of the pupil *decreases* (*sphincter* muscle action predominates).

General Location of Receptors

The receptors (rods and cones) are located in the retina, near the pigmented epithelial cell layer and beneath the other retinal cells (Fig. 72B). Axons of ganglion cells (which relay visual information to the brain) exit the eye in the **optic nerve**, in the region of the **optic disc**, where no receptors are found ("blind spot" of the retina).

The region of greatest visual acuity (**fovea**) receives light more directly than do the other regions of the retina and has the highest density of receptors.

The pigmented epithelial cells minimize reflection of light from the back of the eye and help improve the sharpness of the retinal image. They also remove by phagocytosis material shed from the photoreceptors during renewal of the photoreceptor membranes. In addition, they play a role in regeneration of visual pigment (see Unit 76).

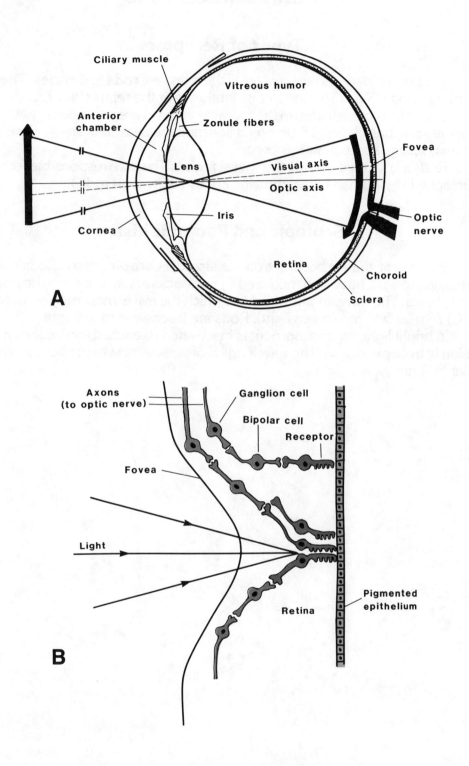

Figure 72 *A*, Structural features of the eye. *B*, General arrangement of receptor elements. (*A*, Modified from Eckert R, Randall D. Animal physiology. New York: WH Freeman, 1978:234. *B*, Modified from Kandel ER, Schwartz JH. Principles of neural science. New York: Elsevier, 1985:345.)

UNIT 73
RETINAL RECEPTORS

Types of Receptors

The two major types of receptors in the retina are **rods** and **cones**. They differ in morphology (Fig. 73A) and in distribution over the retina (Fig. 73B).

Cones are concentrated in the foveal region and are low in density elsewhere. They are responsible for sight in bright light and mediate color vision. (The human retina contains about 3 million cones.)

Rods are located outside the foveal region. They are responsible for sight in dim light. (The human retina contains about 100 million rods.)

Scotopic and Photopic Vision

In dim light, the eye becomes dark-adapted (**scotopic** vision). Rods have high sensitivity to light, but vision mediated by rods lacks acuity since they do not occur in the fovea. The wavelengths of light to which the eye is maximally sensitive (Fig. 73C) lie near 500 nm (green light). Rods are insensitive to red light.

In bright light, the rod pigment is inactivated (bleached) and cones mediate vision (**photopic** vision). The wavelengths of peak sensitivity in photopic vision lie near 560 nm (yellow light).

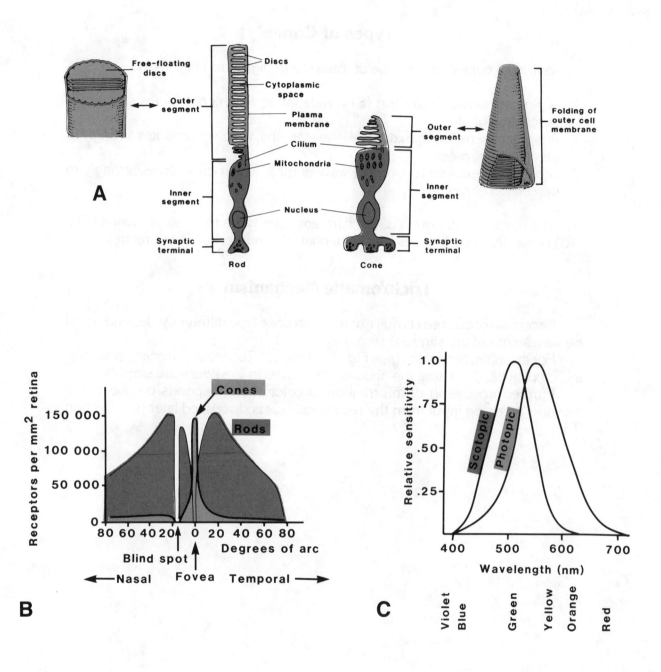

Figure 73 *A,* Structure of the rods and cones. *B,* Distribution of rods and cones over the retina. *C,* Sensitivity to wavelength of light in rods and cones. (*A,* Modified from Kandel ER, Schwartz JH. Principles of neural science. New York: Elsevier, 1985:346. *B,* From Grusser OJ. Vision and eye movements. In: Schmidt RF, Thews G, eds. Human physiology. Heidelberg: Springer-Verlag, 1983:243. With permission from Springer-Verlag, Heidelberg. *C,* From Somjen G. Neurophysiology — the essentials. Baltimore: Williams & Wilkins, 1983:261. With permission from Williams & Wilkins.)

UNIT 74
COLOR RECEPTION

Types of Cones

Individual cones contain one of three visual pigments (Fig. 74A):

1. A pigment sensitive to short (S) wavelengths, which contributes strongly to perception of blue.
2. A pigment sensitive to middle (M) wavelengths, which contributes strongly to perception of green.
3. A pigment sensitive to long (L) wavelengths, which contributes strongly to perception of red.

The overall contribution of the different cone types to photopic vision (Fig. 74B) shows that the S type is less influential (less numerous in the retina).

Trichromatic Mechanism

Reception of colored stimuli excites each cone type differently, depending on the wavelength of the stimulus (Fig. 74C).

For example, Stimulus I (see Fig. 74C) excites Receptor a strongly, b weakly, and c not at all. (Note that the absorbance curves in the figure are simplified.)

Further processing of information in color vision depends on the neural networks receiving input from the receptors. This is discussed later (see Section 15).

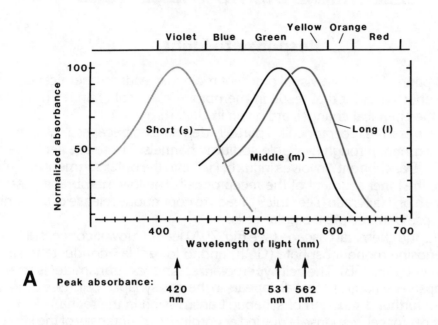

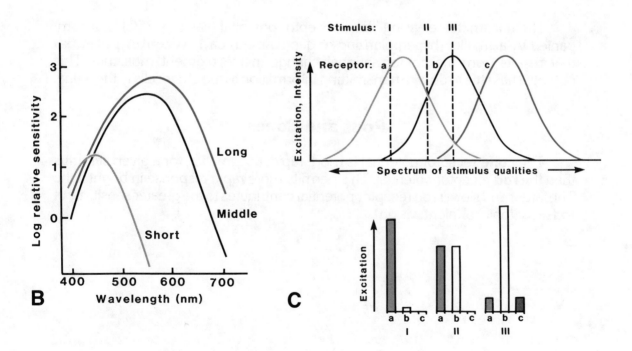

Figure 74 *A,* Absorption spectra of cones. *B,* The relative impact of different cone types on visual function. *C,* Trichromatic mechanism of color reception. (*A,* Modified from Dartnall HJA, Bowmaker JK. Microspectrophotometry of human photoreceptors. In: Mollon JD, Sharpe LT, eds. Colour vision. Physiology and psychophysics. London: Academic Press, 1983:72. *B,* Modified from Kandel ER, Schwartz JH. Principles of neural science. New York: Elsevier, 1985:385. *C,* Adapted from Somjen G. Sensory coding in the mammalian nervous system. New York: Meredith Corp., 1972:154.)

UNIT 75
ELECTRICAL EVENTS IN RECEPTORS

Response to Light

Absorption of light by a visual pigment molecule leads to chemical changes within the photoreceptor that result in membrane potential changes (Fig. 75A). Details of the chemical changes are given in Unit 76.

In *darkness*, the receptor cell is partially depolarized because Na^+ can enter the outer segment through available sodium channels. These are kept open by cyclic AMP. "Dark current" involves influx of Na^+ into the outer segment and efflux of K^+ from the inner segment of the receptor cell. The low membrane potential, caused by a high Na:K ratio (see Unit 9), leads to continuous release of transmitter at the synapse onto recipient bipolar cells.

In *light*, the chemical cascade (see Fig. 75A) leads to lower concentrations of cyclic guanosine monophosphate (GMP) and to lower Na^+ conductance in the outer segment (Fig. 75B). The cell hyperpolarizes, and *less* transmitter is released at the synapse. A synaptic potential appears in the postsynaptic cell. (See Units 113 and 118 for further discussion of synaptic transmission in the retina.)

The receptor cell response is graded according to the intensity of the stimulus (Fig. 75C).

Early and Late Potentials

The transmitter-releasing "late" receptor potential (see Fig. 75C) is accompanied by a smaller (hyperpolarizing or depolarizing) **early receptor potential** that results from the conformational change in the pigment molecule. This potential has little to do with transmitting information to the other cells in the retina.

Rods and Cones

The **cone** receptor potential is more rapid, but smaller, for a given stimulus than the **rod** receptor potential. This permits more rapid response in bright light. The larger and slower rod receptor potential contributes to the greater sensitivity of rods (scotopic, or night, vision).

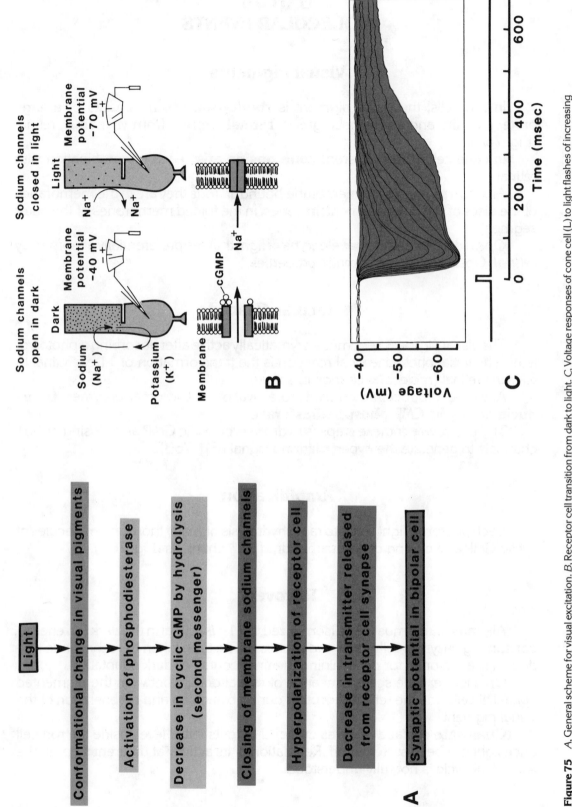

Figure 75 *A,* General scheme for visual excitation. *B,* Receptor cell transition from dark to light. *C,* Voltage responses of cone cell (L) to light flashes of increasing strength. (*B* and *C,* Adapted from Schnaupf JL, Baylor DA. How photoreceptor cells respond to light. Sci Am 1987; 256:43.)

UNIT 76
MOLECULAR EVENTS

Visual Pigments

In rod cells, the visual pigment is **rhodopsin**, which consists of a large protein, **opsin**, and a prosthetic group, **retinal**, derived from vitamin A, retinol (Fig. 76A).

In cone cells, three different **cone opsins** exist, each in combination with retinal.

All visual pigments are membrane-bound. In rods they are in the membranes of the discs of the outer segment; in cones, in the folded membranes of the outer segment.

Opsin determines the wavelengths of light that are preferentially absorbed by *retinal*. Opsin also has enzymatic properties.

Molecular Cascade

The visual pigment becomes enzymatically active after absorbing a photon of light. The initial photochemical reaction is the transformation of 11-*cis* retinal to all-*trans* retinal (molecular change in shape).

Activated *rhodopsin* then leads to activation of two other enzymes, **transducin** and cyclic GMP **phosphodiesterase**.

The end result of these steps is hydrolysis of cyclic GMP and closing of Na^+ channels to generate the hyperpolarizing signal (Fig. 76B).

Amplification

Each photon of light leads to rapid hydrolysis of many thousand molecules of cyclic GMP and closing of several hundred Na^+ channels (Fig. 76C).

Recovery

All-*trans* retinal must be re-isomerized to 11-*cis* retinal in the dark (an energy-consuming enzymatically catalyzed process). The time taken to reconstitute rhodopsin is a major factor determining the time course of dark adaptation.

On a longer time scale, exchange of retinal occurs between the pigmented epithelial cells and the retinal receptors during bleaching and regeneration of the visual pigment.

Guanylate cyclase restores cyclic GMP to its initial level inside the rod cell once light has been switched off. Regulation of its activity at different steps in the light–dark cycle is not fully understood.

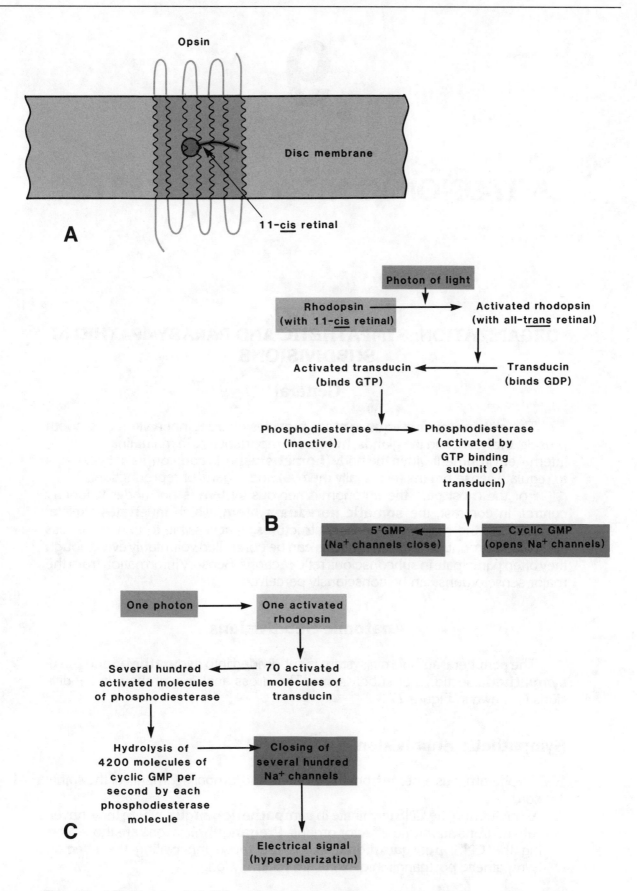

Figure 76 *A*, Rhodopsin in rod cells. *B*, Summary of molecular cascade initiated by light. *C*, Amplification of the effect of a photon.

9

AUTONOMIC NERVOUS SYSTEM

UNIT 77
ORGANIZATION: SYMPATHETIC AND PARASYMPATHETIC SUBDIVISIONS

General

The **autonomic nervous system** provides efferent innervation of smooth muscle, the heart, and the glands. It plays an important role in maintaining a stable internal environment within the body (**homeostasis**). In addition, its activity helps to regulate sense organs (especially the eye) and organs of reproduction.

For the most part, the autonomic nervous system is not under voluntary control. In contrast, the **somatic nervous system**, which innervates skeletal muscles and the majority of sensory structures, is accessible to consciousness and voluntary control. Skeletal muscles can be controlled voluntarily even though they often participate in subconscious reflex actions. Sensory information from the major sense organs can be consciously perceived.

Anatomic Subdivisions

The peripheral autonomic system is subdivided into **sympathetic** and **parasympathetic** sections, or subdivisions. The gross anatomy of the two subdivisions is shown in Figure 77.

Sympathetic Subdivision

1. Peripheral axons emerge from the thoracic and lumbar segments of the spinal cord.
2. Axons leaving the CNS terminate in **sympathetic ganglia**, where they innervate neurons supplying effector organs. **Preganglionic** axons are those leaving the CNS; **postganglionic** axons are those innervating the effector. Sympathetic postganglionic axons are relatively long.

3. Postganglionic neurons supply smooth muscles in all organs (blood vessels, viscera, excretory organs, genitalia, lungs, hair, eyes); the heart; glands (sweat, salivary, digestive); and adipose and liver cells.

Parasympathetic Subdivision

1. Peripheral axons emerge from the brainstem and from the sacral segments of the spinal cord.
2. Axons leaving the CNS go in nerves directly to effector organs, where they innervate neurons *within or close to* the organ. These **postganglionic** neurons innervate the target organs.
3. Postganglionic neurons supply smooth muscles of gastrointestinal organs, excretory organs, genitalia, lungs; glands of these organs; atria of the heart; tear and salivary glands; and intraocular muscles. Most blood vessels (except those of the genitalia and possibly of the brain) do not receive parasympathetic innervation.

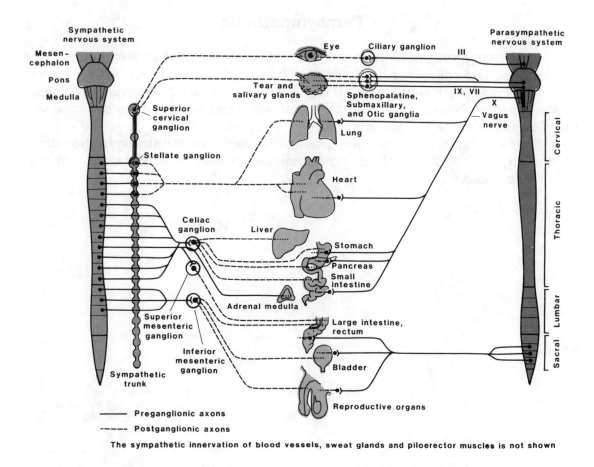

Figure 77 Peripheral autonomic nervous system. (The sympathetic innervation of blood vessels, sweat glands, and piloerector muscles is not shown.) (From Jänig W. The autonomic nervous system. In: Schmidt RF, Thews G, eds. Human physiology. Heidelberg: Springer-Verlag, 1983:112. With permission from Springer-Verlag, Heidelberg.)

167

UNIT 78
PREGANGLIONIC AND POSTGANGLIONIC NEURONS

Sympathetic

Preganglionic neurons (Fig. 78A) originate in the lateral horn of the spinal cord and reach the sympathetic ganglia via the **ventral spinal roots** and the **white ramus communicans** (Fig. 78B). They are mostly small myelinated axons, with a few unmyelinated axons.

Paired **paravertebral ganglia** form the sympathetic trunk. Most neurons synapse with postganglionic neurons here. Unpaired **prevertebral** or **paravisceral ganglia** (celiac, superior mesenteric, inferior mesenteric) are supplied by preganglionic axons that course through the paravertebral ganglia without forming synapses (see Fig. 78B).

Postganglionic neurons have their cell bodies in the sympathetic ganglia and send axons (mostly unmyelinated, a few myelinated) to effectors. Neurons supplying glands and blood vessels of skeletal muscles, skin, and connective tissue send axons through the **gray ramus communicans** to somatic nerves (see Fig. 78B).

Parasympathetic

Preganglionic neurons (see Fig. 78A) with cell bodies located in the brain send axons to cranial nerves. Neurons with cell bodies in the brainstem send their axons through the **vagus nerve** (cranial nerve X) to lungs, heart, and gastrointestinal system. Neurons of the sacral spinal cord send axons out the pelvic nerve. Most of the axons are unmyelinated.

Postganglionic neurons are generally located in **intramural ganglia** within the organs they supply. Thus, postganglionic axons are usually short and are unmyelinated.

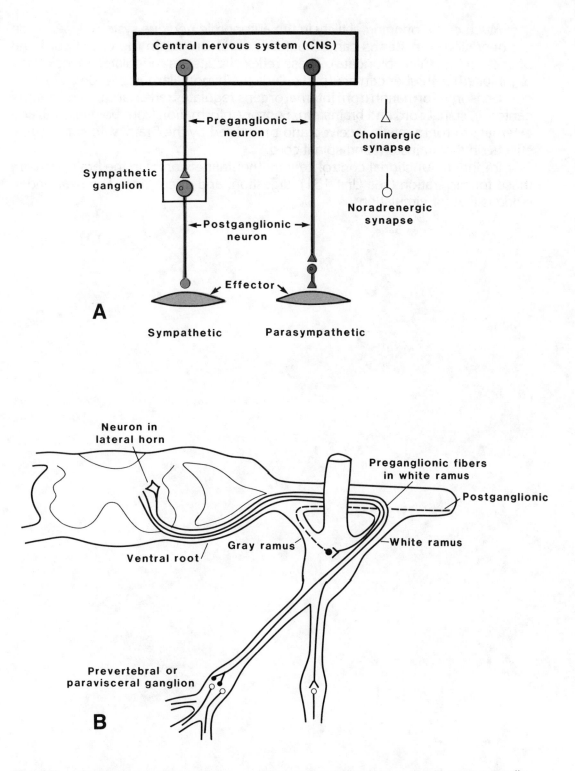

Figure 78 *A*, Preganglionic and postganglionic neurons. *B*, Locations of sympathetic neurons. (*A*, Modified after Jänig W. The autonomic nervous system. In: Schmidt RF, ed. Fundamentals of neuropathy. New York: Springer-Verlag, 1975:234. *B*, Modified after Ranson SW, Clark SL. The anatomy of the nervous system. Its development and function. Philadelphia: WB Saunders, 1959:157; and Somjen G. Neurophysiology — the essentials. Baltimore: Williams & Wilkins, 1983:426.)

UNIT 79
CENTRAL CONTROL OF AUTONOMIC FUNCTION: GENERAL FEATURES

Much of the ongoing activity in the autonomic nervous system depends on the operation of **reflexes** carried out by neural circuits in the spinal cord and brainstem (medulla oblongata). These reflex circuits are modulated (accelerated or inhibited) by higher centers (particularly the hypothalamus; see Unit 91).

Sensory information from internal organs regulates reflex circuits and control centers in spinal cord and brainstem. Sensory information from both internal and external environments is received and processed by the brain, with subsequent effects on the brainstem and spinal cord.

Important functional control centers (neural networks) in the brainstem are those for respiration (see Unit 131), digestion, and circulation. The best understood is that for circulation.

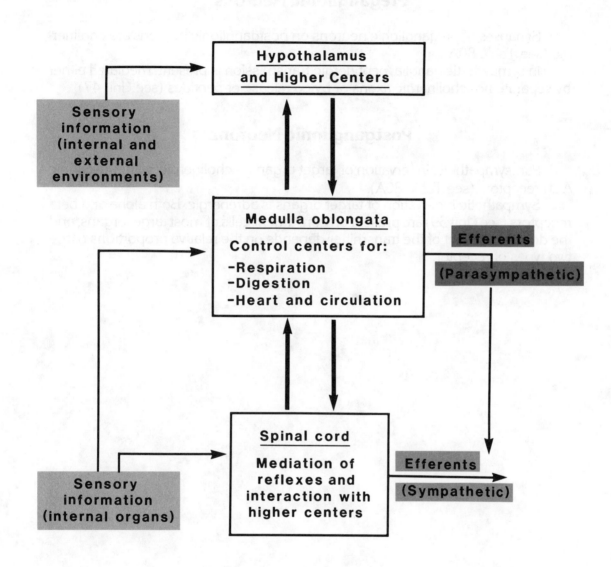

Figure 79 Hierarchy of control in the autonomic nervous system.

UNIT 80
PERIPHERAL AUTONOMIC SYSTEM: RECEPTORS AND TRANSMITTERS

Preganglionic Neurons

Synapses of preganglionic neurons on postganglionic neurons are cholinergic (see Table 80A).

In sympathetic ganglia, peptidergic transmission is present, mediated either by separate noncholinergic axons or by co-release of peptides (see Unit 47).

Postganglionic Neurons

Parasympathetic innervation of target organs is cholinergic, with muscarinic ACh receptors (see Table 80A).

Sympathetic innervation of target organs is adrenergic. Both alpha and beta receptors (see Unit 39) are present on constituent cells of most target organs, and the dominant effect of the transmitter depends on the relative proportions of the two types of receptor.

TABLE 80A Transmitters and Receptors for the Autonomic Nervous System

Synapse	Transmitter	Receptors	Synaptic Action
Sympathetic preganglionic axons to postganglionic neurons	Acetylcholine	Nicotinic ACh receptors	Excitatory (fast potential)
		Muscarinic ACh receptors	Excitatory (slow potential)
		ACh receptors	Inhibitory (slow potential)
	Peptides	Peptide receptors	Excitatory (late slow potential)
Parasympathetic preganglionic axons to postganglionic neurons	Acetylcholine	Nicotinic ACh receptors	Excitatory
Sympathetic postganglionic axons to most target organs	Noradrenaline	Alpha- and/or beta-adrenergic	Excitatory or inhibitory
Sympathetic postganglionic axons to sweat glands	Acetylcholine	Muscarinic ACh receptors	Excitatory
Postganglionic cells of adrenal medulla	Noradrenaline (20%) Adrenaline (80%)	Alpha- and beta-adrenergic receptors (by circulation)	Excitatory
Parasympathetic postganglionic axons to target organs	Acetylcholine	Muscarinic ACh receptors	Inhibitory or excitatory

Predominant Effects on Different Organs

Table 80B shows the effects of sympathetic and parasympathetic innervation on various organs. Generally, the two types of innervation exert opposite effects. The activity of most organs is constantly influenced by tonic discharge of the efferent neurons, with the balance between sympathetic and parasympathetic activity determining the organ's overall performance.

Under steady "resting" conditions, many organs are more strongly regulated by parasympathetic activity.

Functional synergy between the two innervations is achieved by alteration of sympathetic and parasympathetic efferent activity in opposite directions. For example, a decrease in heartbeat frequency and contractility (see Units 58 to 60) is normally brought about by an *increase* in activity of parasympathetic efferents to the heart and a simultaneous *decrease* in activity of sympathetic efferents.

TABLE 80B   Sympathetic and Parasympathetic Actions on Various Target Organs

Organ	Parasympathetic	Sympathetic	Type of Receptor (Sympathetic)
Heart			
Atria	Decreased heart rate	Increased heart rate	Beta
	Decreased contractile force	Increased contractile force	Beta
Ventricles	— —	Increased contractile force	Beta
Blood Vessels			
Vascular smooth muscle	— —	Vasoconstriction	Alpha
Arteriolar smooth muscle, in skeletal muscles	— —	Vasoconstriction; vasodilation (by circulating adrenaline)	Alpha, beta
Gastrointestinal Tract			
Longitudinal and circular muscles	Increased motility	Decreased motility	Alpha, beta
Sphincters	Relaxation	Contraction	Alpha
Urinary bladder			
Detrusor muscle	Contraction	Relaxation	Beta
Lungs			
Tracheal and bronochial musculature	Contraction	Relaxation	Beta
Eye			
Ciliary muscle	Contraction	Slight relaxation	Beta
Iris	Constriction of pupil	Dilation of pupil	Alpha
Hair			
Piloerector muscles	— —	Contraction	Alpha
Exocrine glands			
Salivary	Secretion	Secretion	Alpha
Tear	Secretion	— —	
Sweat	— —	Secretion	ACh
Bronchial	Secretion	— —	
Digestive	Secretion	Decreased secretion	Alpha
Liver	— —	Glycogenolysis, gluconeogenesis	Beta
Genital organs			
Vas deferens	— —	Contraction	Alpha
Uterus	— —	Contraction; relaxation	Alpha; beta
Adipose cells	— —	Liberation of fatty acids to blood	Beta
Pancreas	— —	Reduced secretion of insulin	Alpha

Modified after Jänig W. The autonomic nervous system. In: Schmidt RF, Thews G, eds. Human physiology. Heidelberg: Springer-Verlag, 1983:113.

UNIT 81
REFLEXES: SPINAL AUTONOMIC REFLEX PATHWAY

Reflex

A stereotyped reaction to a specific stimulus is termed a **reflex**. The neural network (circuit) responsible for the action is a **reflex pathway** or **reflex arc** (Fig. 81).

The simplest reflex arcs comprise a sensory element and motor efferent (monosynaptic reflex of the somatic nervous system). In the autonomic nervous system, the simplest circuits also include a spinal interneuron. Altogether, two synapses in the spinal cord and one in the autonomic ganglion intervene between the sensory afferent and the postganglionic efferent axon. Thus, autonomic reflexes generally follow the stimulus with greater delay than somatic reflexes. Slower conduction velocity of impulses in axons of the autonomic nervous system also contributes to slower speed of reflexes.

Segmental Organization

Afferent input for a reflex pathway may come from somatic or visceral afferents, or from higher centers ("descending" input).

Sensory input to the spinal cord activates autonomic reflexes most strongly in the same spinal cord segment.

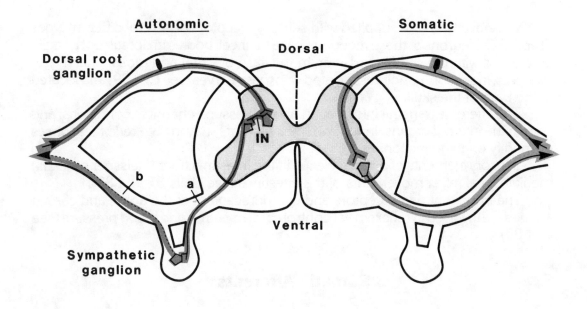

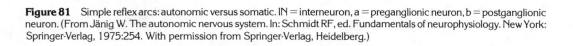

Figure 81 Simple reflex arcs: autonomic versus somatic. IN = interneuron, a = preganglionic neuron, b = postganglionic neuron. (From Jänig W. The autonomic nervous system. In: Schmidt RF, ed. Fundamentals of neurophysiology. New York: Springer-Verlag, 1975:254. With permission from Springer-Verlag, Heidelberg.)

UNIT 82
REFLEXES: AFFERENT INPUT

Visceral Afferents

Visceral organs are supplied with sensory receptors of several different types (Table 82). Neurons of these receptors have their cell bodies in dorsal root ganglia associated with the spinal cord — or, in the case of vagal and glossopharyngeal afferents, in sensory ganglia associated with these nerves (see Unit 99) and located at the base of the skull.

The afferents transmit information about pressure, chemical conditions, and pain in the internal organs. Input from the receptors may initiate reflex responses or modify ongoing responses.

Sensory elements of a nerve plexus in the intestinal tract (Meissner's plexus) mediate local reflex movements of the intestines (see Units 87 and 88).

The important baroreceptors and chemoreceptors of the aortic and carotid arteries are involved in reflexes that control cardiac output and blood pressure (see Unit 85).

Somatic Afferents

Sensory input from peripheral (somatic) sense organs also plays a role in reflex activity of the autonomic nervous system. Thus, for example, thermal and mechanical stimuli in the abdominal region can influence intestinal activity and regional blood flow under certain conditions.

TABLE 82 Visceral Afferents

Sensory Modality	Structures	Locations	Reflex Actions
Mechanoreception	Stretch-sensitive nerve endings in hollow organs; also Pacinian corpuscles	Blood vessels; intestinal tract (Meissner's plexus); bladder	Regulation of blood pressure; regulation of intestinal motility and bladder contraction
Mechanoreception	Baroreceptors (sensitive to distention of blood vessel, signals intra-vascular pressure)	Carotid sinus and aorta (arterial system)	Regulation of cardiac output
Chemoreception	Nerve endings (sensitive to pH, P_{O_2}, etc.)	Intestinal tract and blood vessels	Regulation of blood pressure and intestinal motility
Chemoreception	Carotid body (sensitive to pH, P_{O_2}, P_{CO_2})	Carotid bifurcation (arterial system)	Regulation of blood pressure
Nociception	Nerve endings of C fibers (transmit pain information)	Heart, blood vessels, intestinal tract, most internal structures	Defensive abdominal muscular actions
Thermoreception	Nerve endings	Pharynx and esophagus	Role in swallowing responses

UNIT 83
REFLEXES: DIVERGENCE, CONVERGENCE, RECRUITMENT OF NEURONS

Divergence

Impulse traffic in a reflex pathway may be channeled to many locations from a single neuron as a result of the widespread distribution of nerve terminals (Fig. 83A). Such **divergence** is particularly striking in the sympathetic nervous system. For example, in the superior cervical ganglion there are about 1 million postganglionic neurons innervated by 10,000 preganglionic neurons, so each of the preganglionic neurons diverges to at least 100 postganglionic neurons.

It is apparent that the sympathetic ganglion acts as an "amplifier," since relatively few inputs to it may exert an influence on millions of smooth muscle or other target cells in several parts of the body.

Convergence

In Figure 83A, branches of two preganglionic neurons (A and B) are shown innervating one of the postganglionic neurons (Neuron 5). In Figure 83B, a postganglionic neuron receives converging inputs from preganglionic neurons of its own spinal cord segment and from neurons higher up the sympathetic trunk (see Unit 47). Such **convergence** allows for recruitment of neurons by an adequate stimulus (i.e., one that has made several converging inputs active). Also, convergence of inhibitory inputs to a neuron may *prevent* it from firing impulses even though excitatory inputs to it are active. Thus, the postganglionic neuron acts as a "decision making" unit in the reflex pathway; the relative strength of converging excitatory and inhibitory inputs determines whether the neuron will fire impulses.

Recruitment Mechanisms

In many cases, a single impulse in a presynaptic neuron does not generate a large enough synaptic potential to fire the postsynaptic neuron. Impulses arriving in rapid succession along a single input may generate a suprathreshold potential through **synaptic facilitation** (see Unit 49) or **summation** of successive synaptic potentials (Fig. 83C, 1 and 2). Impulses arriving along two or more inputs (convergence) may also generate a suprathreshold depolarization by summation of synaptic potentials ("spatial facilitation"; Fig. 83C, 3).

Recruitment of neurons is an important mechanism for grading the strength of a reflex response. This is true in both the autonomic and somatic nervous systems.

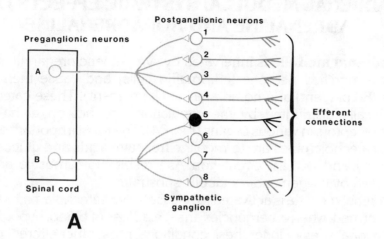

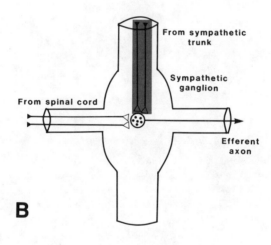

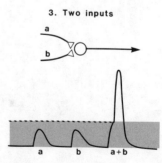

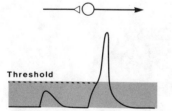

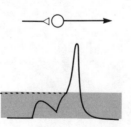

Figure 83 *A,* Divergence of efferent signals. *B,* Convergence of inputs to sympathetic postganglionic neuron. *C,* Recruitment of neurons by facilitation and summation of synaptic potentials.

UNIT 84
ADRENAL MEDULLA: SYSTEMIC EFFECTS OF ADRENALINE AND NORADRENALINE

The **adrenal medulla** is innervated by sympathetic preganglionic neurons that activate modified neurons (chromaffin cells) and cause them to release adrenaline (80 percent) and noradrenaline (20 percent). These catecholamines are systemically distributed by the circulation and act on alpha- and beta-adrenergic receptors in various organs (Fig. 84). The most important effects of the circulating catecholamines are to mobilize free fatty acids and glucose, increase oxygen supply, and increase circulation. As a result, brain, muscle, and heart are better supplied by oxygen and metabolic substrates.

The adrenal medulla is activated to release more catecholamines when heavy work is performed, when emergencies arise (e.g., loss of blood, hypoglycemia), or during emotional stress. Under these conditions, most other efferent pathways of the sympathetic nervous system also become more active than normal. The hypothalamus and associated parts of the central nervous system mediate the general increase in activity.

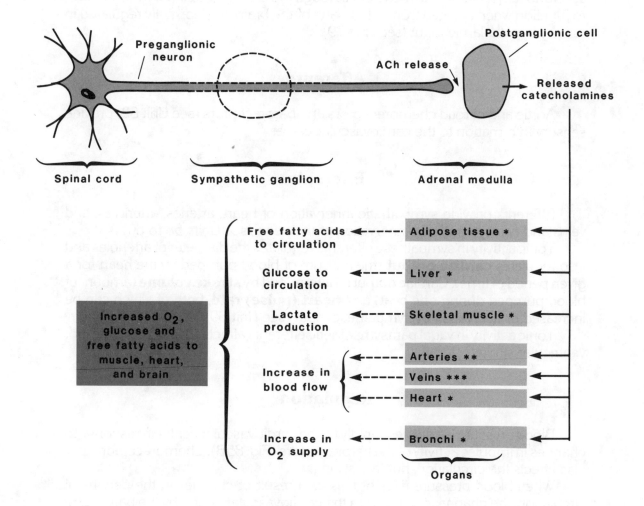

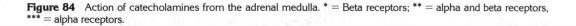

Figure 84 Action of catecholamines from the adrenal medulla. * = Beta receptors; ** = alpha and beta receptors, *** = alpha receptors.

UNIT 85
CIRCULATION: CONTROL OF BLOOD PRESSURE

Central Control

The cardiovascular center of the medulla (Fig. 85A) provides rapid regulation of heart and blood vessels. The neurons responsible for this regulation are found in several locations within the medulla. Although the cardiovascular center continues to function when isolated from other parts of the brain, it is normally regulated in turn by hypothalamic input (see Unit 79).

Afferents

Aortic and carotid chemoreceptors and baroreceptors (see Unit 82) provide sensory information to the cardiovascular center.

Efferents

Efferents provide sympathetic innervation of heart, arteries, arterioles, and veins and parasympathetic innervation of the heart (see Units 58 to 60).

Tonic activity in sympathetic efferents regulates the diameter of arterioles and also regulates **cardiac output** (the amount of blood pumped by the heart for a given period of time). Cardiac output is determined by **stroke volume** (amount of blood pumped during one beat) and **heart (pulse) rate**, both of which can be increased or decreased by sympathetic input (see Unit 60).

Tonic activity in vagal parasympathetic efferents affects mainly heart rate, not ventricular stroke volume.

Regulation

Blood pressure is adjusted rapidly by the cardiovascular center in response to changes in impulse activity of the baroreceptors (Fig. 85B). Chemoreceptor input also affects the circulation, but less strongly.

When blood pressure rises or falls as a result of changes in the peripheral circulation, the change is signaled to the cardiovascular center by the baroreceptors. A counteracting adjustment of efferent output is then made to keep blood pressure near the normal level.

During enhanced muscular activity, peripheral arterioles are dilated by metabolic products of the muscle fibers. This diverts more blood to the active muscles and tends to lower blood pressure. However, blood pressure is maintained at a normal level by two mechanisms: (1) increased cardiac output, and (2) reduction of blood flow to skin and intestinal tract by increased sympathetic output to the arterioles of those organs, with resulting vasoconstriction.

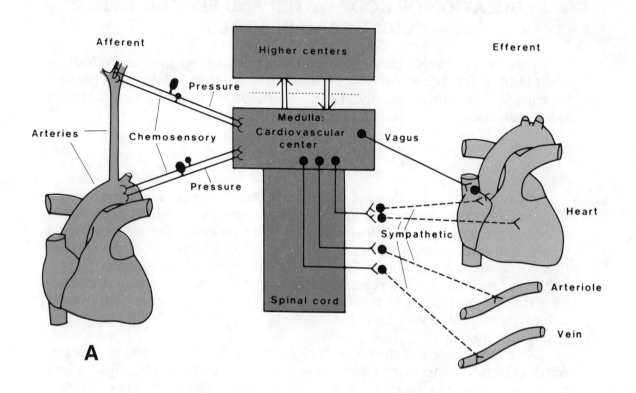

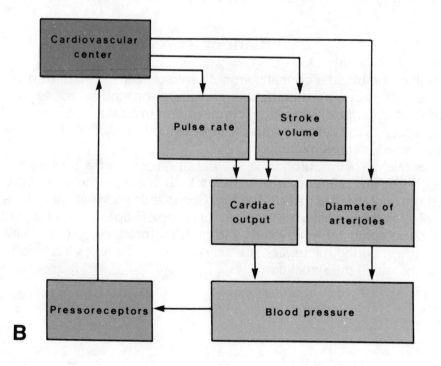

Figure 85 *A,* Control of heart and arteries by the central nervous system. *B,* Control circuit for regulation of blood pressure. (From Jänig W. The autonomic nervous system. In: Schmidt RF, ed. Fundamentals of neurophysiology. New York: Springer-Verlag, 1975:259, 261. With permission from Springer-Verlag, Heidelberg.)

UNIT 86
REGULATION OF BODY WATER AND ELECTROLYTES:
KIDNEY AND BLADDER

Water and electrolyte concentrations of the body are regulated by the **kidney** and **bladder**. The kidney controls the amount of water and electrolytes passing from the bloodstream to the urine. The bladder collects the urine produced by the kidneys and periodically ejects it (**micturition**).

Kidney

Although the kidney receives some sympathetic innervation, the major regulating influences are hormonal (Fig. 86A). Water content of the blood is monitored by osmoreceptors in the hypothalamus and also by mechanoreceptors in blood vessels that respond to blood volume. Low water content increases the firing of magnocellular neurons, which release vasopressin into the circulation in the posterior pituitary (see Unit 92). Vasopressin acts on the kidney to increase water uptake from the glomerular filtrate, thus conserving total body water. High plasma water content inhibits secretion of vasopressin, with the result that more water is passed into the urine.

When salt content of the blood is high, the atria of the heart secrete **atrial natriuretic hormone**, which inhibits re-uptake of Na^+ by the kidney. This leads to greater loss of salt in the urine. In addition, mineralocorticoid hormones of the adrenal cortex play an important role in kidney function (see Unit 95).

Bladder

The wall of the bladder contains smooth muscle cells (**detrusor muscle**). This muscle receives parasympathetic innervation from the sacral spinal cord, along with (less important) sympathetic innervation from the lumbar cord (Fig. 86B). Contraction of the detrusor muscle, coupled with relaxation of internal and external sphincters, causes micturition.

Reflex activation of the autonomic efferents increases as the bladder fills with urine. Stretch-sensitive afferents drive the reflex both directly in the spinal cord and less directly through the brainstem (see Fig. 86B). Under normal conditions, the reflex arc through the brainstem is required for complete operation of micturition.

The external sphincter, innervated by somatic motor axons, is under voluntary control. However, during micturition it is relaxed in part by reflex inhibition of its motor neurons within the spinal cord.

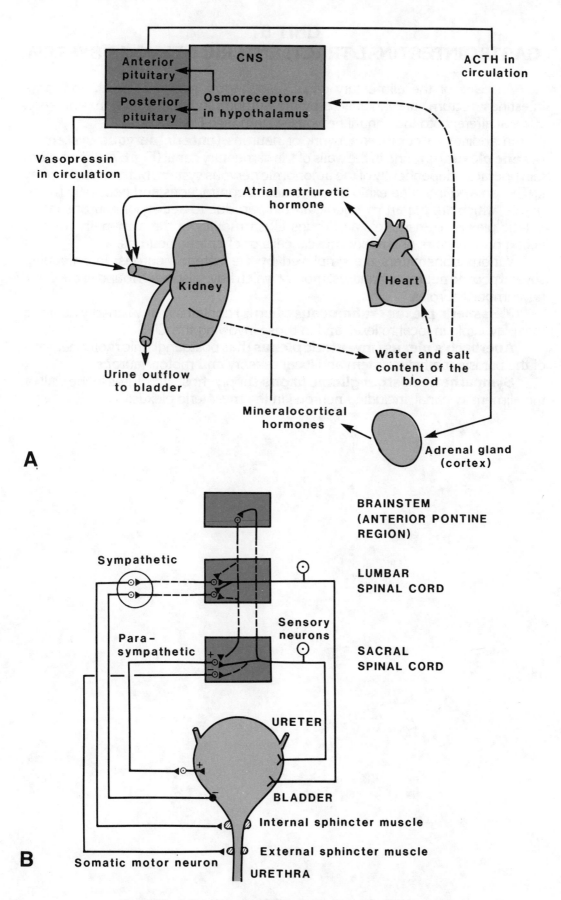

A

B

Figure 86 *A*, Regulation of the kidney. *B*, The micturition reflex.

UNIT 87
GASTROINTESTINAL TRACT: ENTERIC NERVOUS SYSTEM

All parts of the alimentary canal (esophagus, stomach, small and large intestines, rectum) are innervated by the autonomic nervous system and send visceral afferents to the central nervous system (see Unit 77).

In addition, a complex network of neurons (**enteric nervous system** or **enteric plexus**) is found in the walls of the alimentary canal (Fig. 87). This system can operate independently of the autonomic nervous system, but is modulated by it. The isolated intestine exhibits spontaneous contractions and peristaltic movements, which are in part myogenic and in part due to activity of neurons in the enteric plexus. Transmitters and drugs affect motility of the alimentary tract by acting on receptors of smooth muscle cells or of enteric neurons.

Various transmitters are employed by the enteric neurons; in particular, several peptide neurotransmitters, most of which have also been found in the CNS, have important roles.

Meissner's plexus (submucous plexus) contains many sensory neurons that play a role in local reflexes and in those involving the CNS.

Auerbach's plexus (myenteric plexus) has postganglionic motor neurons of the parasympathetic system and local sensory and motor neurons.

Sympathetic postganglionic axons supply most structures in the wall of the alimentary canal, including neurons in the myenteric plexus.

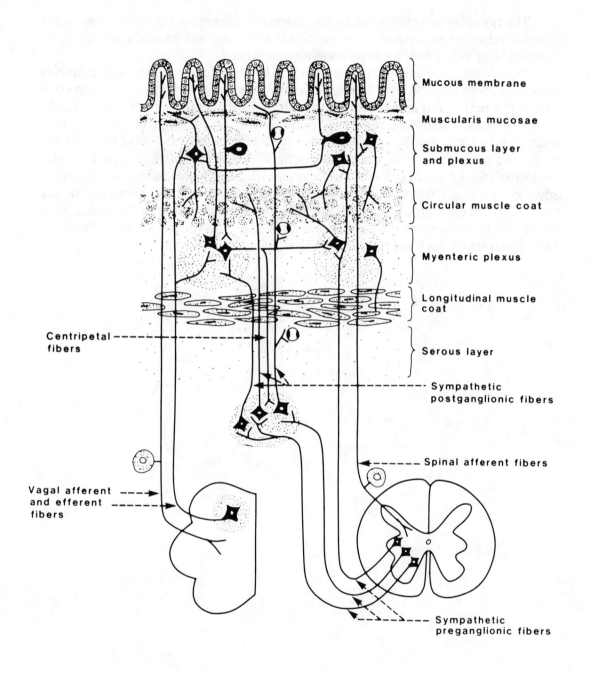

Figure 87 Extrinsic and intrinsic neurons of the enteric plexus. (From Schoefield GC. Anatomy of muscular and neural tissues in the alimentary canal. In: Handbook of physiology. Vol IV, Sect. 6. Bethesda: American Physiological Society, 1968:1611. With permission from the American Physiological Society.)

UNIT 88
GASTROINTESTINAL TRACT: LOCAL REFLEX

The neural connections within the myenteric plexus are complex. However, a general scheme for peristaltic contractions of the gastrointestinal tract has been outlined (Fig. 88). Other local reflexes also occur.

Distention of the wall of the intestine by a bolus of food leads to **relaxation** of the longitudinal muscle layer, **contraction** of the circular muscle layer on the oral side of the bolus, and **relaxation** of the circular muscle layer on the aboral side. Stretch-sensitive afferents respond to distention of the wall of the intestine; impulses in them excite local motoneurons (excitatory and inhibitory) in the myenteric plexus. Inhibitory neurotransmitters (probably ATP and peptides) relax the longitudinal muscle layer and the circular muscle layer downstream from the advancing bolus. Excitatory neurotransmitters (ACh and possibly others, including serotonin) excite the circular muscle layer on the oral side of the bolus. As a result, the bolus is moved in the aboral direction. The reflex "travels" down the intestinal tract as the food bolus moves.

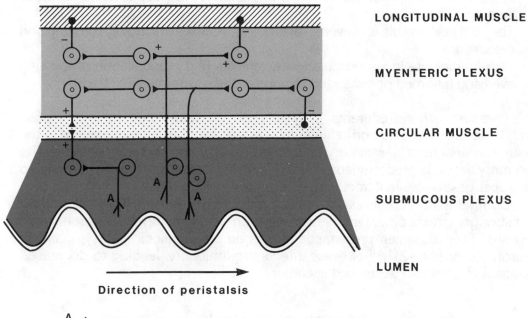

LONGITUDINAL MUSCLE

MYENTERIC PLEXUS

CIRCULAR MUSCLE

SUBMUCOUS PLEXUS

LUMEN

Direction of peristalsis

A ⊸ Afferent

⊸ Cholinergic

⊸ Purinergic or other transmitters

Figure 88 The peristaltic reflex.

UNIT 89
GASTROINTESTINAL TRACT: AUTONOMIC INFLUENCES

Efferent Control

Autonomic efferents (Fig. 89A) have several actions on the gastrointestinal tract:

1. They modulate (increase or decrease) the neural activity in the enteric nervous system. An example of autonomic modulation is inhibition of intestinal motility during exercise.
2. They are responsible for several "overriding" reflexes (including vomiting and defecation).
3. They participate in viscerocutaneous reflexes (e.g., vasodilation of the skin overlying inflamed or distended regions of the gastrointestinal tract).

Parasympathetic efferents activate both excitatory and inhibitory postganglionic neurons. The normal influence of the parasympathetic system in the gastrointestinal tract is excitatory (increased motility and secretory activity). The excitatory action is predominantly cholinergic. Hyperactivity of vagal efferents to the upper gastrointestinal tract can initiate the vomiting reflex.

Sympathetic efferents exert a weak direct action on intestinal smooth muscle and stronger effects on enteric neurons and on parasympathetic postganglionic neurons. They also exert presynaptic effects on preganglionic parasympathetic neurons (see Unit 42). All of these effects are inhibitory, leading to decreased intestinal motility and decreased secretion.

Levels of Control

Several parts of the CNS, as well as the enteric nervous system and the smooth muscle cells themselves, contribute to gastrointestinal motility and secretory activity (Fig. 89B).

Smooth muscle cells are spontaneously active electrically and mechanically even when neural effects are blocked with tetrodotoxin (see Unit 57). They generate "slow waves" and action potentials, and they respond to stretch with increased electrical activity.

The enteric nervous system and the autonomic nervous system modulate and sometimes dominate the spontaneous activity of the smooth muscle cells.

Reflex circuits governing the activity of the autonomic nervous system are present in spinal cord and brainstem.

The hypothalamus provides descending input to circuits in the brainstem and spinal cord. Emotional and physical stress exert influences on the gastrointestinal tract via the hypothalamus.

The control of gastrointestinal function is extremely complex and not yet fully understood.

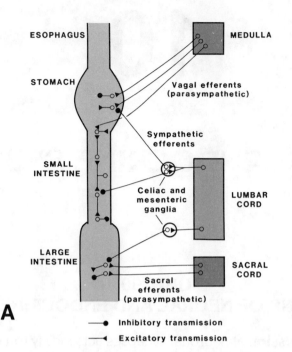

ESOPHAGUS

MEDULLA

STOMACH

Vagal efferents
(parasympathetic)

Sympathetic
efferents

SMALL
INTESTINE

LUMBAR
CORD

Celiac and
mesenteric
ganglia

LARGE
INTESTINE

SACRAL
CORD

Sacral
efferents
(parasympathetic)

A

●── Inhibitory transmission

◄── Excitatory transmission

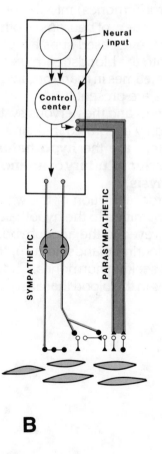

Neural
input

Control
center

SYMPATHETIC

PARASYMPATHETIC

B

HYPOTHALAMUS

- neuroendochrine control center
- general regulation of other CNS
  centers

BRAINSTEM

- neural control center for
  gastrointestinal function
- parasympathetic efferent control
  via vagus nerve

SPINAL CORD

- accepts visceral sensory input
- contains circuits for local reflexes
- accepts input from higher centers

**SYMPATHETIC AND
PARASYMPATHETIC**

- exert general excitatory and
  inhibitory effects
- trigger dominant reflexes in
  certain parts of the tract

ENTERIC NERVOUS SYSTEM

- modulates smooth muscle activity
- local reflexes
- accepts and transmits signals from
  sympathetic and parasympathetic
  nervous systems

SMOOTH MUSCLE CELLS

- generate and conduct "slow waves"
- generate and conduct action
  potentials
- respond to transmitters and
  hormones
- respond to stretch

Figure 89   *A,* Outline of autonomic input to the gastrointestinal tract. *B,* Levels of control of the gastrointestinal tract.

10

NEUROENDOCRINE SYSTEM

UNIT 90
INTERACTIONS OF NEURAL AND ENDOCRINE SYSTEMS

Neurotransmission at neuronal synapses acts locally (on other nerve cells or specific target organs).

Neurosecretion of substances (neurohormones) into the bloodstream by neurons (see Unit 61) can influence large numbers of neurons or other target cells if the latter are endowed with receptors for the released substance(s).

Endocrine secretion of hormones into the bloodstream (see Unit 61) also influences large numbers of target cells, sometimes in many organs, provided that the appropriate receptors for the hormones are present.

Interaction between the endocrine system and the nervous system occurs in many ways, so that the two systems are highly integrated in their activities.

The key elements in the control system are the **hypothalamus** and the **pituitary** or **hypophysis** (comprising **anterior pituitary** or **adenohypophysis**, and **posterior pituitary** or **neurohypophysis**).

Neural influences signaling the need for regulation of the whole body or of specific target organs by hormones are transmitted to the hypothalamus. Releasing or release-inhibiting hormones are conveyed to the adenohypophysis, which secretes hormones whose targets are endocrine glands. In turn, the endocrine glands are stimulated to secrete their target-seeking hormones. Endocrine glands may also respond to the levels of substances in the blood that are generated by, or used by, target organs.

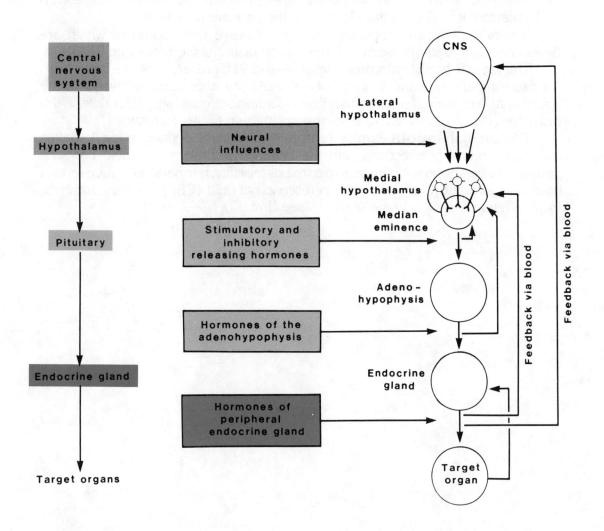

Figure 90 Flow of information in the neuroendocrine system. (Adapted from Jänig W. The autonomic nervous system. In: Schmidt RF, Thews G, ed. Human physiology. Heidelberg: Springer-Verlag, 1983:133.)

UNIT 91
HYPOTHALAMUS: INPUT AND OUTPUT

Anatomic Features

The hypothalamus is located above the brainstem and below the cerebrum and thalamus; it is closely associated with the pituitary (Fig. 91A).

Several functionally important groups of nerve cells, some of which are designated as hypothalamic nuclei, have been distinguished (see Fig. 91A).

The **lateral hypothalamus** (Fig. 91A and 91B) receives neural input from brainstem, thalamus, and limbic system and from ascending pathways of the spinal cord. It makes efferent connections to autonomic and somatic nuclei in the brainstem (through multisynaptic pathways in the reticular formation).

The **medial hypothalamus** (comprising several defined nuclei) makes reciprocal neural connections with the lateral hypothalamus. It also contains neurons that respond to changes in plasma osmolality, temperature, glucose, and hormonal content. Changes in the cerebrospinal fluid (CSF) are also detected. Major efferent output is to the pituitary (see Unit 92).

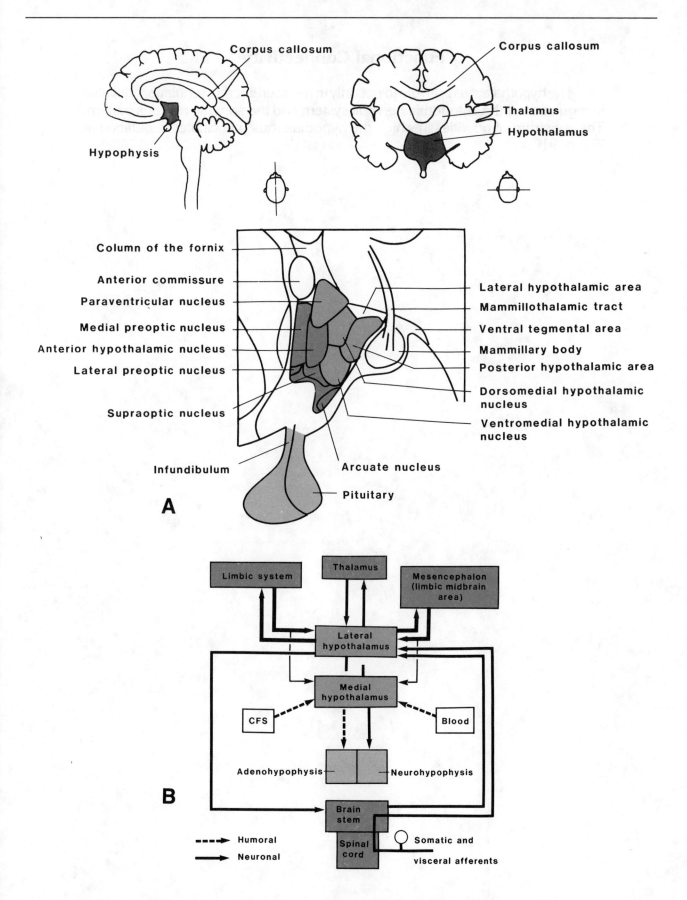

Figure 91 *A,* The hypothalamus and its constituent nuclear groups. *B,* General scheme of afferent and efferent connections of the hypothalamus. *Figure continues.*

Functional Connectivity

The hypothalamus is involved not only in neuroendocrine regulation, but also in regulation of the autonomic nervous system and the somatic nervous system. The spectrum of activities in which the hypothalamus participates is outlined in Figure 91C.

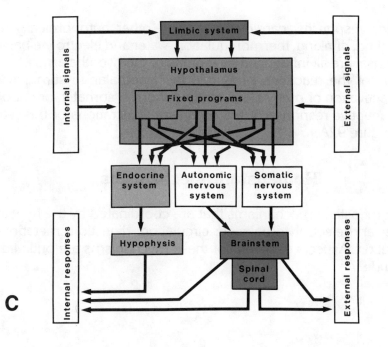

Figure 91 *(continued)* C. Functional organization of hypothalamic activity. (*A, Top* from Jänig W. The autonomic nervous system. In: Schmidt RF, ed. Fundamentals of neurophysiology. New York: Springer-Verlag, 1975:264. With permission from Springer-Verlag, Heidelberg. *Bottom,* Modified from Kandel ER, Schwartz JH. Principles of neural science. New York: Elsevier, 1985:615. *B* and *C,* Adapted from Jänig W. The autonomic nervous system. In: Schmidt RF, Thews G, ed. Human physiology. Heidelberg: Springer-Verlag, 1983:132, 136.)

UNIT 92
HYPOTHALAMUS: HOMEOSTASIS, APPETITES

The connection of neural centers in the hypothalamus to autonomic, somatic, and endocrine systems (see Unit 91) provides for regulation of activities that involve all of these systems, or selected elements of them.

Stimulation and Lesion

An initial approach to the functions of the hypothalamus is obtained by selectively stimulating or "lesioning" small areas with implanted electrodes (Table 92).

Endocrine responses, cardiovascular and other autonomically regulated responses, eating, drinking, thermoregulation, water and electrolyte balance, and degree of arousal are all influenced by regions of the hypothalamus.

A feature of the reactions produced by hypothalamic stimulation is the coordinated activation of many elements (autonomic, somatic, or endocrine) to produce an adaptive response of the organism. Illustrations of this feature are provided in Figure 92A.

Homeostatic Mechanisms

Major homeostatic mechanisms that are coordinated by the hypothalamus include water and electrolyte balance, circulation, digestion, metabolism, and thermoregulation. Aspects of several of these mechanisms are outlined in Units 85, 86, 96, and 97.

TABLE 92 Stimulation and Lesion of Hypothalamic Areas

Nucleus or Area	Effect of Stimulation	Effect of Lesion
Supraoptic nucleus, paraventricular nucleus	Release of vasopressin and/or oxytocin	Diabetes insipidus
Medial hypothalamic areas	Secretion of releasing factors into portal circulation	Various endocrine deficiencies
Preoptic nuclei, anterior nucleus	Cutaneous vasodilation, sweating (heat loss)	Hyperthermia in warm environment
Posterior hypothalamic area	Cutaneous vasoconstriction, increased muscle tone, shivering (heat production), general arousal, rage	Loss of thermoregulation
Area dorsolateral to para-ventricular nucleus	Drinking	
Ventromedial nucleus	Cessation of eating, placidity	Voracious eating, obesity; aggressive behavior
Areas in lateral hypothalamus and near ventromedial nucleus	Voracious eating	Weight loss due to lack of food intake
Area lateral to mammilothalamic tract	Defensive behavior, rise in arterial pressure, increased cardiac output and vasodilation in muscle	Hypoactivity

Adapted from Somjen G. Neurophysiology—the essentials. Baltimore: Williams & Wilkins, 1983:440.

Thermoregulation

The hypothalamus receives information about environmental and body temperature from cutaneous and central thermoreceptors, respectively. Through the autonomic nervous system and the endocrine system, the hypothalamus also adjusts heat production (by regulation of metabolic rate — see Unit 97 — and by somatic control of muscular activity, as in shivering). Heat production and heat loss are balanced to maintain brain temperature at a constant level.

Behavior

Various patterns of behavior are elicited by hypothalamic stimulation. These are generally concerned with functions essential to self-preservation (eating, drinking, defense; also sexual activity). Normally, interaction of the hypothalamus with the limbic system (see Unit 146) determines when these behavioral activities are called forth.

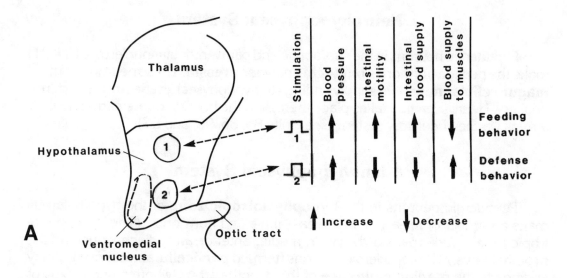

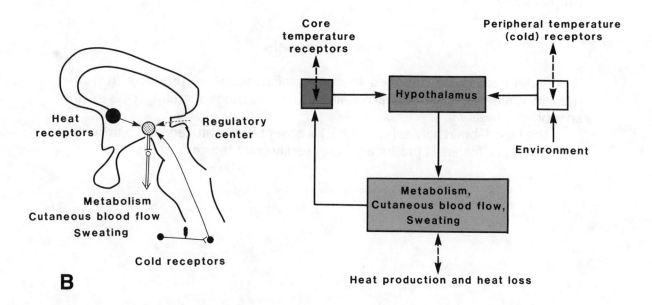

Figure 92 *A*, Autonomic responses to hypothalamic stimulation: feeding and defense behavior. *B*, Thermoregulation. (*A*, From Jänig W. The autonomic nervous system. In: Schmidt RF, Thews G, ed. Human physiology. Heidelberg: Springer-Verlag, 1983:134. With permission from Springer-Verlag, Heidelberg. *B*, From Jänig W. The autonomic nervous system. In: Schmidt RF, ed. Fundamentals of neurophysiology. New York: Springer-Verlag, 1975:266, 267. With permission from Springer-Verlag, Heidelberg.)

UNIT 93
HYPOTHALAMIC-HYPOPHYSEAL SYSTEM

Neurohypophyseal System

Peptidergic neurons in the supraoptic and paraventricular nuclei (see Unit 91) make the peptide hormones **oxytocin** and **vasopressin**. These neurons (termed **magnocellular neurons**) supply endings to hypophyseal arteries in the posterior pituitary. Neurosecretion takes place there, and the hormones are carried to their targets via the circulatory system (see Units 85, 86, 96, and 97).

Adenohypophyseal System

Peptidergic neurons in the **hypophysiotropic zone** of the hypothalamus make a number of releasing and release-inhibiting hormones. (The hypophysiotropic zone includes parts of the ventromedial, anterior, and adjacent nuclei of the hypothalamus.) The peptidergic neurons (termed **parvicellular neurons**) supply endings to the **median eminence** of the hypothalamus, where a fine plexus of capillaries is present. Neurosecretion provides hormones to the portal vessels, in which they are conveyed to the secretory cells of the adenohypophysis. Tropic hormones of the adenohypophysis reach their targets (endocrine glands) via the circulatory system.

Portal Vessels

Portal vessels are designed to convey neurosecretory products from the median eminence (and pituitary stalk) to the hormone-secreting cells of the adenohypophysis.

The blood-brain barrier (see Unit 2) is absent in the pituitary and parts of the hypothalamus. Materials produced there readily enter the circulation.

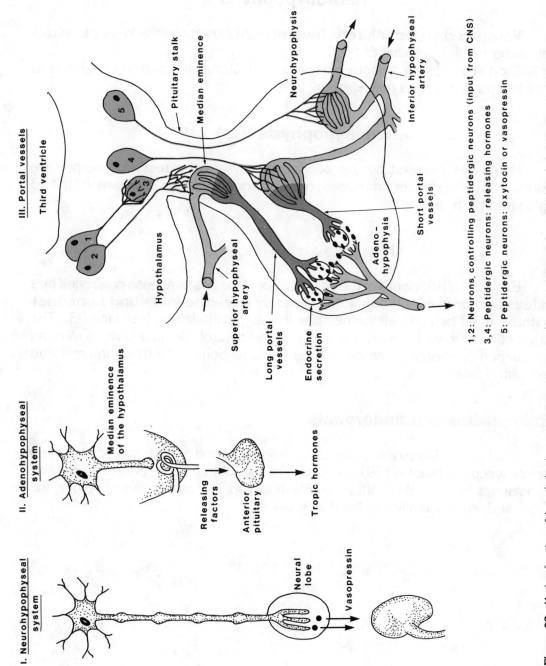

Figure 93 Mode of action of hypothalamic neurosecretory neurons. (*I* and *II*, Adapted from Reichlin S. Introduction. In: Reichlin S, Baldessarini RJ, Martin JB, eds. The hypothalamus. New York: Raven Press, 1978:5. *III*, Modified after Kandel ER, Schwartz JH. Principles of neural science. New York: Elsevier, 1985:618.)

I. Neurohypophyseal system

Neural lobe

Vasopressin

II. Adenohypophyseal system

Median eminence of the hypothalamus

Releasing factors

Anterior pituitary

Tropic hormones

III. Portal vessels

Third ventricle

Pituitary stalk

Median eminence

Neurohypophysis

Inferior hypophyseal artery

Hypothalamus

Short portal vessels

Adeno-hypophysis

Superior hypophyseal artery

Long portal vessels

Endocrine secretion

1,2: Neurons controlling peptidergic neurons (input from CNS)

3,4: Peptidergic neurons: releasing hormones

5: Peptidergic neurons: oxytocin or vasopressin

UNIT 94
HORMONES OF HYPOTHALAMUS AND PITUITARY

Neurohypophysis

Vasopressin or **antidiuretic hormone** (ADH) acts on the kidney to stimulate water uptake (see Unit 86).

Oxytocin acts on smooth muscles of the uterus and mammary glands to facilitate parturition and milk ejection.

Adenohypophysis (Table 94A)

Hormones released by the adenohypophysis act directly on responsive somatic targets (effector hormones) or on endocrine glands as shown in Unit 93 (glandotropic hormones).

Hypothalamus (Table 94B)

Each of the hormones of the adenohypophysis has its release controlled by a **releasing hormone** (and in some cases by a **release-inhibiting hormone**), manufactured by parvicellular neurons in the hypothalamus (see Unit 93). The production of these hormones is under neural control. Neural activity governing production of hypophysiotropic hormones is responsive to many internal and external signals.

Enkephalins and Endorphins

The hypothalamus also produces enkephalins and endorphins, which act on opiate receptors (see Unit 39) of neurons and smooth muscle. Secretion of these substances is thought to influence intestinal motility, perception of pain in the CNS, and other neurally regulated processes.

TABLE 94A Hormones Released in the Adenohypophysis

Glandotropic hormones
    Follicle-stimulating hormones (FSH)   } Gonadotropic
    Luteinizing hormone (LH) = interstitial cell-stimulating hormone (ICSH) }   hormones
    Thyrotropin = thyroid-stimulating hormone (TSH)
    Adrenocorticotropic hormone (ACTH)
Effector hormones
    Growth hormone (GH) = somatotropic hormone (STH)
    Prolactin (PRL) = luteotropic hormone
    Melanocyte-stimulating hormone (MSH)

From Bruck K. Functions of the endocrine system. In: Schmidt RF, Thews G, eds. Human physiology. Heidelberg: Springer-Verlag, 1983:664. With permission from Springer-Verlag, Heidelberg.

TABLE 94B Hypophysiotropic Hormones

Name	Acts on*
Releasing hormones	
Thyrotropin releasing hormone (TRH)	TSH
Chemically: tripeptide	
Luteinizing hormone releasing hormone (LH-RH)	LH, FSH
Chemically: decapeptide	
Corticotropin releasing hormone (CRH)	ACTH
Growth hormone releasing hormone (GH-RH)	GH
Prolactin releasing hormone (PRL-RH)	PRL
Melanocyte-stimulating hormone releasing hormone (MSH-RH)	MSH
Inhibitory hormones	
Growth-hormone inhibitory hormone (GH-IH) = somatostatin	GH
Chemically: tetradecapeptide	
Melanocyte-stimulating hormone inhibitory hormone (MSH-IH)	MSH
Prolactin inhibitory hormone (PRL-IH)	PRL

* See Table 94A.
From Bruck K. Functions of the endocrine system. In: Schmidt RF, Thews G, eds. Human physiology. Heidelberg: Springer-Verlag, 1983:664. With permission from Springer-Verlag, Heidelberg.

UNIT 95
ENDOCRINE GLANDS: FUNCTIONAL ROLES

Hormones

Effector hormones act directly on the target organ. They are usually produced by an endocrine gland.

Tropic (or **glandotropic**) **hormones** act on glands to regulate synthesis and/or secretion of effector hormones. They are usually produced by the adenohypophysis (see Units 93 and 94).

Releasing and release-inhibiting hormones act on the hormone-secreting cells of the adenohypophysis to regulate synthesis and/or release of the hormones of the adenohypophysis (see Unit 94).

Effector Hormones

Effector hormones participate in neuroendocrine control circuits in which hormone secretion is regulated to control a physiological parameter within certain limits (Fig. 95A). Examples include regulation of water and salt output by the kidney, regulation of contraction in uterine smooth muscle, and others.

Releasing and Tropic Hormones

Releasing and tropic hormones participate in neuroendocrine control circuits that sense the level of a hormone and regulate this level within certain limits (Fig. 95B).

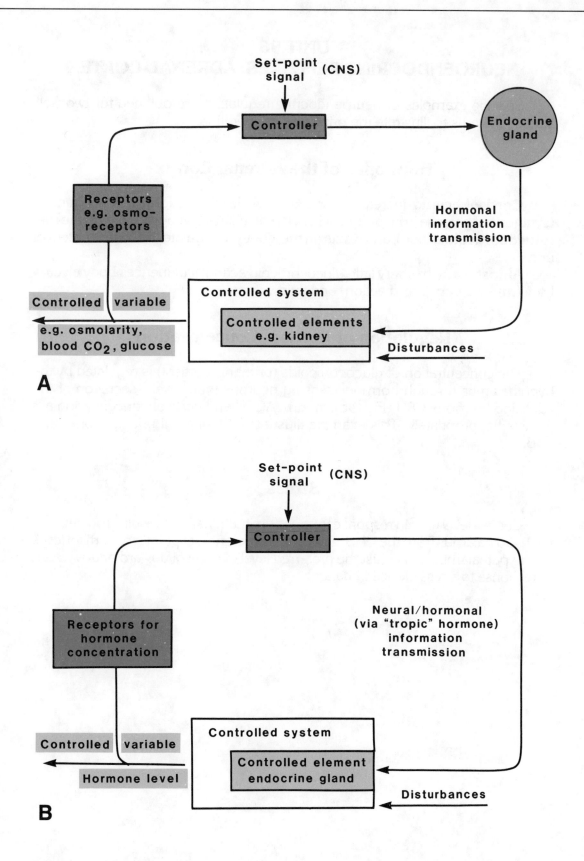

Figure 95 *A*, Hormonal control of physiological performance. *B*, Neural control of hormone level. (From Bruck K. Functions of the endocrine system. In: Schmidt RF, Thews G, eds. Human physiology. Heidelberg: Springer-Verlag, 1983:660. With permission from Springer-Verlag, Heidelberg.)

UNIT 96
NEUROENDOCRINE REFLEXES: ADRENAL CORTEX

Specific examples of neuroendocrine regulation are outlined for two well-studied systems to illustrate the principles of operation.

Hormones of the Adrenal Cortex

Cortisol acts to increase blood glucose level through gluconeogenesis (synthesis of glucose from amino acids). It replenishes glycogen stores in the liver (**glucocorticoid** action), and it acts on the kidney to regulate the water content of urine.

Aldosterone has very little glucocorticoid action; it influences body electrolytes (**mineralocorticoid** action) and fluid volume.

Regulation of Cortisol Concentration

The concentration of glucocorticoids (primarily cortisol) is regulated by the hypothalamus through hormone-sensing neurons that govern secretion of the releasing hormone CRH (Fig. 96). In turn, ACTH and cortisol concentration are adjusted appropriately. This example illustrates the general principle of Figure 95B.

Stress

Cortisol level rises in response to stressful situations. This results from input to the hypothalamus from the CNS leading to a different "set point" for cortisol level. The hypothalamus can adjust the preferred level of cortisol upward or downward in response to stress-induced changes.

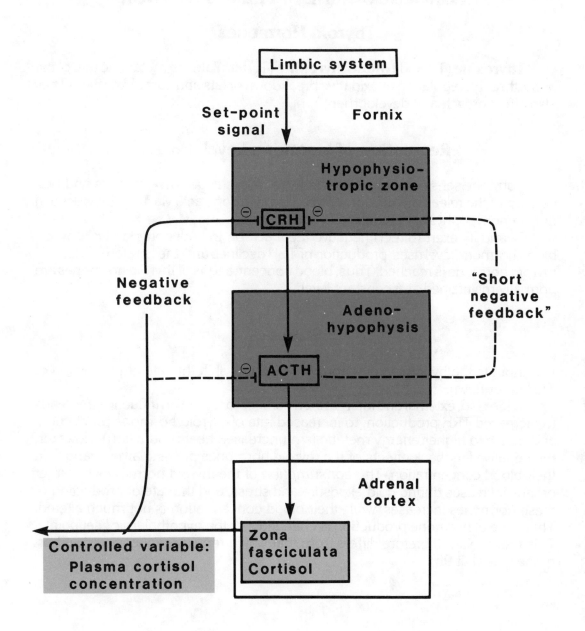

Figure 96 Control of glucocorticoid secretion. (From Bruck K. Functions of the endocrine system. In: Schmidt RF, Thews G, eds. Human physiology. Heidelberg: Springer-Verlag, 1983:669. With permission from Springer-Verlag, Heidelberg.)

UNIT 97
NEUROENDOCRINE REFLEXES: THYROID

Thyroid Hormones

Thyroxine (T_4) and **triiodothyronine** (T_3) regulate the metabolic rate of the body, through regulation of oxidative breakdown of fats and carbohydrates. (They also affect growth and development.)

Regulation of Hormone Level (Fig. 97)

Hormone-sensing neurons in the hypothalamus govern synthesis and production of the releasing hormone TRH. This hormone acts via TSH, produced in the adenohypophysis, to regulate T_3 and T_4 levels.

T_3 and T_4 exert (direct) negative feedback on the adenohypophysis. When blood hormone level rises, production of TSH declines until the "preferred" level of thyroid hormone is reached. Thus, blood concentrations of thyroid hormones are normally maintained at a constant level.

Stress

Input to the hypothalamus from the CNS can shift the rate of production of TRH up or down.

In the cold, external and internal thermoreceptors exert an influence that leads to increased TRH production, to increased rate of thyroid hormone production, and hence to higher energy metabolism (increased heat production). However, the negative feedback effects of the thyroid hormones prevent large changes in their blood concentration. The *consumption* of the thyroid hormones by target organs increases during cold exposure and stress, and the rate of production of these hormones increases, while their blood concentration is not much altered. Thus, rate of hormone production is changed, not the hypothalamic "set point." This mechanism therefore differs from that which regulates glucocorticoid hormone (see Unit 96).

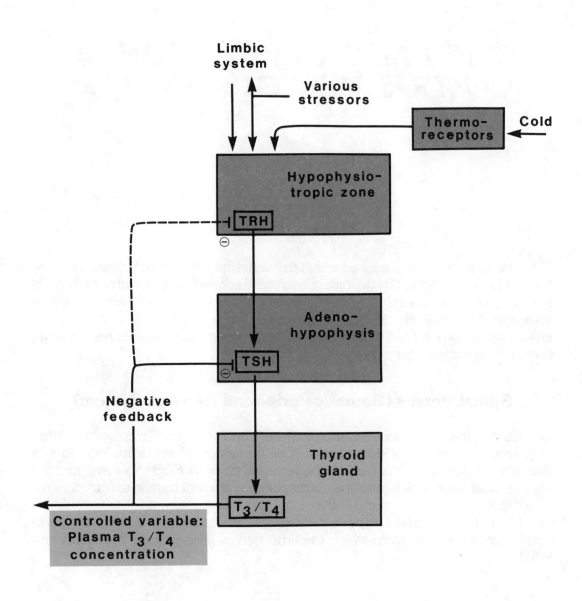

Figure 97 Regulation of thyroid hormone levels. (From Bruck K. Functions of the endocrine system. In: Schmidt RF, Thews G, eds. Human physiology. Heidelberg: Springer-Verlag, 1983:673. With permission from Springer-Verlag, Heidelberg.)

11

GENERAL ORGANIZATION OF CENTRAL NERVOUS SYSTEM

UNIT 98
SPINAL CORD

The spinal cord is enclosed within the vertebral column but extends only to the first lumbar vertebra. By definition, each cord segment is the source of a pair of spinal nerves (one on each side): The nerves exit sequentially between successive vertebrae (Figs. 98A and 98B) and are named according to their exit point. The enlargements of the cord at cervical and lumbosacral segments serve the large arm and leg nerves, respectively.

Spinal Nerves (Somatic Peripheral Nervous System)

Each spinal nerve contains motor *efferent* and sensory *afferent* axons. Afferents enter the cord via a **dorsal root**: Cell bodies of afferents are located in a **dorsal root ganglion**, just outside the vertebral column. Efferents leave the cord via a **ventral root**, which joins the corresponding afferent bundle to form a nerve (Fig. 98C).

In the brachial and lumbosacral regions, the spinal nerves intermingle in complicated plexuses from which the limb nerves emerge (see Figs. 98A and 98B).

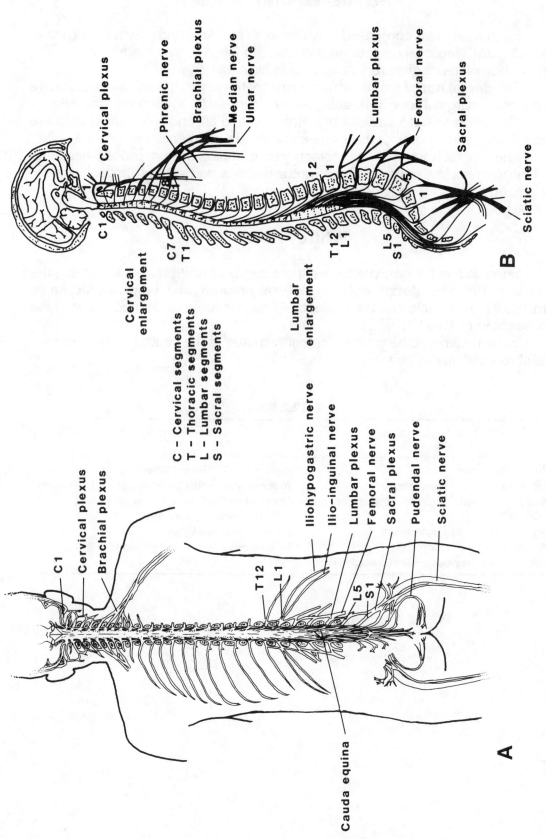

Figure 98 Spinal nerves. *A,* dorsal view and *B,* lateral view. *Figure continues.*

Cervical plexus
Phrenic nerve
Brachial plexus
Median nerve
Ulnar nerve

C 1
C 7
T 1

Lumbar plexus
Femoral nerve
Sacral plexus

T 12
L 1

L 5
S 1

Sciatic nerve

B

Cervical
enlargement

C – Cervical segments
T – Thoracic segments
L – Lumbar segments
S – Sacral segments

Lumbar
enlargement

C 1
Cervical plexus
Brachial plexus

Iliohypogastric nerve
Ilio–inguinal nerve
Lumbar plexus
Femoral nerve
Sacral plexus
Pudendal nerve
Sciatic nerve

T 12
L 1

L 5
S 1

Cauda equina

A

Segmental Gray Matter

Each segment is composed of white (axon bundles) and gray matter (neuronal somata). Neuronal somata are collected in layered gray matter comprising dorsal horn, intermediate zone, and ventral horn (see Fig. 98C).

The **dorsal horn** receives sensory afferent terminals. It is subdivided into five laminae: I, marginal zone; II-III, substantia gelatinosa; IV-V, nucleus proprius.

The **intermediate zone** of propriospinal and ascending neurons links the dorsal and ventral horns of the same and different segments.

The **ventral horn** contains motor nuclei, groups of motoneurons innervating a common skeletal muscle. One motor nucleus can extend through several segments.

White Matter

Surrounding the gray matter are three bands of white matter stretching the length of the cord: **dorsal column**, **lateral column**, and **ventral column**. A **dorsolateral fascicle** and **anterolateral fascicle** are also defined between the three columns (see Fig. 98C).

In the midline, at the center of the gray matter, is the central canal filled with cerebrospinal fluid (CSF).

TABLE 98

Peripheral Nervous System (PNS)	Central Nervous System (CNS)
No bony protection	Protected by skull or vertebrae
Axons in cranial and spinal *nerves*	Axons in white matter *tracts* (spinal cord and brain)
Neuronal cell bodies in *ganglia* (dorsal root, autonomic)	Neuronal cell bodies in gray matter *nuclei*
	CNS surrounded by dura mater
Nerves surrounded by perineurium	Myelin formed by *oligodendroglia*
Myelin formed by *Schwann cells*	Includes retina (see Units 103 and 104)
Includes enteric nervous system (see Unit 87)	

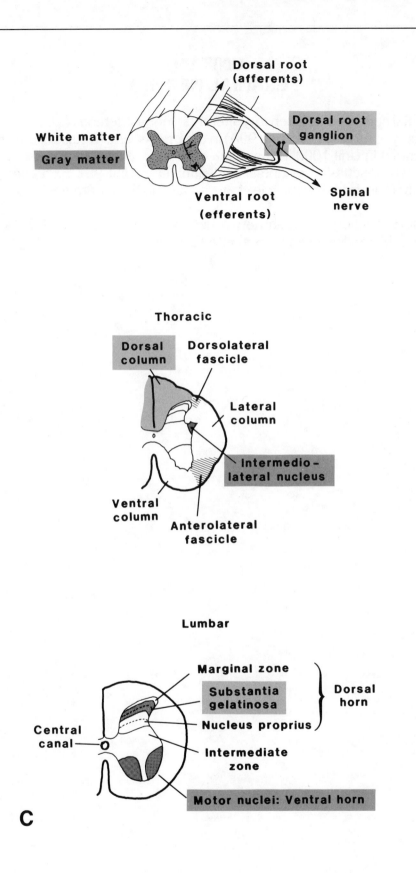

Dorsal root (afferents)

White matter

Gray matter

Dorsal root ganglion

Ventral root (efferents)

Spinal nerve

Thoracic

Dorsal column

Dorsolateral fascicle

Lateral column

Intermedio-lateral nucleus

Ventral column

Anterolateral fascicle

Lumbar

Marginal zone

Substantia gelatinosa

Nucleus proprius

Dorsal horn

Central canal

Intermediate zone

Motor nuclei: Ventral horn

C

Figure 98 *(continued)* *C,* Spinal cord. (*A,* Modified after Netter FH. The nervous system. In: The CIBA collection of medical illustrations. Vol. I. Summit, NJ: CIBA Pharmaceutical, 1980:49. *B,* Adapted from Gardner E. Fundamentals of neurology. Philadelphia: WB Saunders, 1963:35.)

UNIT 99
CRANIAL NERVES

Cranial nerves contain sensory afferents, motor efferents, or both, associated with sensory or motor nuclei (Fig. 99A) in the **brainstem**. (Details of the brainstem are described in Unit 100.) The somata of sensory axons are located in sensory *ganglia* (see discussion of dorsal root ganglia in Unit 98). *Exception*: Muscle spindle afferents from jaw muscles have somata in the trigeminal mesencephalic nucleus.

General positions of cranial nerve nuclei are shown in Figure 99B. Nerve exits from the CNS are illustrated in Figure 99C.

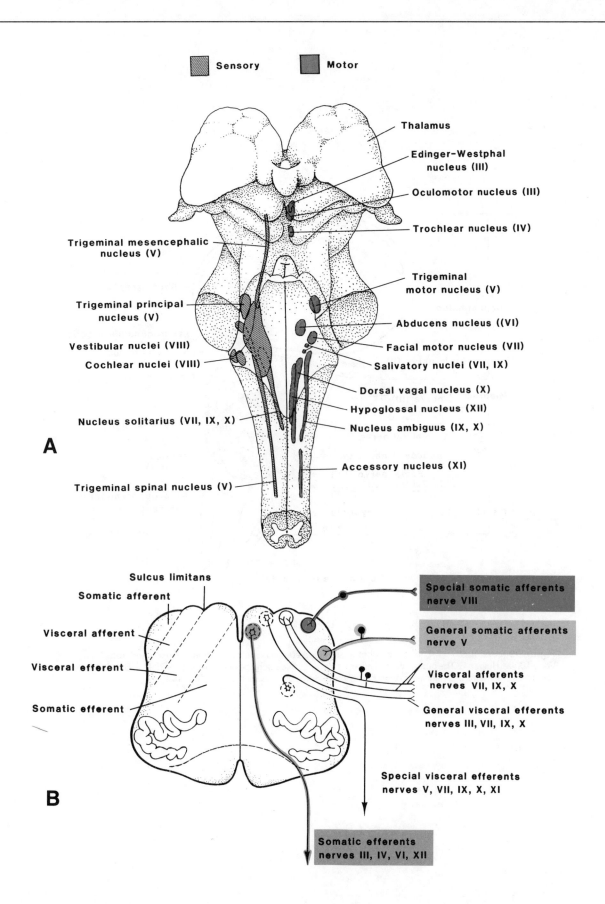

Figure 99 *A*, Cranial nerve nuclei. *B*, Positions of cranial nerve nuclei in medulla (schematic frontal section). *Figure continues.*

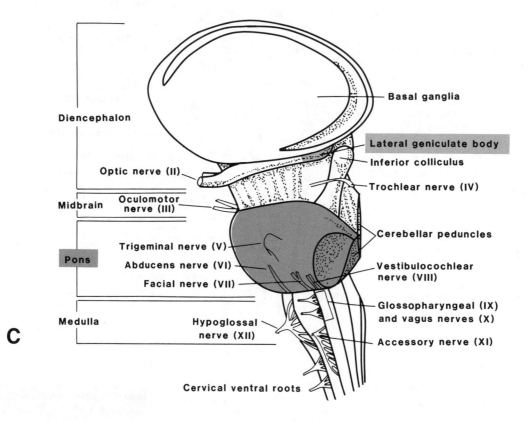

Figure 99 *(continued)*   C, Lateral view of brainstem and cranial nerve connections. (*A*, Adapted from Nieuwenhuys R, Voogd J, van Huijzen C. The human central nervous system. Heidelberg: Springer-Verlag, 1981:114. *B* and *C*, Adapted from Kandel ER, Schwartz JH. Principles of neural science. New York: Elsevier, 1985:546, 544.)

TABLE 99 Peripheral Origins and Targets of Cranial Nerve Axons

| No. | Name | Ganglia [Para-sympathetic] | Somatic, Special Senses | | Autonomic | |
			Afferent	Efferent	Afferent	Efferent
I	Olfactory	Olfactory mucosa	Olfactory cells	—	—	—
II	Optic	Retina	Ganglion cells	—	—	—
III	Oculomotor	[ciliary]	—	Extraocular, eyelid muscles	—	Iris (circular muscle); ciliary muscle
IV	Trochlear	—	—	Superior oblique	—	—
V	Trigeminal	Semilunar (gasserian)	Face, mouth somatic receptors	Mastication muscles	—	—
VI	Abducens	—	—	Lateral rectus	—	—
VII	Facial	Geniculate	Taste (anterior 2/3 of tongue)	Facial expression muscles	—	Lacrimal, sub-maxillary, sublingual glands
VIII	Vestibulo-cochlear	Vestibular or scarpae (2); spiral	Labyrinth hair cells	Hair cells	—	—
IX	Glosso-pharyngeal	Superior, petrous	Taste (posterior tongue)	Swallowing muscles	Carotid body receptors	Parotid gland
X	Vagus	Jugular, nodose	Taste (epiglottis)	Speech (muscles of larynx, pharynx)	Pharynx, larynx, GI tract, lungs	Heart, trachea, bronchi, GI tract
XI	Spinal accessory	—	—	Trapezius, sternocleido-mastoid	—	Pharynx, larynx, soft palate
XII	Hypoglossal	—	—	Tongue	—	—

UNIT 100
BRAINSTEM AND DIENCEPHALON

The brainstem is composed of three parts: **medulla**, **pons**, and **mid-brain** (or **mesencephalon**) (Figs. 100A and 100B; also see Fig. 99C). The **diencephalon** caps the brainstem, providing an interface between it and the cerebrum (**telencephalon**).

Medulla

The structure of the medulla may be likened to an "exploded" spinal cord. The central canal enlarges abruptly to form the fourth ventricle. The dorsal and ventral horns become sensory and motor nuclei located lateral and ventral, respectively, to the ventricle (Fig. 100C). The **reticular formation**, an expanded intermediate zone, makes up the core of the entire brainstem. It is a lattice-like mix of axon bundles and clumps of neurons; nuclei are poorly defined.

Pons

The pons is structurally similar to the medulla; the massive **pontine nuclei** are added on the ventral side (see Fig. 100C). These nuclei receive input from the cerebral cortex and transmit it to the cerebellum, which sits astride the fourth ventricle over pons and medulla.

Mid-brain

Here the fourth ventricle reverts to a canal, the "cerebral aqueduct" (see Figs. 100A and 100C), surrounded by neurons comprising **periaqueductal gray (PAG)** matter, where autonomic behavioral patterns are organized. On the dorsal surface sit the **superior** and **inferior colliculi** (see Figs. 100A and 100B), "little hills" of layered gray matter where spatial maps of visual and auditory data are represented. The **red nuclei** (see Unit 121) are located ventrally. Next to the descending cortical efferents (basis pedunculi) is another nucleus associated with motor control, the **substantia nigra** (see Unit 138).

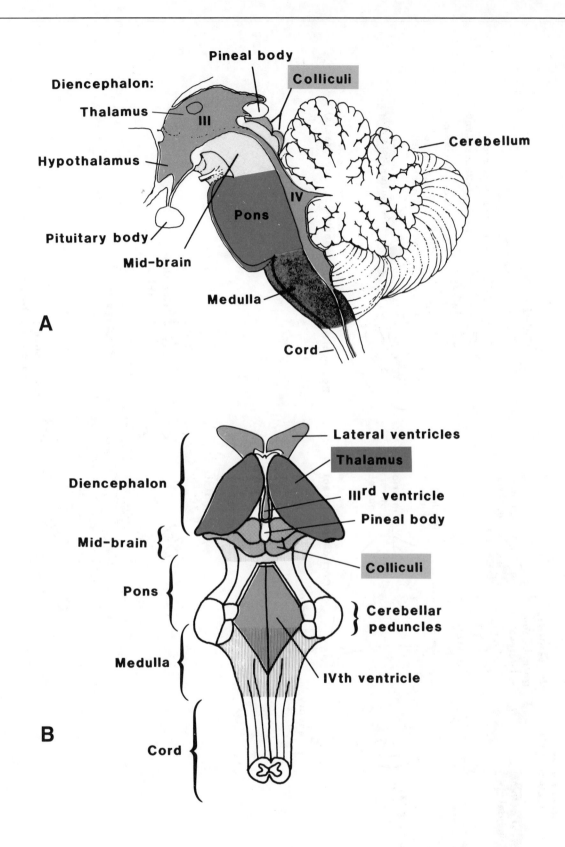

Figure 100 *A,* Midsagittal section of brainstem. *B,* Dorsal view of brainstem. *Figure continues.*

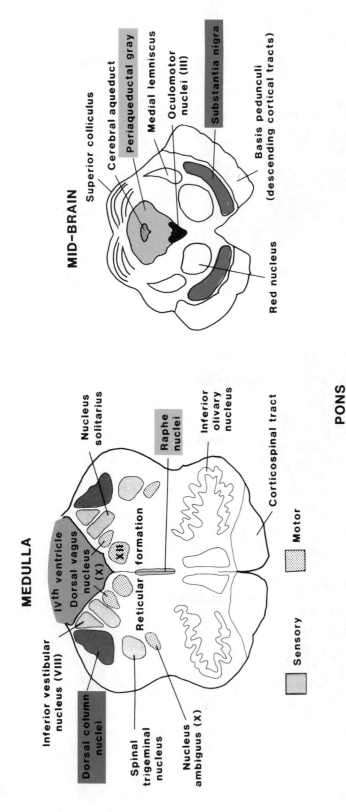

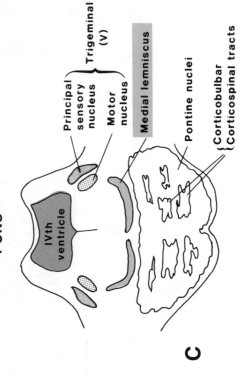

MID-BRAIN

Superior colliculus
Cerebral aqueduct
Periaqueductal gray
Medial lemniscus
Oculomotor nuclei (III)
Substantia nigra
Basis pedunculi (descending cortical tracts)
Red nucleus

MEDULLA

Inferior vestibular nucleus (VIII)
Nucleus solitarius
IVth ventricle
Dorsal vagus nucleus (X)
Raphe nuclei
Inferior olivary nucleus
XII
Reticular formation
Corticospinal tract
Dorsal column nuclei
Spinal trigeminal nucleus
Nucleus ambiguus (X)

Sensory   Motor

PONS

Principal sensory nucleus
Motor nucleus
Trigeminal (V)
Medial lemniscus
IVth ventricle
Pontine nuclei
Corticobulbar Corticospinal tracts

C

Figure 100 *(continued)* C, Transverse sections of brainstem. *Figure continues.*

Thalamus

The diencephalon is split into two major structures, **thalamus** and **hypothalamus**. The thalamus is subdivided into many nuclei (Fig. 100D), each one projecting to a specific cerebral territory. The projection may be discrete (primary sensory pathways) or rather diffuse (ventrolateral nucleus to motor cortex). Inputs to the thalamus arise from each sensory system, from the entire cerebral cortex, from cerebellum (to ventrolateral nucleus), basal ganglia (to ventroanterior nucleus), hypothalamus (to anterior and mediodorsal nuclei), and reticular formation (to centromedian nucleus).

Hypothalamus

The hypothalamic nuclei serve as a neuroendocrine interface (see Units 90 to 93). By axonal projections or "releasing factors" they control the secretion of hormones from the pituitary body (see Fig. 100A). Extensive interconnections exist with PAG, reticular formation, and limbic areas of the cerebrum.

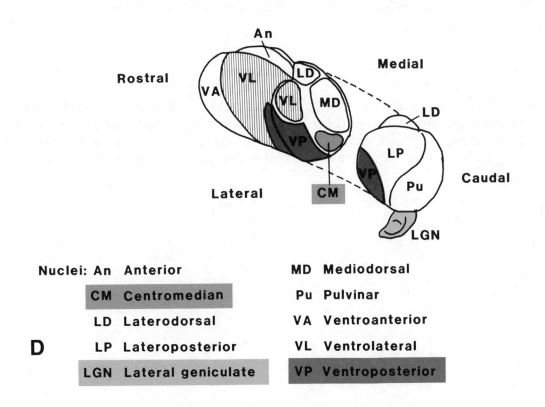

Nuclei: An Anterior

CM Centromedian

LD Laterodorsal

D   LP Lateroposterior

LGN Lateral geniculate

MD Mediodorsal

Pu Pulvinar

VA Ventroanterior

VL Ventrolateral

VP Ventroposterior

Figure 100 *(continued)*   *D,* Thalamic nuclei: side view section.

UNIT 101
CEREBRUM

The **cerebrum** or **telencephalon** is divided bilaterally into two hemispheres. Each consists of a heavily folded **cerebral cortex** (outer "bark" of gray matter) and a complex of nuclei deep inside the white matter surrounding the diencephalon.

Cerebral Cortex

In each hemisphere the cortex is morphologically divisible into four lobes of functional significance: **frontal**, **parietal**, **occipital**, and **temporal** (Fig. 101A). A fold in the cortex is called a **sulcus**; the crest between sulci is a **gyrus**.

Throughout most of its extent, the cortex is six layers deep (**neocortex**). **Allocortex** or primitive cortex can have as few as three layers. Each layer serves a specific function in terms of receiving synaptic inputs and distributing projection axons to other cortical or subcortical areas (Fig. 101B).

The fine histologic appearance of the six cortical laminae ("cytoarchitectonics") changes from one functional patch of cortex to the next. Each distinguishable region of cortical surface area has been assigned a number; these numbers range from 1 to 47.

Claustrum

An enigmatic adjunct of the cortex, this extensive shell of gray matter lies just beneath the lateral cortex (Fig. 101C). Each major region of cortex (visual, somatosensory, motor, and so forth) reciprocally interconnects with a specific region of the claustrum. (See discussion of end-stopped cells in Unit 117).

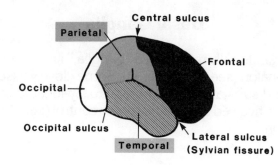

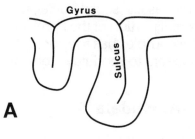

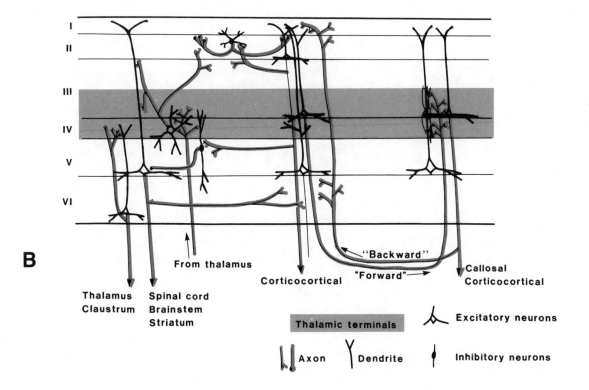

Figure 101 *A*, Lobes of the cerebral cortex. *B*, Inputs and outputs of the cortical layers. *Figure continues.*

Basal Ganglia

These nuclei, traditionally mislabeled "ganglia," line the lateral ventricles and encircle the diencephalon (see Fig. 101C, D). Some closely associated nuclei (subthalamic nucleus and substantia nigra) are actually located in the diencephalon and mid-brain. All are involved in somatic motor control (see Units 138 and 139) or autonomic regulation.

Basal Forebrain

This group of nuclei (nucleus basalis, septal nuclei, nucleus of the diagonal band) lies at the bottom of the frontal portion of the hemispheres, underneath the basal ganglia (see Fig. 101C). The complex has a topographic cholinergic projection to the cerebral cortex and appears to modulate cortical activity.

Amygdala

A complex of nuclei within the tip of the temporal lobe (see Fig. 101D), the amygdala regulates the autonomic nervous system and is very important in memory consolidation (see Unit 143).

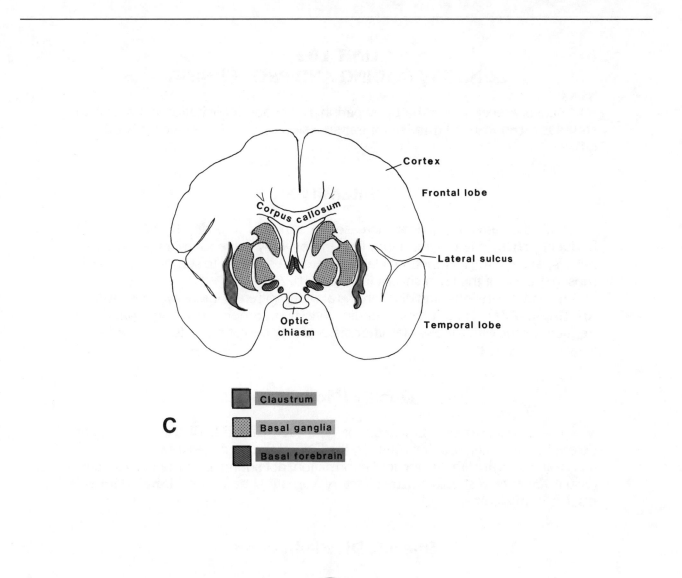

C

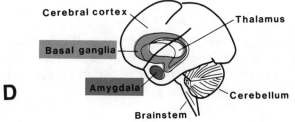

D

Figure 101 *(continued)* *C,* Frontal section of hemispheres. *D,* Deep nuclei of the cerebrum.

UNIT 102
SENSORY CODING AND PROCESSING

Sensory receptors in the body periphery encode information pertaining to stimulus **intensity** and **quality** for transmission into the CNS (see Units 62 and 64).

Intensity

Individual afferents signal increases in stimulus intensity by higher spike frequency rates up to the frequency limit imposed by nerve membrane refractoriness (see Unit 13). The function relating afferent responses to stimulus intensity is most generally of the form shown in Figure 102A.

Individual afferents start discharging at widely different intensity levels (**stimulus thresholds**). Thus intensity coding has two components (Fig. 102B): (1) frequency code within individual afferents, and (2) population code, i.e., number of activated afferents.

Quality (Modality)

The physical origin and receptor type (see Unit 62) of a given afferent determines the interpretation made by the CNS of the mediated information; e.g., retinal afferents are labeled for light information, not sound. Each sensory system (visual, auditory, vestibular, taste, olfactory, somatic) has its own "**labeled lines**" distinct from all others.

Specific Discrimination

Location

The labeled line strategy is used to signal where the stimulus arises in the periphery. Each somatosensory (visual) afferent has a discrete **receptive field** or body region (visual space) in which afferent activity can be elicited. Activity in the afferent is always referred to that field.

Feature

In general there are too many stimulus qualities and submodalities (e.g., colors, surface textures, odors) to design specific receptors for each. A **population code** is used, whereby a number of receptors respond to different segments of the discriminable stimulus range (Fig. 102C). Specific stimuli are coded by the profile of relative discharge rates across the afferent population. (Absolute discharge rates depend on stimulus intensity.)

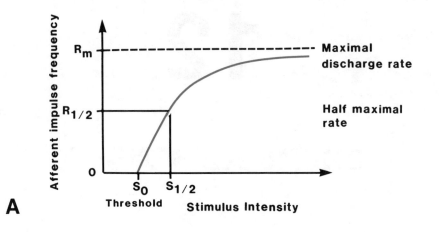

A

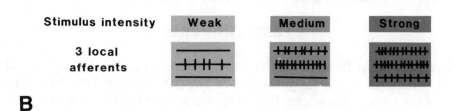

B

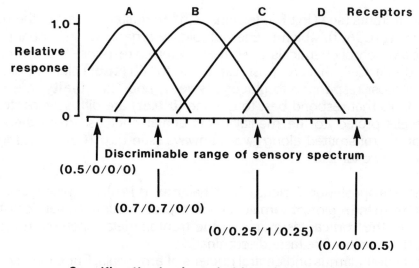

C

Figure 102 *A*, General stimulus-response function. *B*, Intensity coding. *C*, Population code for specific stimuli.

12

CHEMICAL SENSES

UNIT 103
CENTRAL PATHWAYS FOR TASTE

Taste Afferents

Branches of the facial nerve (VII) innervate taste cells in the palate, and in the anterior two-thirds of the tongue (chorda tympani nerve). The lingual nerve, a branch of the glossopharyngeal (IX), innervates the posterior tongue, and a vagal (X) branch, the superior laryngeal nerve, innervates taste receptors of the pharynx and larynx.

Pathways

Taste afferents (see Unit 65) terminate in the gustatory part of the nucleus solitarius (Fig. 103A, i), which is chemotopically organized. Individual neurons respond to a variety of chemicals, but have a preferred response to one molecular type (Fig. 103B). Cells that are most responsive to HCl (**sour**) cluster posteriorly, while those most responsive to glucose (**sweet**) and NaCl (**salty**) are located anteriorly. Cells that respond best to quinine (**bitter**) are diffusely located. The solitarius cells project to the medial parabrachial nucleus. From there, taste information is transmitted along two pathways (see Fig. 103A, i and ii); note bifurcation) to two targets:

1. Medial ventroposterior nucleus of the thalamus (VPm), a parvocellular region distinct from the region of somatosensory representation. Thalamic taste cells project to the cortical taste area in the frontoparietal operculum (see Fig. 103A, l). Function: fine taste discrimination.
2. Lateral hypothalamus and central nucleus of amygdala. Function: regulation of feeding behavior.

Because of the almost direct access of taste signals to the limbic system, taste stimuli are readily conditioned to serve a reinforcing or aversive role, e.g., eliciting appetite or nausea.

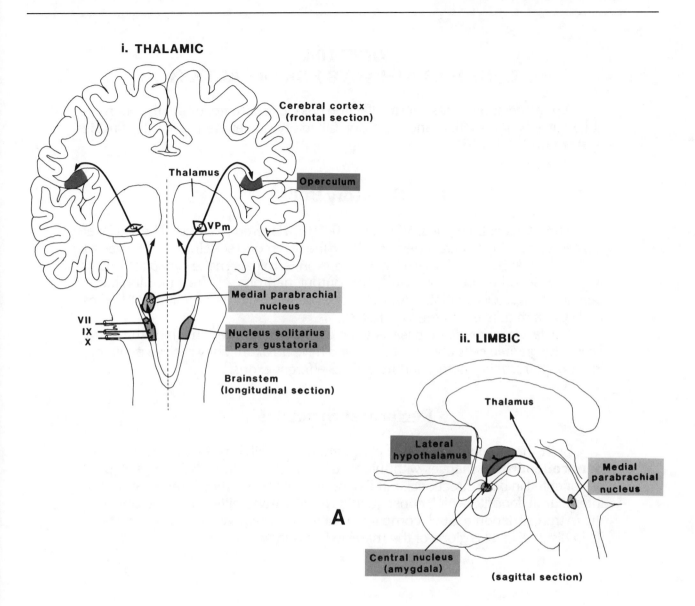

i. THALAMIC

Cerebral cortex
(frontal section)

Thalamus

Operculum

VPm

Medial parabrachial
nucleus

Nucleus solitarius
pars gustatoria

VII
IX
X

Brainstem
(longitudinal section)

ii. LIMBIC

Thalamus

Lateral
hypothalamus

Medial
parabrachial
nucleus

Central nucleus
(amygdala)

(sagittal section)

A

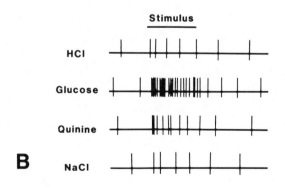

Stimulus

HCl

Glucose

Quinine

NaCl

B

Figure 103 *A*, Schematic representation of taste pathways. *B*, Selective taste response (nucleus solitarius).

233

UNIT 104
CENTRAL PATHWAYS FOR OLFACTION

A primordial sensory system, olfaction has close connections to the brain circuits subserving emotion and memory. Olfactory nuclei are part of the **limbic system** (see Unit 146).

Olfactory Bulb

The olfactory bulb (Figs. 104A and 104B) is a layered structure. The first layer contains incoming olfactory nerves (I) from the receptors (see Unit 65). The nerves terminate in spherical glomeruli, in which axon terminals make synaptic contact with the dendrites of mitral cells, the output neurons of the bulb. Inhibitory periglomerular cells mediate lateral inhibition between glomeruli. Mitral cell bodies make up a middle layer (see Fig. 104B).

The last layer of the bulb is made up of granule cells which inhibit the mitral cells. The granule cells are nonspiking and have no axon. They receive excitatory input both from the mitrals and from CNS efferent axons.

Reciprocal Synapses

Both the granule cells and periglomerular inhibitory interneurons make **dendrodendritic** synapses with mitral cell dendrites (Fig. 104C). The synapses are oriented in both directions: mitral dendrite transmitter release depolarizes the interneuron dendrite, which consequently releases transmitter that hyperpolarizes the mitral cell dendrite. Such compact circuits rapidly regulate the level of excitability in discrete local regions of the mitral cell dendritic tree.

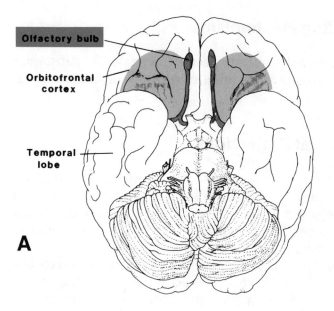

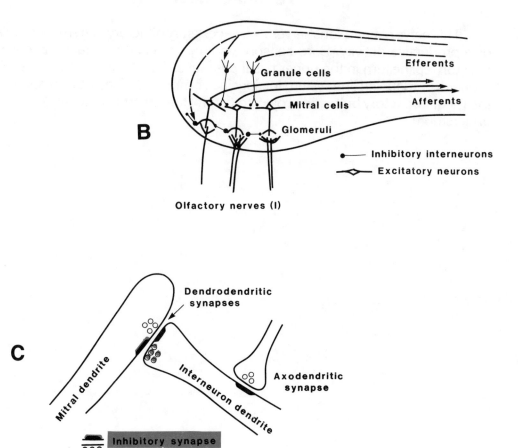

Figure 104 *A*, Olfactory neocortex. *B*, Olfactory bulb. *C*, Reciprocal synapses. *Figure continues.*

Coding Mechanisms

Odors are spatially coded within the olfactory bulb. Each specific substance elicits activation of olfactory bulb neurons in a unique "mosaic" distribution (Fig. 104D).

Central Projections

The olfactory bulb projects to the anterior olfactory nucleus, the olfactory tubercle, the prepyriform cortex, and cortical and medial nuclei of the amygdala (Fig. 104E). These are all limbic structures which regulate autonomic behaviors organized within the hypothalamus-PAG-reticular axis. The prepyriform cortex is three-layered allocortex with afferents entering the superficial layer.

The first three regions (above) project to the mediodorsal (MD) nucleus of the thalamus and thence to the orbitofrontal cortex. The posterior part of the orbitofrontal cortex (see Fig. 104A) serves as a zone for fine odor discriminations.

Terminal Nerve

This nerve of fine axons serves as an accessory olfactory system for regulation of reproductive activity. Bare sensory endings innervate surface epithelia and olfactory epithelium in the upper nasal passages. They respond to sexual pheromones, i.e., a labeled-line system for specific compounds. The cell bodies lie along the medial olfactory bulb and project to central targets (this mechanism is poorly understood).

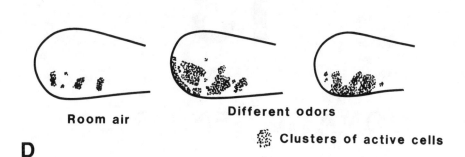

D

Room air

Different odors

🌑 Clusters of active cells

E

Orbitofrontal cortex

Olfactory bulb

Reticular formation

1. Olfactory tubercle
2. Prepyriform cortex
3. Amygdala
4. Thalamus: medial dorsal nucleus (MD)

Figure 104 *(continued)* D, Spatial coding of odors. E, Olfactory pathways. (E, Adapted from Nieuwenhuys R, Voogd J, van Huijzen C. The human central nervous system. Heidelberg: Springer-Verlag, 1981:215.)

13

SOMATIC SENSATION

UNIT 105
LEMNISCAL PATHWAY

Somatosensory Modalities

There are four primary somatosensory modalities:

1. Tactile sensation (cutaneous)
2. Proprioception (position sense and kinesthesia) } Mechanoreception
3. Thermal sensation
4. Nociception (pain)

There is considerable interaction within the CNS among these modalities; they are not entirely separate sensory systems.

Lemniscal Composition

Only myelinated, large-diameter **mechanoreceptor** afferents (see Unit 67) take the fast lemniscal route to the cerebral cortex. **Cutaneous** and **proprioceptive** mechanoreceptor afferents are segregated. Cutaneous rapidly (fast) and slowly adapting (FA and SA) afferents (see Unit 66) are also kept apart.

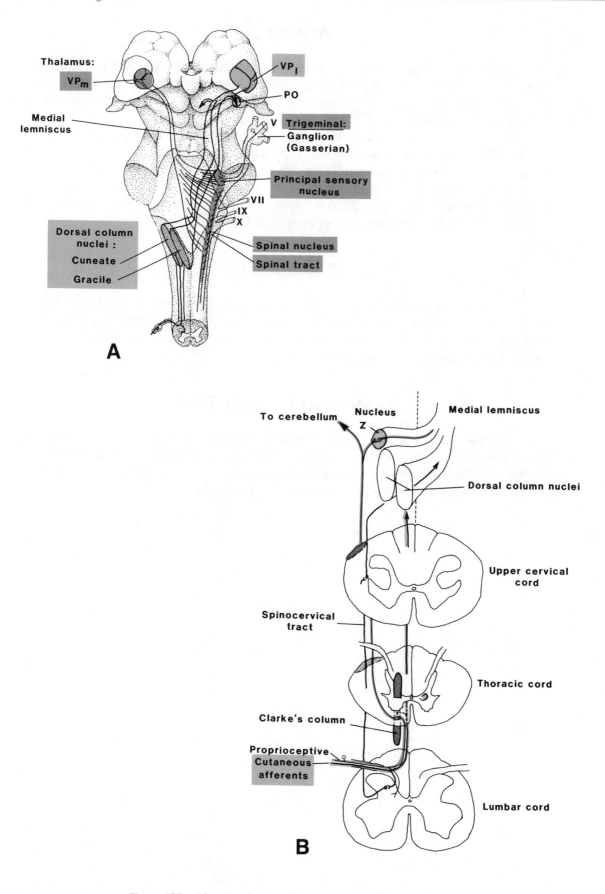

Figure 105 *A,* Lemniscal system. *B,* Accessory paths. *Figure continues.*

Anatomy

The **lemniscal pathway** comprises the **dorsal columns, medial lemniscus**, and **thalamocortical projection** to the somatosensory cortex (S1). The trigeminal nerve and trigeminothalamic tract mediate face and mouth inputs in a parallel compartment (Fig. 105A).

Afferents ascending in the dorsal columns terminate in the **dorsal column nuclei (DCN)** on lemniscal neurons. The **gracile nucleus** serves leg and lower trunk afferents; the **cuneate nucleus** serves those of the arms, chest, neck, and back of the head. Cutaneous afferents lie in a more dorsal position than the proprioceptive afferents. Leg proprioceptive afferents ascend in the dorsolateral column (Fig. 105B) and synapse in their own DCN (nucleus Z).

Somatotopy

Neurons are spatially organized according to the order of their peripheral connections (**somatotopic order**). Receptive fields gradually enlarge for successive neurons in the pathway, because of convergence of inputs, but they are well defined and confined to a single territory.

Spinocervicothalamic Tract

This tract carries second-order mechanoreceptor signals (mostly cutaneous) from dorsal horn neurons, up the lateral column, to synapse on diffusely scattered neurons in the lateral column at the level of the DCN (see Fig. 105B). The ascending projection joins the medial lemniscus in the medulla.

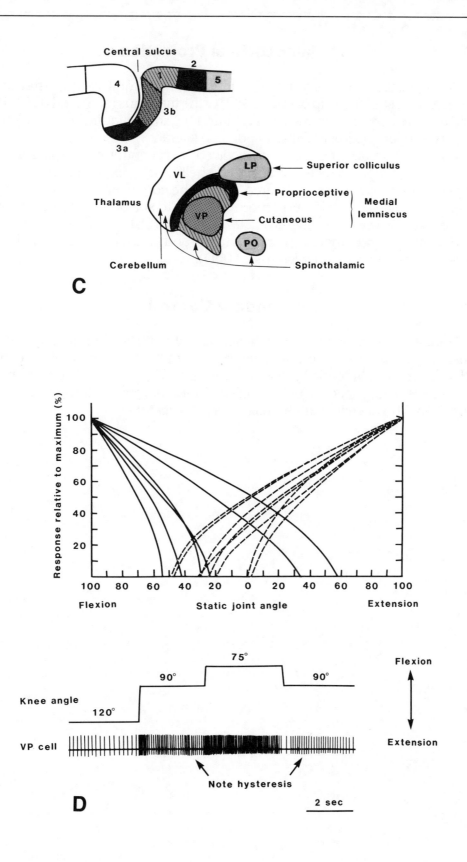

Figure 105 *(continued)*   C, Thalamocortical projection. *D*, Proprioceptive VP cells. *Figure continues.*

Thalamocortical Projection

The medial lemniscus terminates in the contralateral ventroposterior (VP) nucleus and posterior group of nuclei (PO) of the thalamus (see Fig. 105A). Spinal inputs are directed to the lateral VP (VP_1) and trigeminal inputs to the medial VP (VP_m). The trigeminothalamic projection is bilateral.

Within VP, cutaneous input is received in a central core zone, whereas proprioceptive input is directed to a rostral "shell" (Fig. 105C). Both zones project to the cerebral cortex, the shell to area 3a and the core to area 3b, making up S1 proper. VP also projects, although more sparsely, to surrounding cortical areas 1 and 2, and to S2 within the lateral sulcus (see Unit 108).

VP cells respond either to cutaneous touch and pressure in specific fields or to muscle tensions and joint angles (Fig. 105D).

Descending Control

Transmission of signals along the lemniscal route is controlled by descending axons from layer V of somatosensory (and motor) cortex to the level of the DCN, or from layer VI to the VP thalamus (Fig. 105E). The major effect on DCN appears to be presynaptic inhibition (via local interneurons) of currently unwanted information. The net effect at the thalamus is facilitatory.

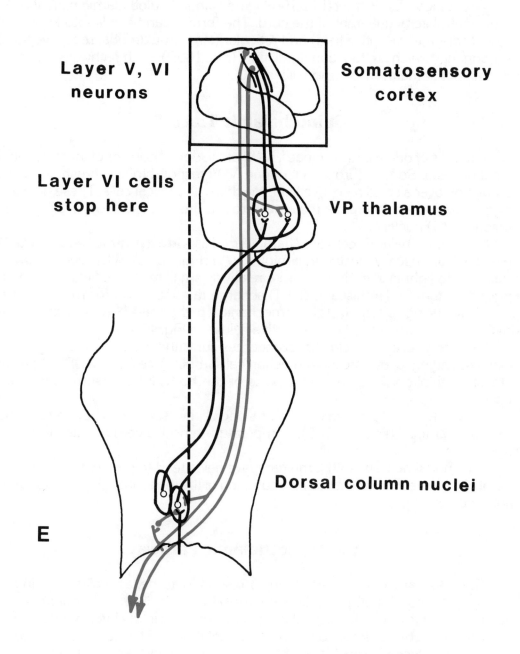

Layer V, VI neurons

Somatosensory cortex

Layer VI cells stop here

VP thalamus

Dorsal column nuclei

E

Figure 105 *(continued)* E, Descending control. (*A* and *E*, Adapted from Nieuwenhuys R, Voogd J, van Huijzen C. The human central nervous system. Heidelberg: Springer-Verlag, 1981:122, 124, 123. *C*, Adapted from Jones EG, Friedman DP. Projection pattern of functional components of thalmic ventrobasal complex on monkey somatosensory cortex. J Neurophysiol 1982; 48:542. *D, Top,* Adapted from Mountcastle VB, Poggio GF, Werner G. The relation of thalmic cell response to peripheral stimuli varied over an intensive continuum. J Neurophysiol 1963; 26:828.)

UNIT 106
SPINOTHALAMIC AND RETICULAR PATHWAYS

The spinothalamic tract (Fig. 106A) and spinoreticulothalamic path ascend in the ventrolateral quadrant of the cord. The former can be split into lemniscal adjunct (discrete receptive field) and reticular (large, multimodal receptive field) components, which are functionally distinct (Fig. 106B). Both pathways serve the full range of somatosensory modalities.

Spinothalamic Tract

The cells of origin lie in laminae I, IV–VI of the dorsal horn, or of the trigeminal spinal nucleus. Some neurons in laminae IV–VI respond to low-threshold tactile stimulation over a small receptive field, much like lemniscal cells. These neurons project to the contralateral VP thalamus around the lemniscal focus, and to the posterior (PO) nuclei.

Many spinothalamic cells are characterized as **wide dynamic range (WDR)** cells. They are usually located in laminae IV–VI (Fig. 106C). WDR cells respond phasically to light tactile stimuli from a relatively small receptive field (but much larger than that for lemniscal cells). Discharge rate increases for more intense stimuli into the noxious range (either mechanical or thermal). Noxious stimulation drives the cell from a very large receptive field (see Fig. 106C).

Excitatory receptive fields are sometimes surrounded by an inhibitory zone, both responding to low-threshold mechanical stimuli. More often WDR cells have extensive inhibitory fields on other parts of the body: Intense stimulation can suppress firing.

Only a few spinothalamic cells are nociceptive-specific. They tend to be located in lamina I (see Unit 109). Temperature-sensitive cells are also found in lamina I.

Multimodal neurons with large receptive fields tend to project to the centro-lateral (CL) nucleus of the intralaminar division of the thalamus. CL projects to the motor cortex.

Spinoreticulothalamic Pathway

The reticular route is specialized to discriminate behaviorally meaningful sensory patterns. Spinal projection neurons to the ipsilateral or contralateral reticular formation lie in the base of the dorsal horn and in the intermediate zone.

The cells receive highly convergent afferent inputs in terms of body location and modality. Receptive fields may cover up to half the body and are not confined to one side. Both cutaneous and proprioceptive components may be present; the cell may respond to an overall body posture or to a phase of a movement (e.g., locomotion). Other neurons respond to intense or noxious stimuli.

Spinothalamic cells of the reticular type (large receptive fields, convergent modalities) contribute to this pathway by synapsing onto reticular formation neurons via collaterals, en route to the CL thalamus (see Fig. 106B). The reticular formation projects to the centromedian (CM) nucleus of the intralaminar thalamus, which projects in turn to the basal ganglia (Fig. 106D).

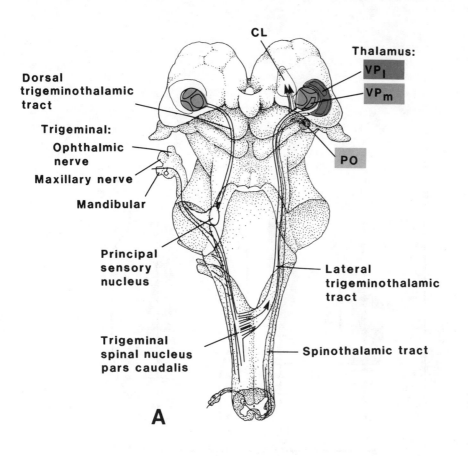

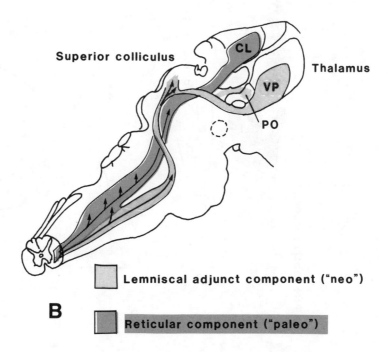

Figure 106 *A,* Spinothalamic system. *B,* Components of the spinothalamic tract. *Figure continues.*

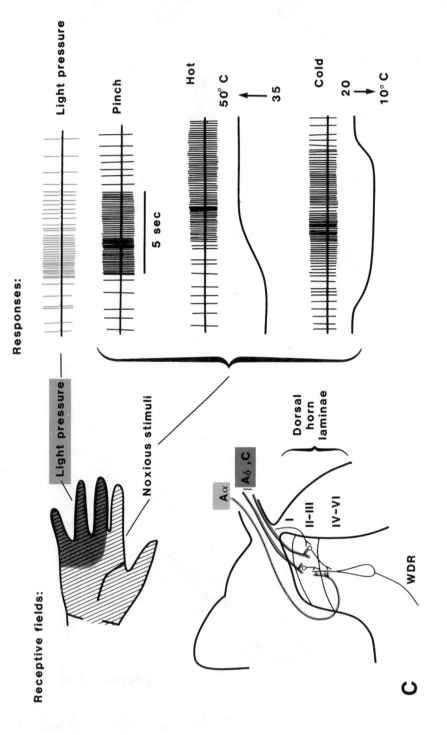

Figure 106 *(continued)*   C, Wide dynamic range (WDR) cell. *Figure continues.*

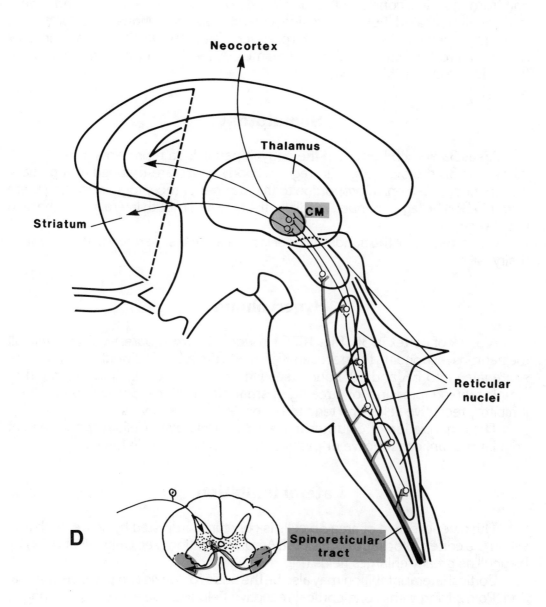

Figure 106 *(continued)*   *D*, Spinoreticulothalamic tract. (*A* and *D*, Adapted from Nieuwenhuys R, Voogd J, van Huijzen C. The human central nervous system. Heidelberg: Springer-Verlag, 1981:120, 124, 151. *B*, Adapted from Mountcastle VB, ed. Pain and temperature sensibilities. In: Medical physiology. 14th ed. St. Louis: CV Mosby, 1980:406.)

UNIT 107
SOMATOSENSORY CORTEX (S1)

S1, the region of the cortex receiving input from the surface of the body and from muscles, consists of areas 3a and 3b (Fig. 107A). (Areas 1 and 2 were traditionally included, but they provide separate representations of the body with different properties.) Area 3a receives proprioceptive (and vestibular) input in layer IV from the rostral "shell" of the VP thalamus. Area 3b receives cutaneous input from VP (see Unit 105).

Somatotopy

Areas 3a and 3b both map the body in parallel: 3a represents muscles and joints, and 3b the overlying skin regions. Body zones are mapped in a partially discontinuous fashion, in proportion to the number of receptors originating there (Fig. 107B). The leg is mapped medially, the face and mouth laterally, and the arm in between.

Glabrous skin of the hands and feet is represented separately from the dorsal (hairy) skin.

Hypercolumn

A block of cortex in 3b (Fig. 107C), roughly 1 mm square, would contain all the neurons responding to one receptive field on the skin. The inputs to layer IV are segregated into FA and SA bands (see Unit 105). Most cells in 3b respond to simple tapping, pressing, or stroking of small skin regions. Some neurons have inhibitory receptive fields and tend to be located in deep layers.

The organization of columns in area 3a is unknown. Cells respond to joint angular motion, either active or passive, and to active muscle forces.

Lateral Inhibition

The receptive field of area 3b cells is constantly adjusted by active inhibition within the cortex. Blockage of this GABAergic inhibition (see Units 38 and 39) by bicuculline greatly enlarges fields (Fig. 107D).

Cortical lateral inhibition may also be the basis for tactile two-point discrimination. Points lying within one cortical receptive field may be easily discriminated: The limit is set by the size and density of primary afferent receptive fields. Because of lateral inhibition, within the lemniscal pathway and at the cortex, the populations of neurons activated from two nearby points on the skin do not merge into one (Fig. 107E).

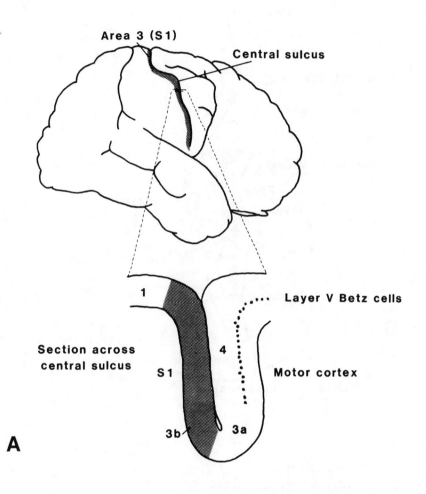

Figure 107 *A*, Primary somatosensory cortex (S1). *Figure continues.*

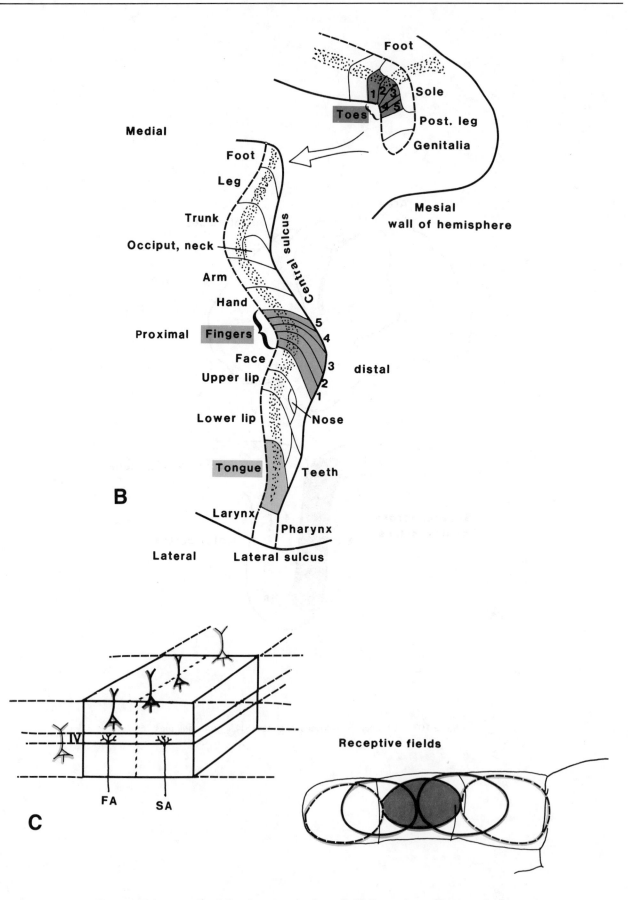

Figure 107 *(continued)* *B*, Somatotopic map of area 3b. *C*, Hypercolumn. *Figure continues.*

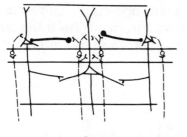

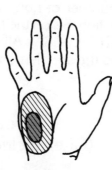

●——— **GABAergic inhibitory interneuron**

D

▨ **Receptive field with inhibition**

▨ **Receptive field with inhibition blocked (bicuculline)**

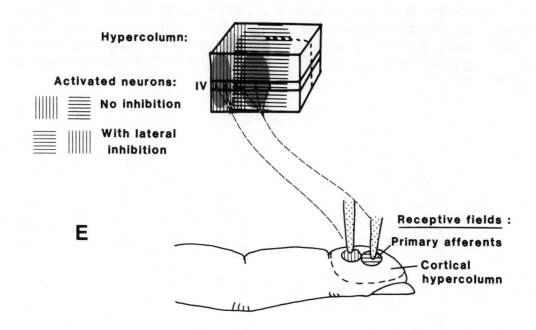

Hypercolumn:

Activated neurons:

‖‖ ☰ **No inhibition**

☰ ‖‖ **With lateral inhibition**

IV

Receptive fields :

Primary afferents

Cortical hypercolumn

E

Figure 107 *(continued)* *D*, Modifiability of the receptive field. *E*, Two-point discrimination.

UNIT 108
SOMATOSENSORY ASSOCIATION CORTEX

There are a large number of nonprimary body representations, varying in complexity and specialization. S2 on the frontoparietal operculum and areas 1, 2, and 5 are the best known (Fig. 108A). All receive input from the thalamus and S1 (Fig. 108B); all project to the supplementary motor area and motor cortex (see Units 135 and 136).

Area 1
(Often included in S1)

The body surface is remapped in area 1 as a mirror image of the area 3b representation but with more emphasis on FA responses. Receptive fields are larger and more integrated (see Fig. 108B), with some neurons receiving proprioceptive input. Pacinian corpuscle input, excluded from area 3b, projects here. Neurons tend to respond to moving stimuli; some have a preferred direction (Fig. 108C, i). Overt inhibitory receptive fields are often demonstrable (Fig. 108D), with "OFF" responses appearing when a stimulus is removed.

Area 2

Somatotopy becomes generalized as receptive fields become increasingly large; body zones and modalities are integrated into complex response patterns. Cutaneous receptive fields may be expressed by neural activity only if the body part is in a particular posture (Fig. 108E) or if the stimulus has a specific form or orientation.

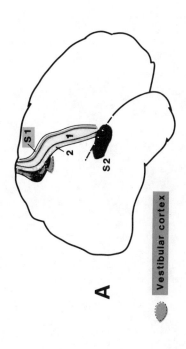

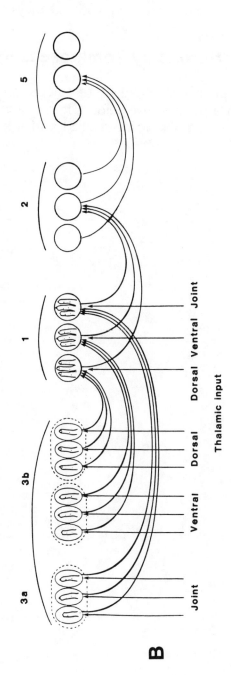

Figure 108 *A,* Somatosensory association areas. *B,* Corticocortical projections. *Figure continues.*

Area 5

The highest level of proprioceptive integration is achieved in area 5. Postural information arrives via area 2, the lateroposterior (LP) thalamus and the posterior (PO) nuclei. The latter includes a vestibular component. Neurons respond to static angles and/or dynamic motion, usually of several joints. Motion-sensitive cells (the majority) are directional (see Fig. 108C, ii); they code velocity well and force poorly.

Secondary Somatosensory Cortex (S2)

On the upper bank of the lateral sulcus (see Fig. 108A), S2 maps the entire body but with large receptive fields. Often regions on both sides are included. S2 receives the same thalamic input as S1 and areas 1 to 5 combined, plus callosal input.

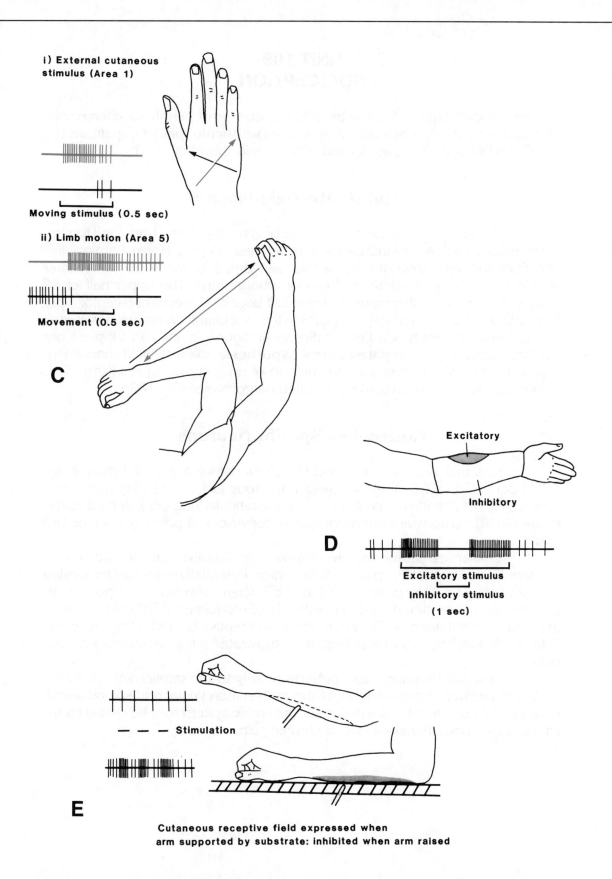

i) External cutaneous stimulus (Area 1)

Moving stimulus (0.5 sec)

ii) Limb motion (Area 5)

Movement (0.5 sec)

C

Excitatory

Inhibitory

D

Excitatory stimulus

Inhibitory stimulus

(1 sec)

– – – Stimulation

E

Cutaneous receptive field expressed when
arm supported by substrate: inhibited when arm raised

Figure 108 *(continued)* C, Directional specificity. D, Inhibitory surround field (area 1). E, Cutaneous-proprioceptive interaction (area 2). (B, Adapted from Iwamura Y, Tanaka M, Sakamoto M. Converging patterns of finger representation and complex response properties of neurons in area 1 of the first somatosensory cortex of the conscious monkey. Exp Brain Res 1983; 51:335.)

UNIT 109
NOCICEPTION

Pain signals are mediated mainly by two classes of peripheral afferents: (1) mechanoreceptive Aδ nociceptors, associated with acute "pricking" pain, and (2) C polymodal nociceptors, associated with chronic "burning" pain.

Substantia Gelatinosa

Small afferents terminate in superficial layers of the dorsal horn (and trigeminal spinal nucleus): Aδ in laminae I-V, C in laminae I-III (Fig. 109A). Laminae II-III constitute the substantia gelatinosa (SG; see Unit 98), made up of tiny interneurons with dense dendritic and axonal arborizations. The upper half of SG receives *cutaneous* C fiber input, the lower half large fiber mechanoreceptor input. Many SG cells have reciprocal responses to light mechanical and noxious stimuli.

Different afferent modalities are directly antagonistic and can suppress one another. According to the **gate control hypothesis**, low-threshold mechanoreceptor input to SG suppresses transmission of nociceptive signals from SG to spinothalamic and spinoreticular projection neurons (see Fig. 109A).

Nociceptive-Specific Neurons

Neurons that selectively respond to painful stimuli are uncommon. In the spinal cord (Fig. 109B) they are most numerous in laminae I (spinothalamic neurons) and X (beside the central canal: spinoreticular neurons). Wide dynamic range (WDR) neurons are the more typical conveyors of pain signals (see Unit 106).

In the thalamus, neurons receiving lamina I nociceptive-specific input may be clustered in the ventral VP, a parvocellular region. Potentially important for localization of acute pain, they project to S1 and S2 where nociceptive responses are uncommon and scattered among low-threshold modalities. WDR cells project to the intralaminar thalamus (CL) where some nociceptive cells with large receptive fields are found. They may be an important substrate for the sensation of chronic pain.

The reticular formation also projects heavily to the intralaminar thalamus (CM) and receives convergent input from both spinoreticular and spinothalamic neurons. Reticular input to the thalamus and limbic system may be critical for the affective and motivational aspects of chronic pain.

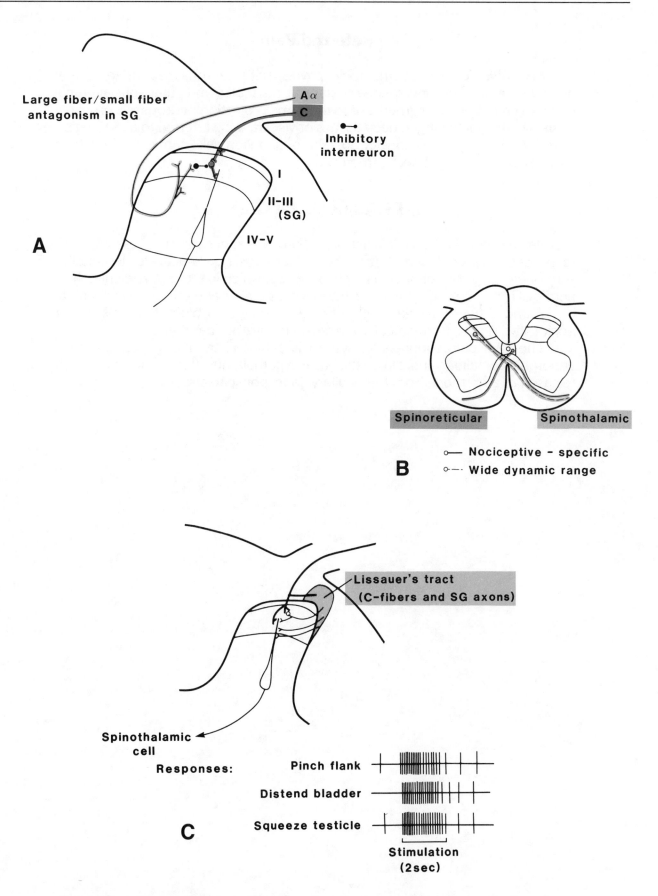

A

Large fiber/small fiber
antagonism in SG

Aα

C

Inhibitory
interneuron

I

II–III
(SG)

IV–V

B

Spinoreticular   Spinothalamic

○— Nociceptive – specific
○--- Wide dynamic range

Lissauer's tract
(C–fibers and SG axons)

Spinothalamic
cell

Responses:

Pinch flank

Distend bladder

Squeeze testicle

C

Stimulation
(2sec)

Figure 109 *A*, Gate control hypothesis. *B*, Projection cells. *C*, Convergence of nociceptive input. *Figure continues.*

Referred Pain

Many WDR cells and some nociceptive-specific neurons respond to visceral noxious stimuli. The convergence of visceral, muscular, and cutaneous afferents from several adjacent segments onto the same projection neurons is a probable basis for pain originating in deep tissues or viscera to be referred to a skin region (Fig. 109C). (Peripheral axons of dorsal root ganglion cells can also bifurcate to innervate both skin and deep structures.)

Periaqueductal Gray

Periaqueductal gray (PAG) activity in particular zones can suppress WDR cell responses to noxious stimuli (Fig. 109D). The PAG cells activate descending serotonergic neurons of nucleus raphe magnus, which in turn activate enkephalinergic SG interneurons. The opioid transmitter **enkephalin** presynaptically inhibits $A\delta$ and C fiber terminals within SG. PAG may also block transmission of nociceptive signals from reticular formation to intralaminar thalamus.

The PAG pain suppression system is activated by another opioid: beta-endorphin-containing fibers from the basal hypothalamus. Beta-endorphin is also released as a hormone from the pituitary, in response to stress.

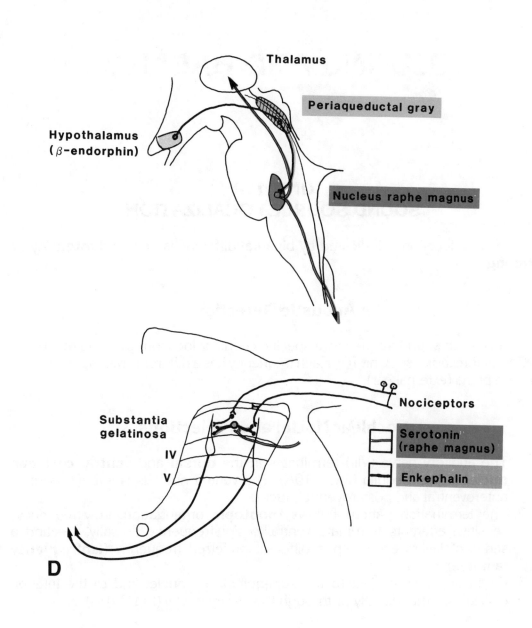

Thalamus

Periaqueductal gray

Hypothalamus
(β-endorphin)

Nucleus raphe magnus

Nociceptors

Substantia
gelatinosa

IV

V

Serotonin
(raphe magnus)

Enkephalin

D

Figure 109 *(continued)* *D,* Control of pain transmission.

14

HEARING AND BALANCE

UNIT 110
SOUND SOURCE LOCALIZATION

Sound location is indicated by binaural differences in sound **intensity** or **timing**.

Acoustic Detection

For each sound frequency, a specific cochlear location gives the minimum afferent threshold (see Unit 70). Each frequency has a different "best spot" relative to the pinna (external ear).

Cochlear Nuclei and Projections

1. The auditory nerve (VIII) terminates in the **dorsal** and **ventral cochlear nuclei** in the medulla (Fig. 110A). The ventral nucleus is subdivided into anteroventral and posteroventral nuclei.
2. The termination pattern follows **tonotopic** organization: Low-frequency-sensitive afferents terminate ventrally, high-frequency dorsally, creating a series of layers each with a different preferred frequency (**isofrequency laminae**).
3. Cochlear nuclei project to the superior olivary nuclei and to the inferior colliculus, either directly or through the olivary nuclei (Fig. 110B).

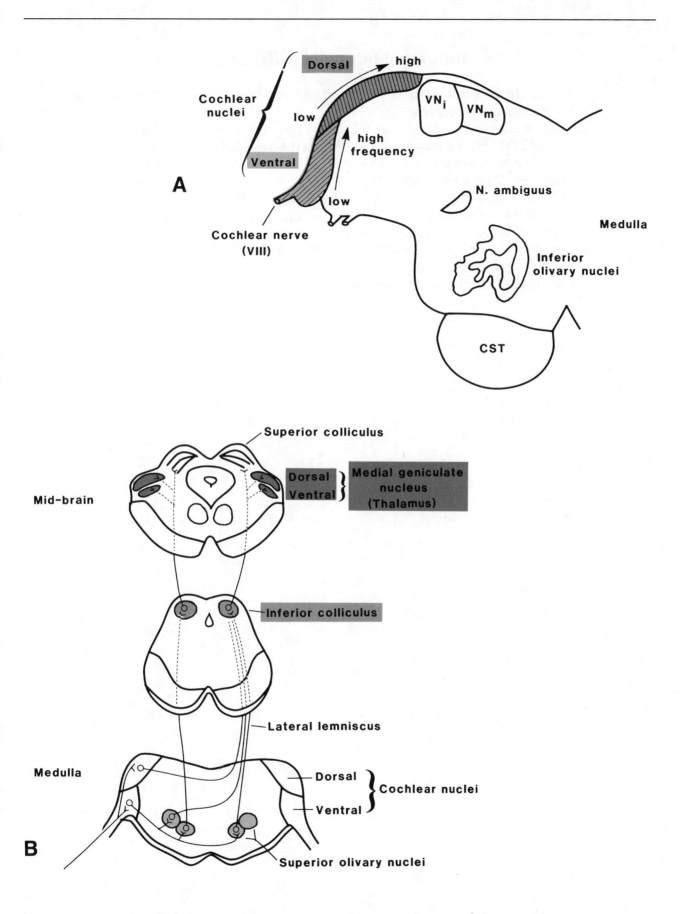

Figure 110 *A*, Cochlear nuclei. *B*, Brainstem auditory pathway. *Figure continues.*

Interaural Intensity Difference

1. The cochlea ipsilateral to the sound source is more strongly stimulated than the contralateral cochlea.
2. Interaural intensity difference (IID) is frequency dependent. Frequencies *above* 2,000 Hz are increasingly attenuated across the head.
3. For each frequency band above 2,000 Hz, IID is computed in the **lateral superior olivary nucleus** (LSO).
4. LSO neurons excited from the ipsilateral ventral cochlear nucleus are inhibited from the contralateral (via the interneuron) in the medial nucleus of the trapezoid body (Fig. 110C).
5. LSO cells signal IID independent of overall intensity level: IID threshold varies systematically across the nucleus.
6. LSO projects to the contralateral inferior colliculus.

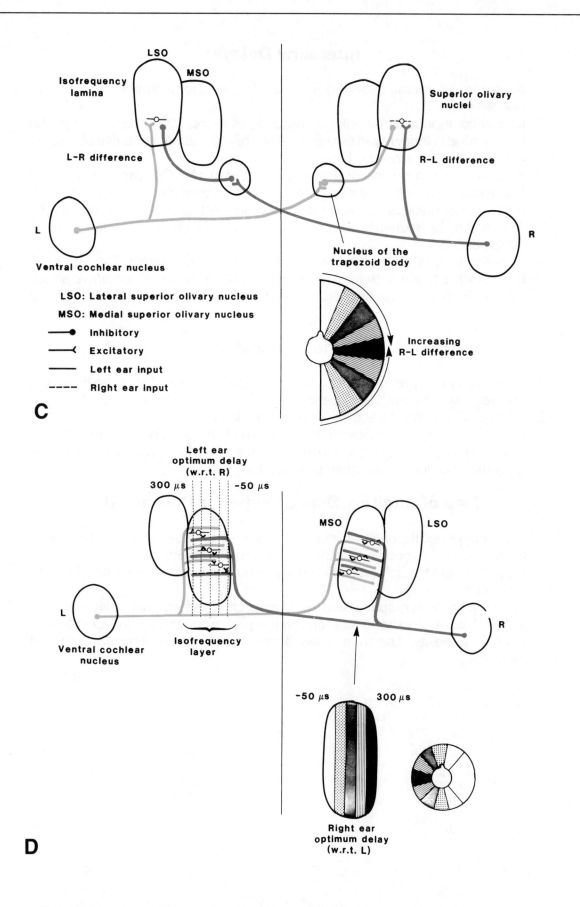

Figure 110 *(continued)*   C, Interaural intensity difference. D, Computation of interaural delay. *Figure continues.*

Interaural Delay

1. Maximum interaural delay (ID) is about 600 μsec, for a source maximally to one side.
2. ID computation is made only for frequencies *below* 2,000 Hz, i.e., when the cycle period is longer than 600 μsec. A second pulse will not arrive at one ear before the first has reached the other.
3. ID is mapped in the **medial superior olivary (MSO) nucleus** for each frequency separately. The sets of frequency-matched afferents from the ventral cochlear nucleus on each side make up a series of isofrequency layers. Across an isofrequency layer (Fig. 110D), the preferred delay varies systematically.
4. Optimal delay is determined by interaural latency difference: The MSO cell fires maximally when excitatory synaptic inputs from each side arrive simultaneously. (See discussion of summation of excitatory potentials, Units 49 and 83.)

Inferior Colliculus

1. Cells respond to preferred locations on the contralateral side of the head, but only for a specific frequency band.
2. Maps of ID are aligned across isofrequency laminae.
3. ID maps at low frequencies are aligned with IID maps at high frequencies.
4. The inferior colliculus projects to the superior colliculus (deep) and the medial geniculate nucleus of the thalamus (see Fig. 110B).

Map of Auditory Space (Superior Colliculus)

1. Frequency-specific binaural cues correspond to a *set* of possible source locations. *Unique* coding of the source requires mapping in at least three frequency bands, each with different maximum sensitivity locations relative to the pinna.
2. The map of auditory space is in the lower layers of the superior colliculus (Fig. 110E). Neurons respond to sound in the preferred location independent of pitch or intensity. The map is two-dimensional, representing azimuth and elevation.

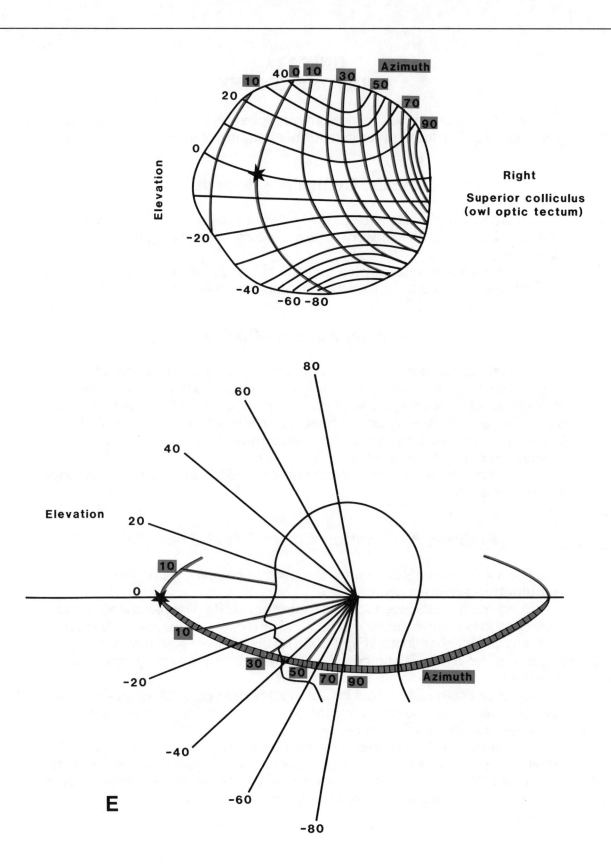

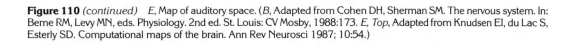

Figure 110 *(continued)* *E*, Map of auditory space. (*B*, Adapted from Cohen DH, Sherman SM. The nervous system. In: Berne RM, Levy MN, eds. Physiology. 2nd ed. St. Louis: CV Mosby, 1988:173. *E, Top*, Adapted from Knudsen El, du Lac S, Esterly SD. Computational maps of the brain. Ann Rev Neurosci 1987; 10:54.)

UNIT 111
AUDITORY CORTEX

Auditory regions in the superior temporal lobe are responsible for recognition of sound patterns, allowing interpretation of environmental sounds and of speech.

Medial Geniculate Nucleus

The medial geniculate nucleus (MGN) is the thalamic interface between the inferior colliculus and the auditory cortex. It retains tonotopic organization of the colliculus.

The laminated ventral division projects to the primary auditory cortex (A1). Other divisions project to surrounding auditory association areas (Fig. 111A).

Primary Auditory Cortex

The primary auditory cortex is a small area deep within the lateral sulcus. It is divided into a series of isofrequency strips along one axis (Fig. 111B). Along the orthogonal axis, the cortex is divided into alternating bands of binaural summation (contralateral + ipsilateral) and subtraction (contralateral − ipsilateral). Isofrequency strips may be graded: sharply tuned to a given frequency at one end, more broadly responsive at the other (see Fig. 111B).

Layer V pyramidal cells project to the inferior colliculus and aid in formation of the map of auditory space.

Auditory Association Cortex (Mustached Bat)

The auditory association cortex is the site of complex sound processing by **combination-sensitive** neurons.

Echo-locating bats detect specific **frequency shifts** (Doppler shifts) between emitted sounds and the returning echo: Cortical regions are mapped in frequency versus frequency coordinates (Fig. 111C, i) to discriminate systematically a range of precise frequency differences. Any delay, 0 to 10 msec, for the echo is permitted.

Other cortical regions (Fig. 111C, ii) map the **time delay** between successive sounds within a specific frequency range. Preferred delays vary systematically along the long axis of a "hypercolumn."

Similar neuronal processes in the human auditory cortex may underlie discrimination of complex sounds, especially of particular voices in a crowd (cocktail party effect). Perception of phonemes makes use of the discrimination both of intervals between tonal events and of frequency combinations.

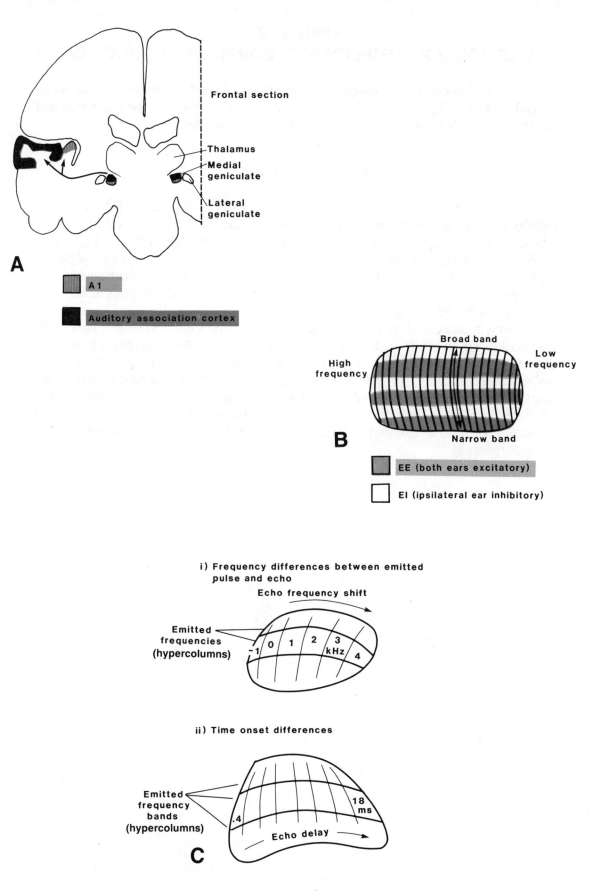

Figure 111 *A*, Thalamocortical projection. *B*, Auditory cortex. *C*, Auditory association cortex of the mustached bat.

UNIT 112
VESTIBULAR COMPLEX AND CORTICAL PROJECTION

Most of the central connections of the vestibular afferents are part of reflex loops (see Units 125 and 126). An ascending sensory pathway to the thalamus and cerebral cortex is treated as part of the proprioceptive system.

Vestibular Nuclei

There are 4 major vestibular nuclei (VN): superior (SVN), lateral (LVN), medial (MVN), and inferior (IVN) (see Figs. 112B and 112D). The vestibular afferents (cell bodies in the two ganglia of Scarpa) provide one major input (Figs. 112A and 112B). The fastigial nucleus of the cerebellum is another source of excitatory input, and the cerebellar cortex, of inhibitory input. Trunk and limb somatosensory pathways send collaterals to LVN, MVN, and IVN. Visual motion signals also arrive, possibly via the accessory optic system.

Semicircular canal afferents terminate in SVN, MVN, and LVN (see Fig. 112B), and otolith organ afferents in LVN, MVN, and IVN (the utricle projects mainly to LVN, the saccule to IVN). Secondary vestibular neurons responding to canal inputs are classified as type 1 or type 2 (Fig. 112C). Type 1 cells respond best to head rotation in the plane of a particular canal, in a direction that excites ipsilateral canal afferents (ipsilateral excitatory input). Type 2 cells respond to oppositely directed rotations, i.e., those exciting afferents from contralateral canals (contralateral excitatory input).

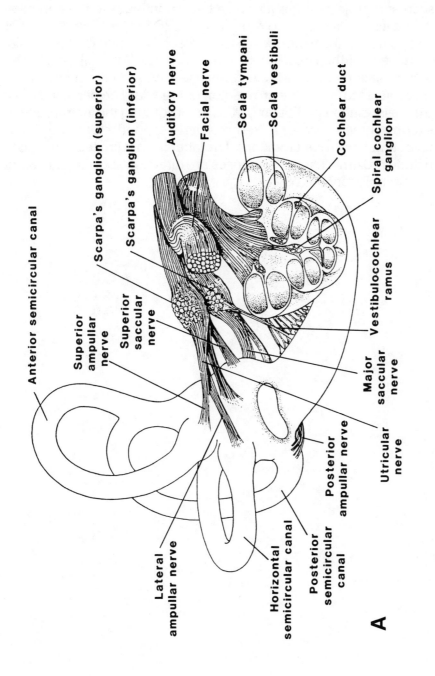

Anterior semicircular canal

Superior ampullar nerve

Scarpa's ganglion (superior)

Scarpa's ganglion (inferior)

Auditory nerve

Facial nerve

Scala tympani

Scala vestibuli

Superior saccular nerve

Cochlear duct

Spiral cochlear ganglion

Vestibulocochlear ramus

Major saccular nerve

Utricular nerve

Posterior ampullar nerve

Posterior semicircular canal

Horizontal semicircular canal

Lateral ampullar nerve

A

Figure 112 *A,* Peripheral vestibular apparatus. *Figure continues.*

269

Cortical Projection

The vestibular nuclei project to the deep layers of the superior colliculus, alongside neck proprioceptive inputs. The colliculus is provided with full information about the relative position and motion of the head.

A small ascending projection (largely from LVN) continues to the contralateral thalamus, where it terminates in two zones (Fig. 112D): (1) the inferior part of the proprioceptive "shell" in the ventroposterior nucleus (VP), and (2) the medial (magnocellular) nucleus of the medial geniculate complex (MGN_m), part of the posterior group. Stimulation of either locus gives rise to vestibular sensations.

The VP zone projects to S1, in the arm region of area 3a. The parallel MGN_m zone projects to the association vestibular cortex, incorporating the lateral edge of area 5 and neck representation of area 2. Neurons here respond to both vestibular and proprioceptive stimulation (joint rotation). The latter are not limited to the neck and trunk but include proximal joints. Responses are direction-specific: excitatory for rotation one way, inhibitory the other.

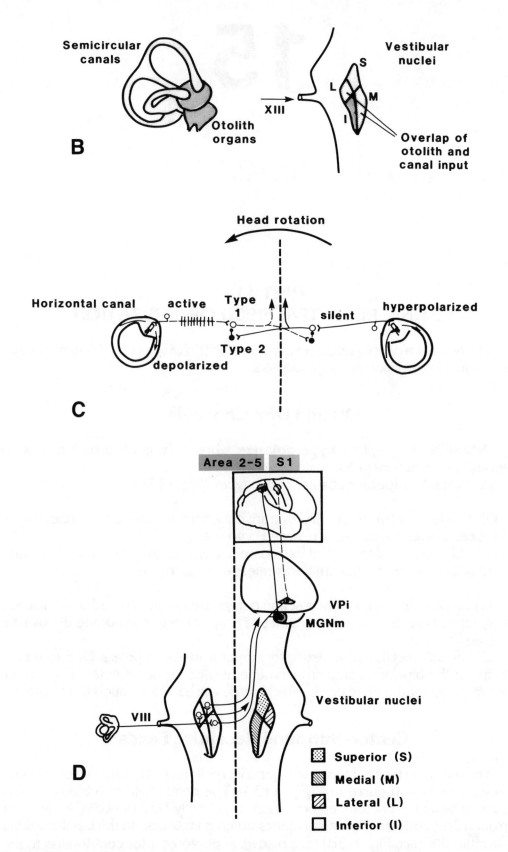

Figure 112 *(continued)* B, Vestibular nuclei. C, Bilateral interaction. D, Vestibular sensory pathway. (A, From Cohen DH, Sherman SM. The nervous system. In: Berne RM, Levy MN, eds. Physiology. 2nd ed. St. Louis: CV Mosby, 1988:181. With permission from the CV Mosby Company. B and D, Adapted from Nieuwenhuys R, Voogd J, van Huijzen C. The human central nervous system. Heidelberg: Springer-Verlag, 1981:137.)

15

VISION

UNIT 113
RETINA: RECEPTIVE FIELD ORGANIZATION

The retina is a peripheral extension of the CNS in which considerable processing of visual information is accomplished.

ON and OFF Channels

Retinal photoreceptors **hyperpolarize** when light is absorbed; they stop releasing the transmitter glutamate (see Unit 75).
Postsynaptic **bipolar cells** are of two types (Fig. 113A):

1. ON bipolars are hyperpolarized by transmitter; hence, they *depolarize in light* (because less transmitter is released onto them).
2. OFF bipolars are depolarized by transmitter; hence, they *depolarize in darkness* (because more transmitter is released onto them).

Bipolar cells do not generate action potentials: Passive spread of summated postsynaptic potentials releases vesicles in proportion to membrane depolarization (see Unit 32).
ON ganglion cells receive excitatory input from ON bipolars, OFF ganglion cells from OFF bipolars. Ganglion cells generate action potentials (see Fig. 113A). Their axons enter the optic nerve, which carries visual information to the brain.

Center-Surround Receptive Fields

The receptive field of bipolar and ganglion cells is made up of two concentric regions, **center** and **surround** (Fig. 113B). The center field of a bipolar cell is mediated by all the photoreceptors synapsing directly onto the cell. The annular surround field consists of photoreceptors which gain access to the bipolar cell via horizontal cells (see Fig. 113B) (see below). A photoreceptor contributing to the center field of one bipolar cell also contributes to the surround fields of other bipolar cells via horizontal cells.

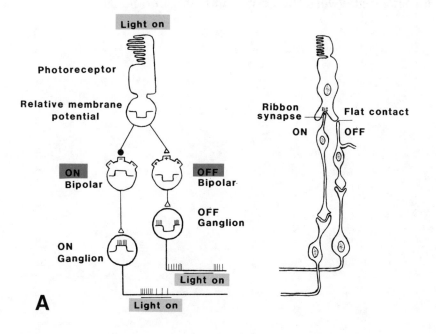

Figure 113 *A*, ON and OFF channels. *Figure continues.*

Lateral Inhibition (Horizontal Cells)

Horizontal cells are nonspiking inhibitory interneurons. They make complex synaptic connections with neighboring photoreceptors and bipolar cells. Horizontal cells are hyperpolarized when light stimulates input photoreceptors. When they depolarize (i.e., release transmitter), they *inhibit* photoreceptors (Fig. 113C).

If the center field of a bipolar or ganglion cell is ON, the surround field is OFF and vice versa. Simultaneous stimulation by light of both fields gives no net response, since the antagonistic excitatory and inhibitory inputs neutralize each other. Because of center-surround antagonism, ganglion cells monitor *differences* in luminance between the center and surround fields.

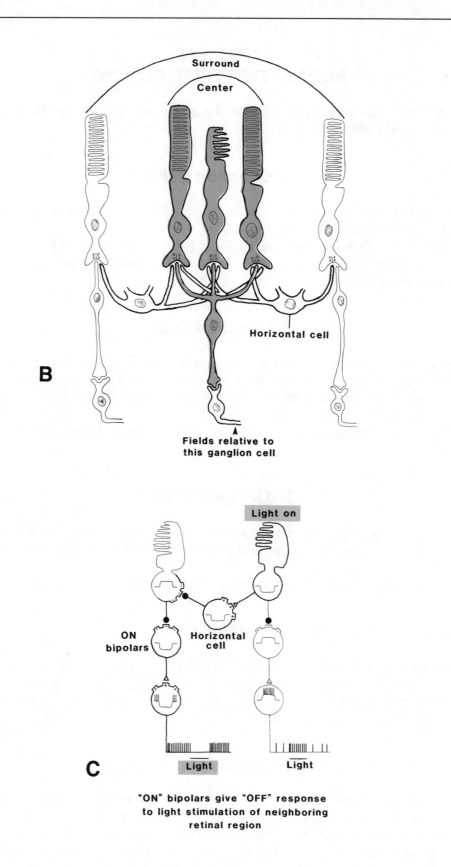

Surround

Center

Horizontal cell

B

Fields relative to
this ganglion cell

Light on

ON
bipolars

Horizontal
cell

C

Light

Light

"ON" bipolars give "OFF" response
to light stimulation of neighboring
retinal region

Figure 113 *(continued)*   *B*, Center-surround receptive fields. *C*, Lateral inhibition. (*A* and *C*, Modified after Kandel ER, Schwartz JH. Principles of neural science. New York: Elsevier, 1985:350, 354.)

UNIT 114
RETINA: TEMPORAL CODING

As with other sensory modalities, the visual system has rapidly and slowly adapting channels (see Unit 64).

X Ganglion Cells

1. Receive input mostly from bipolar cells; relatively small somata with slow axonal conduction velocity (Fig. 114A).
2. *Sustained* ON or OFF responses (Fig. 114B) to light stimuli (slowly adapting).
3. Linear summation of responses to stimuli in various parts of center and surround fields.

Y Ganglion Cells

1. Receive input mostly from **amacrine cells** (see Fig. 114A); larger receptive fields than X cells, large somata, and fast axonal conduction velocity.
2. *Transient* responses (rapidly adapting) to changes in illumination: respond best to *moving* stimuli (see Fig. 114B).
3. Nonlinear summation of responses in various parts of center and surround fields.

W Ganglion Cells

1. Smallest cell bodies, slowest conduction velocity; functionally heterogeneous.
2. Many lack center–surround antagonistic fields; they act as light intensity detectors.
3. Some respond to large field motion; they can be direction-specific.

Amacrine Cells

1. Receive input from bipolar cells, project to ganglion cells (see Fig. 114A); several subtypes with different transmitters (GABA, dopamine, and so on).
2. Transform sustained ON or OFF depolarizing potentials of bipolars into *transient* depolarizations and action potentials.

Receptive Field Size

In fovea and parafoveal retina the ratio of cones to bipolar cells to ganglion cells can be as low as 1:1:1, and receptive field centers 1 minute of arc.

At the retinal periphery, hundreds of rods supply a single bipolar cell and many bipolars are connected to one ganglion cell. Some ganglion cells have mixed cone and rod input. Receptive fields subtend 1 degree or more.

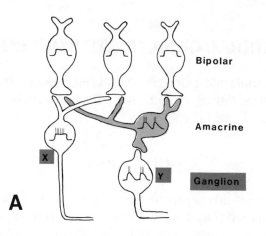

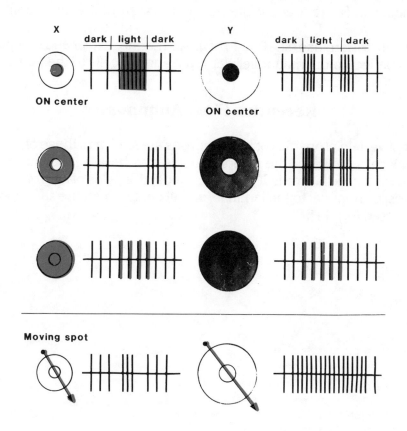

Figure 114 *A,* Ganglion cell inputs. *B,* X and Y cell responses. (*B,* Modified after Kuffler SW, Nicholls JG, Martin AR. From neuron to brain. Sunderland, MA: Sinauer, 1984:27.)

UNIT 115
LATERAL GENICULATE NUCLEUS

As the primary thalamic nucleus for retinal inputs, the lateral geniculate nucleus (LGN) organizes retinal afferents from both eyes in terms of receptive field location and in terms of class (X, Y).

Optic Chiasm

Ganglion cell axons arising from the "nasal" half of each retina cross the midline in the optic chiasm (Fig. 115A). Afferents from either retina, responding to the same side of the visual field, project to the same side of the brain: The right visual hemifield is transmitted to the left half of the brain (see Fig. 115A).

Ocular Layering

Each LGN receives afferents from both retinae. Those from the contralateral side terminate in layers roughly alternate to those from the ipsilateral side (Fig. 115B).

There are six laminae (see Fig. 115B): two magnocellular and four parvocellular. Y cells project to the magnocellular layers, and X cells to the parvocellular.

Receptive Field Alignment

Receptive field properties of LGN neurons are similar to those of corresponding X and Y cells. However, the receptive fields may be larger because of convergence of ganglion cells onto LGN neurons. Receptive fields of neurons lying along a radial axis, orthogonal to the laminae, are all centered on the same point in the visual field (see Fig. 115B).

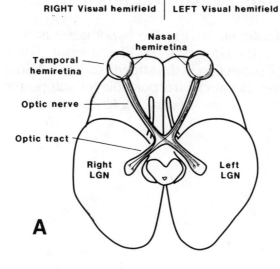

RIGHT Visual hemifield | **LEFT Visual hemifield**

Nasal hemiretina

Temporal hemiretina

Optic nerve

Optic tract

Right LGN

Left LGN

A

Common receptive field for neurons along one radial axis through LGN

Radial axis

6
5
X ➤ Parvocellular laminae
4
3
Y ➤ Magnocellular laminae
1

Ipsilateral retina

Contralateral retina

B

Figure 115   *A*, Optic nerve and tract. *B*, Lateral geniculate nucleus. *Figure continues.*

Extrageniculate Targets (Fig. 115C)

The suprachiasmatic nucleus of the hypothalamus is a circadian rhythm generator entrained to the light cycle by W cell input. The superior colliculus receives a heavy Y cell projection in the superficial layer. Also in the mid-brain, W cells project to the pretectal nuclei (responsible for autonomic eye reflexes) and the accessory optic nucleus (involved in optokinetic nystagmus).

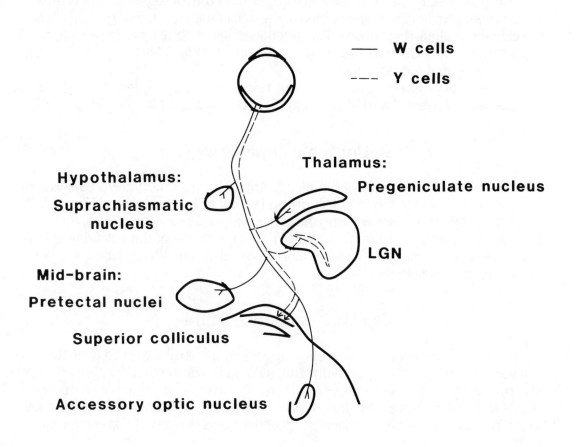

— W cells

--- Y cells

Thalamus:

Pregeniculate nucleus

Hypothalamus:

Suprachiasmatic nucleus

LGN

Mid-brain:

Pretectal nuclei

Superior colliculus

Accessory optic nucleus

C

Figure 115 *(continued)* *C,* Nongeniculate retinal targets. (*B* and *C,* Modified after Cohen DH, Sherman SM. The nervous system. In: Berne RM, Levy MN, eds. Physiology. 2nd ed. St. Louis: CV Mosby, 1988:115, 114.)

UNIT 116
PRIMARY VISUAL CORTEX

Cortical area 17, or V1, is the primary sensory area for visual input. It is mostly on the medial wall of the hemispheres at the occipital pole, covering both sides of the calcarine sulcus (Fig. 116A). The functional unit of cortex is a "hypercolumn," a block through all six layers roughly 1 mm square (Fig. 116B). It is the territory serving one visual receptive field.

V1 is distinguished by having about twice the neuronal density of all other cortical areas. Layers III and IV are expanded into many sublaminae (Fig. 116C).

Retinotopic Organization

The retina is mapped logarithmically onto V1: Proportionately less and less cortical area is devoted to increasingly peripheral retinal zones (see Fig. 116A). The horizontal meridian falls along the calcarine sulcus, and the vertical meridian falls along the border with area 18 (V2). The upper bank of the calcarine sulcus maps the upper hemiretina (lower half of the visual hemifield), and the lower bank maps the lower hemiretina.

Ocular Dominance Bands

LGN inputs from alternate layers (opposite eyes) terminate in adjacent bands in layer IV, dividing each hypercolumn into two halves dominated by the ipsilateral and the contralateral eye, respectively (see Fig. 116B). These ocular dominance bands are continuous across long rows of hypercolumns. Layer IV stellate cells, receiving LGN inputs, have concentric receptive fields similar to LGN and ganglion cells.

Magnocellular (Y) and parvocellular (X) LGN terminals are strictly segregated into separate sublaminae of layer IV (see Fig. 116C).

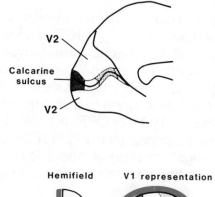

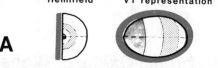

Hemifield   V1 representation

A

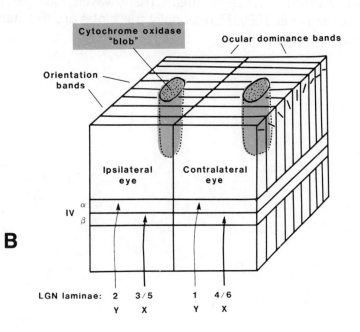

B

Figure 116   *A*, Retinotopic organization of V1. *B*, Hypercolumn (V1). *Figure continues.*

Simple Cells

Above and below layer IV are "simple cells" (see Fig. 116C): They integrate concentric receptive fields into linear bars (Fig. 116D), and they exhibit varying degrees of binocularity; i.e., they respond to visual input via either eye. Simple cell input derives from X cells.

A simple cell responds to a bar of light (or darkness) within the receptive field, if the bar has a specific orientation (see Fig. 116C). The sharpness of orientation specificity depends on local inhibitory mechanisms. Simple cells of similar orientation preference are found together in narrow bands running orthogonal to the ocular dominance bands (Fig. 116E). Orientation bands are systematically ordered so that successive bands respond to a slightly more rotated bar.

The excitatory receptive field (ON or OFF) is flanked by two inhibitory fields that antagonize the central response (see Fig. 116D). Simple cells may also respond to oriented "gratings" *moving* at about 2 degrees per second in a direction orthogonal to the grating orientation. (Spatial frequency of grating is 0.5 cycle per degree.)

Cytochrome Oxidase "Blobs"

At the center of each ocular dominance band in a hypercolumn are regions rich in cytochrome oxidase (see Fig. 116B). These blobs extend through the superficial and deep layers but not through layer IV. Neurons in the blobs have concentric, not oriented bar, receptive fields; many wavelength-specific responses are found here (see Unit 109). Functionally the blobs are the starting point of cortical *color* processing.

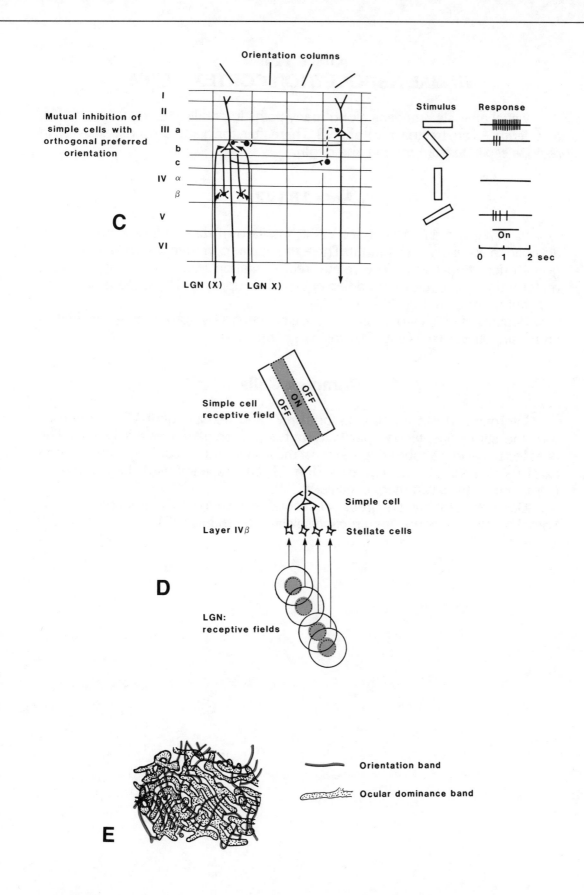

Figure 116 *(continued)* C, Simple cell (V1). *D*, Synthesis of response properties of a simple cell. *E,* Ocular dominance and orientation bands.

285

UNIT 117
VISUAL ASSOCIATION CORTEX: FORM

Visual analysis proceeds along many paths in parallel: form, color, motion, and depth. All are treated in V1 and V2. Thereafter, form and color are analyzed in regions separate from motion and depth.

Area 18 (V2)

V2 repeats many aspects of V1. It has its own direct input from LGN, in addition to pulvinar and V1 input. There are ocular dominance bands and orthogonal orientation bands. The retinal representation is a mirror image of V1, matched along the vertical meridian but split into upper and lower parts along the horizontal meridian (Fig. 117A).

Regions of high cytochrome oxidase concentration form alternating "thick" and "thin" stripes (see Unit 120), instead of blobs as in V1.

Complex Cells

Intermingled with simple cells, both in V1 and increasingly in V2, are neurons with the same orientation specificity but a motion-dependent response. The oriented bar (width about 1 degree) must move in a direction orthogonal to its long axis to elicit a complex cell response (Fig. 117B). The response is largely derived from Y cell signals (via magnocellular LGN).

Bar motion (about 2 degrees per second) can be in either direction for many complex cells, but some are direction-selective (see Unit 120).

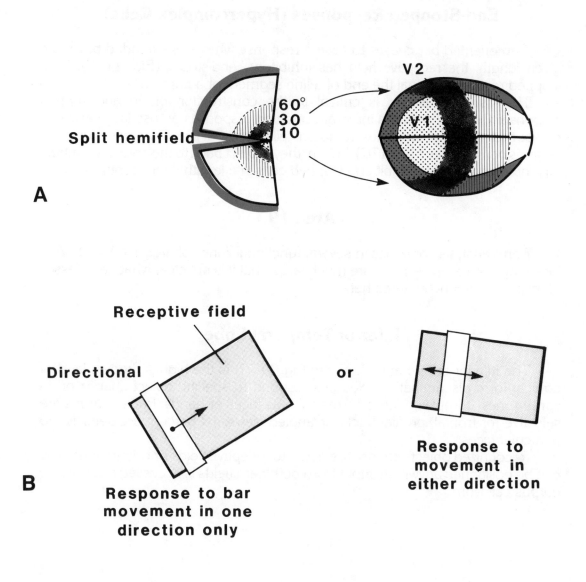

A

Split hemifield

60°
30
10

V 2

V 1

B

Receptive field

Directional   or

**Response to bar
movement in one
direction only**

**Response to
movement in
either direction**

Figure 117 *A*, Area 18 hemifield map. *B*, Complex cell. *Figure continues.*

End-Stopped Responses (Hypercomplex Cells)

If an oriented bar ceases to elicit a response when it is extended beyond a given length, the receptive field has inhibitory "end-stops" (Fig. 117C). End-stopped responses signal the end of a line segment or a corner.

The visual claustrum is critical to the construction of an end-stopped response. Claustral neurons integrate oriented responses across large areas of cortex; their response increases monotonically as the bar length increases up to 40 degrees or more (see Fig. 117C). In turn, they project back to the cortex. Via inhibitory interneurons they inhibit end-stopped cells in a length-dependent manner.

Area 19

Form analysis continues in several functional zones of area 19 (Fig. 117D), including V3. Receptive fields are much larger, but it is not clear what new classes of response are encountered here.

Inferior Temporal Lobe

The inferior temporal region (see Fig. 117C) is the highest known level of cortical form discrimination. Neurons respond to specific object shapes or, in some zones, complex generic forms such as faces or hands. Face neurons are selective for frontal, profile, back, or angled views; 10 percent are sensitive to particular faces.

Recognized objects are not restricted to receptive fields or orientation: They can be positioned anywhere. Input from both hemifields is accessed through the corpus callosum.

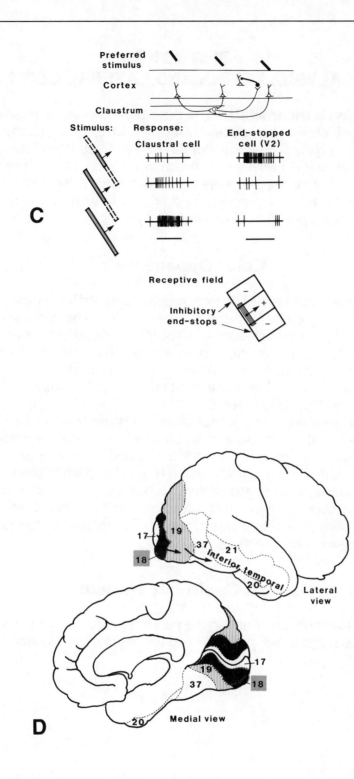

Figure 117 *(continued)*   *C*, End-stopped receptive field (hypercomplex). *D*, Visual areas: form analysis. (*D*, Adapted from Nieuwenhuys R, Voogd J, van Huijzen C. The human central nervous system. Heidelberg: Springer-Verlag, 1981:10.)

UNIT 118
COLOR ANALYSIS: RETINA AND LATERAL GENICULATE

Human vision is **trichromatic**. The three pigments that mediate color perception have absorption maxima at about 420 to 440 nm, 530 to 535 nm, and 560 to 570 nm (Fig. 118A). The corresponding cone types constitute a short (S), medium (M), and long (L) wavelength mechanism, respectively (see Unit 74).

In the fovea all photoreceptors are cones, 3 percent of them of the S type and the rest of M and L types. Cone density drops off toward the retinal periphery. Outside the fovea, 10 percent of cones are S type.

Color Opponency

Every perceived hue (including extraspectral hues such as purple) is coded by the relative activity it elicits in the three cone types. This population code is implemented using the center-surround receptive field antagonism of ganglion cells: One cone type supplies the center, another the surround. Color-selective ganglion cells are maximally responsive to a narrower range of the spectrum ("action spectrum") than either of the input cone types, because one inhibits part of the range of the other (Fig. 118B).

The center-surround cone signal inhibition is the basis of perceived color opponency—red and green, blue and yellow, white and black antagonize one another. Red-green opponency stems from M and L cone antagonism; blue-yellow from S and M + L cone antagonism (Fig. 118C); white-black from achromatic ganglion cells responding to center-surround luminance differences. (Red-cyan and green-magenta opponencies also exist, but are much rarer.)

Chromatic ganglion cells make up 60 to 75 percent of the ganglion cell population. They all belong to the X cell class.

Lateral Geniculate Nucleus

Color-sensitive cells are found in the parvocellular layers of LGN. They have the same spectral response properties as color-sensitive ganglion cells (Fig. 118D).

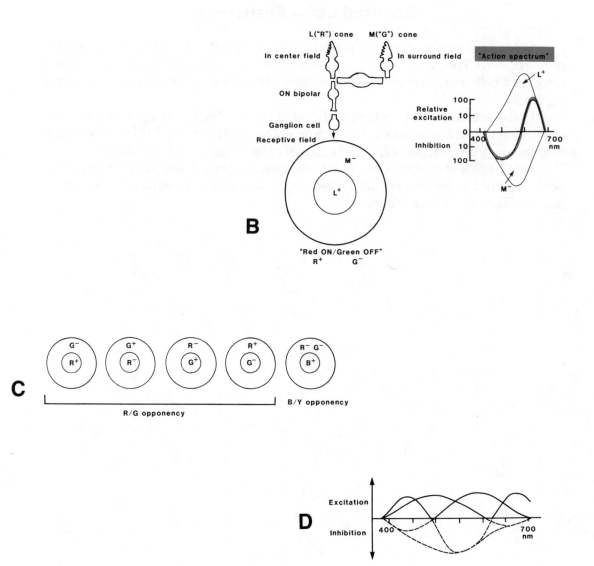

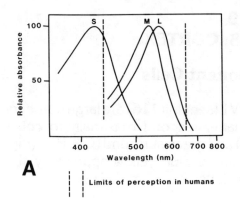

Figure 118 *A*, Cone absorbance spectra. *B*, Color-opponent ganglion cells. *C*, Common color-opponent combinations. *D*, Common action spectra (ganglion cells and LGN). (*A*, Modified after Bowmaker JK. Trichromatic colour vision: Why only three receptor channels? Trends Neurosci 1983; 6:42.)

UNIT 119
COLOR ANALYSIS: CORTEX

Color Double-Opponent Cells

Within the cytochrome oxidase blobs of V1 (see Unit 116) are large numbers of single and double-opponent cells. The latter respond maximally to **color contrasts** in space, e.g., red center (R+, G−) and green surround (G+, R−) (Fig. 119A). Individual blobs specialize in red–green or blue–yellow opponency; the former is three times more common than the latter.

Oriented Color Responses

Color-selective simple cells (Fig. 119B) are found in V1 at the edges of the blob regions. The simple cells are essentially a linear composite of double-opponent cells along a preferred orientation. They detect oriented bars of spectral contrast.

Color-selective complex cells respond to an oriented bar of light, in a specific spectral range, which moves across the receptive field (see Fig. 119B). Movement may be in either direction or, for directional cells, in one preferred direction.

In V1, color-selective cells are usually within layers III and IV. The response peak may occur for any specific wavelength, but most commonly it occurs at about 450, 506, 577, or 656 nm.

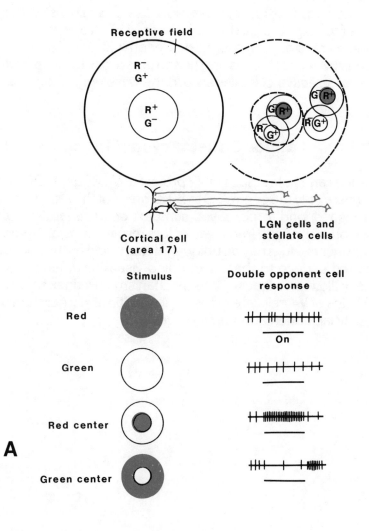

Figure 119 *A*, Double-opponent cell. *Figure continues.*

V2 Color Cells

In V2, end-stopped color-selective cells are found (see Fig. 119B). The stimulus bar must have the correct orientation, move across the receptive field, be in the right spectral range, and not extend beyond a critical length.

In V2, cortical hypercolumns are functionally subdivided into a **stripe** organization that is continuous over many columns.

Most color-opponent cells without orientation selectivity in V2 are located within the **thin** cytochrome oxidase stripes (Fig. 119C). V1 blobs project directly to these thin stripes (see Fig. 119C); nonblob zones of V1 project to the **pale stripe** zones of V2, where end-stopped responses predominate.

Spectral sensitivities of V2 cells are the same as those in V1. In both areas, the responses of color-selective cells depend on the wavelength composition of the stimulus.

Color Constancy in V4

The thin stripes and pale stripes of V2 project to V4 (Figs. 119C and 119D), a part of area 19 where only the central 20 to 30 degrees of the retina is represented. Some V4 neurons respond to perceived stimulus *color* regardless of the wavelength composition of the light. Perceived colors remain constant over a wide mix of spectral components. Hue may be uniquely determined by the spectral relationship of the colored surface to the surrounding visual field, as assessed by the red–green, blue–yellow, and black–white mechanisms (Retinex theory).

Receptive fields of V4 cells are on average four times larger than those of V1 cells and generally lack orientation preferences.

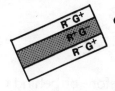
Simple (V1)

Oriented color contrast

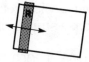

Complex (V1, V2)

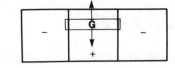

End-stopped (hypercomplex; V2)

B

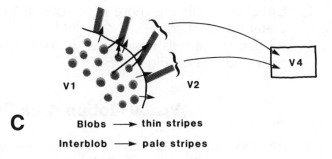

C

Blobs ⟶ thin stripes

Interblob ⟶ pale stripes

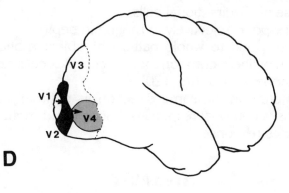

D

Figure 119 *(continued)* *B*, Color-selective receptive fields. *C*, Cytochrome oxidase regions. *D*, Color analysis. (*D*, Adapted from Nieuwenhuys R, Voogd J, van Huijzen C. The human central nervous system. Heidelberg: Springer-Verlag, 1981:10.)

UNIT 120
MOTION AND DEPTH ANALYSIS

Stereoscopic Depth Mechanisms (V1, V2)

1. Depth is estimated from **binocular disparity**: Points before or behind the focal plane do not project to the same relative position in each retina (Fig. 120A).
2. Binocular disparity neurons in V1 (layer IIIc) respond to the difference in retinal image position in two eyes; mismatch is averaged over a wide retinal area. Disparity cells are also found in *thick* cytochrome oxidase stripes of V2 (Fig. 120B).
3. Binocular **velocity disparity** codes motion in depth (Fig. 120C). Some V1 and V2 motion-sensitive cells detect disparities in retinal image velocity.
4. Binocular latency differences may code motion in planes parallel to the fixation plane.

Direction-Specific Cells (V1, V2)

1. Many complex cells in V1 respond best to bar motion in one direction (see Unit 117): located in layer IIIc, project to V5 (MT), and thick cytochrome oxidase stripes of V2 (see Fig. 120B).
2. Directional cells are more numerous in V2; they lie in bands of the same preferred direction.
3. V2 directional cells congregate in thick cytochrome oxidase stripes, which project to V5 (see Fig. 120B).

Visual Motion Area (V5 or MT)

1. All cells respond to moving stimuli, usually in a preferred direction; color, shape, and orientation are not important.
2. Preferred directions are systematically ordered within a hypercolumn serving one patch of visual field (see Fig. 120B). Receptive fields are about 100 times larger than those of V1 directional cells.
3. Some V5 cells respond selectively to motion in depth.
4. Many V5 cells respond to whole pattern or object motion, not the often divergent motion of linear components. V1 complex cells respond to isolated motion of component lines (Fig. 120D).
5. *Background* motion in the same direction as optimally directed stimulus motion suppresses neuronal responses; background motion in the opposite direction facilitates response.

Area MST

1. Neurons may respond selectively to rotatory motion (clockwise, anticlockwise, or in depth) or to changing size of objects.
2. Area MST projects to area 7 (Fig. 120E) where optic flow patterns are discriminated (Unit 137).

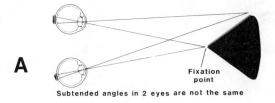

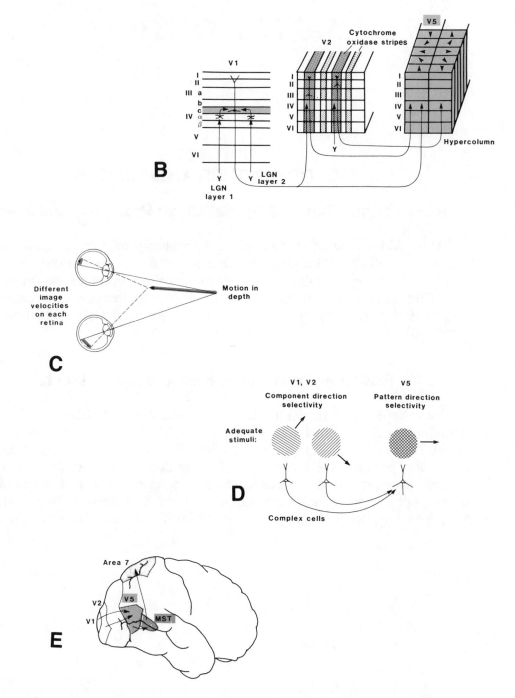

Figure 120 *A,* Depth perception (stereopsis). *B,* Directional responses. *C,* Detection of motion in depth. *D,* Hierarchy of directional responses. *E,* Visual motion analysis. (*A,* Adapted from Poggio T. Vision by man and machine. Sci Am 1984; 250:109. *D,* Adapted from Maunsell JHR, Neusome WT. Visual processing in monkey extrastriate cortex. Ann Rev Neurosci 1987; 10:327. *E,* Adapted from Nieuwenhuys R, Voogd J, van Huijzen C. The human central nervous system. Heidelberg: Springer-Verlag, 1981:10.)

16

MOTOR OUTPUT

UNIT 121
MOTOR CENTERS AND TRACTS

Intermediate Zone of Spinal Cord: Propriospinal Tracts

The middle laminae of the spinal gray matter provide an interface between both sensory afferents and descending tracts and the spinal motor nuclei. Neurons from one segment can project to many other segments via propriospinal tracts (Fig. 121A). The function of the propriospinal tracts is to organize spinal reflexes and muscle synergies of posture and locomotion (with the reticular formation).

Reticular Formation: Reticulospinal Tracts

Four large-celled nuclei in the medial reticular formation of the pons and medulla project to cranial and spinal motor nuclei and intermediate zone (Fig. 121B). Their function is to organize cranial reflexes and synergies of mastication, swallowing, posture, and locomotion. The modulatory **raphe** nuclei (serotonergic) and **locus ceruleus** (noradrenergic) project diffusely to the spinal motor nuclei (raphe) and dorsal horn (raphe and locus ceruleus). Their function is autonomic regulation of motor activity and somatosensory transmission.

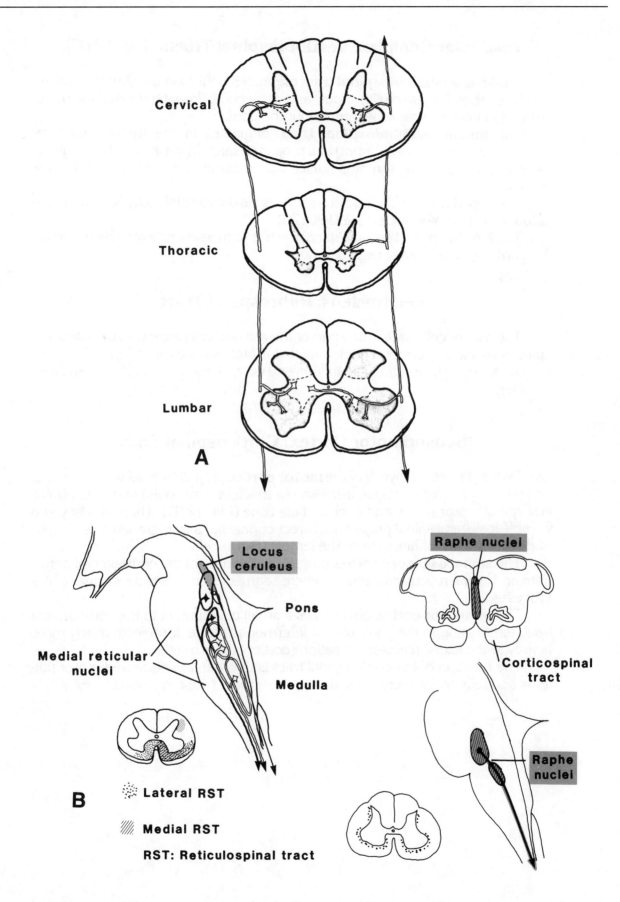

Figure 121 *A*, Propriospinal tracts. *B*, Reticulospinal tracts. *Figure continues.*

Vestibular Complex: Vestibulospinal Tracts (Fig. 121C).

The **lateral vestibulospinal tract** originates in the lateral vestibular nucleus, which receives largely otolith input, and projects to ipsilateral extensor motor nuclei and intermediate zone throughout the cord.

The **medial vestibulospinal tract** originates in the medial vestibular nucleus (semicircular canal input) and projects bilaterally via the medial longitudinal fasciculus to cervical motor nuclei. Some axons are inhibitory and some excitatory.

The superior vestibular nucleus projects via the **medial longitudinal fasciculus** to oculomotor nuclei (see Unit 126).

The function of the vestibulospinal tracts is to mediate reflexes which stabilize the trunk, head, and eyes, respectively.

Red Nucleus: Rubrospinal Tract

The magnocellular (caudal) part of the red nucleus projects to the contralateral cranial and spinal motor nuclei and to the intermediate zone (Fig. 121D). This tract is very small in humans. Its function is to control discrete sets of limb and face muscles.

Sensorimotor Cortex: Corticospinal Tract

Pyramidal cells in layer V of the **motor cortex** project to cranial motor nuclei and reticular formation (bilaterally with contralateral emphasis) and to contralateral spinal motor nuclei and intermediate zone (Fig. 121D). There is a tiny and variable ipsilateral spinal projection. Direct connections to motoneurons, usually of distal muscles, originate from the largest (**Betz**) cells.

The **somatosensory cortex** projects to the base of the contralateral dorsal horn and lateral reticular formation, where segmental and cranial sensory input is processed.

The **premotor cortex** also makes a small contribution to the corticospinal tract, terminating in the contralateral intermediate zone. It projects much more heavily to the lateral reticular formation (corticobulbar tract).

The function of the corticospinal tract is to organize specialized motor patterns and regulate sensory influx during movement (see Fig. 105E).

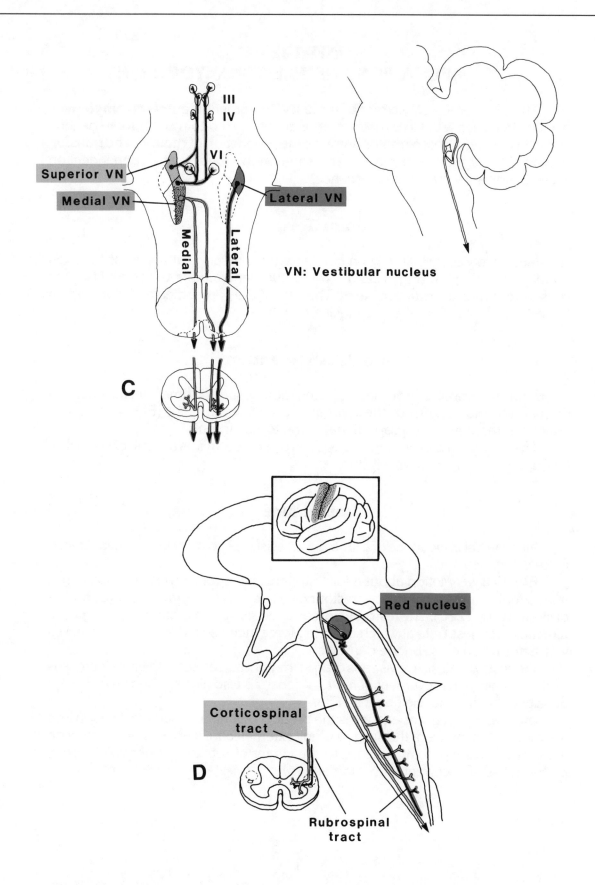

Figure 121 *(continued)* C, Vestibulospinal and vestibulo-ocular tracts. D, Corticospinal and rubrospinal tracts. (Adapted from Nieuwenhuys R, Voogd J, van Huijzen C. The human central nervous system. Heidelberg: Springer-Verlag, 1981:108, 151, 137, 157, 184.)

UNIT 122
LIMB MECHANICS AND ELECTROMYOGRAPHY

The gross electrical activity of a muscle, recorded in an **electromyogram** (EMG), increases with CNS motor output and is related to muscle force generation. But a general goal of motor output is the production of motion. The transformation of linear muscle forces into angular motions about joints is dependent on muscle properties and joint impedance.

Joint Torque

Muscle forces pull directly on bones to generate angular forces or **torques** about a specific joint (Fig. 122A). The torque generated is the product of the muscle force and the **moment-arm**. The latter is the perpendicular distance from the center of rotation to the muscle line of action.

Impulse-Momentum

A torque "impulse" (torque integrated within a specific time interval) changes the angular momentum of the limb about the relevant joint (Fig. 122B). The change in momentum is proportional to the torque impulse.

The change in momentum is opposed by and decays as a result of viscoelastic impedance and often gravity.

Impedance

Mechanical impedance of a limb is the resistance to motion. It is measured in three categories:

Elasticity. Motion about a joint stretches antagonist muscles, ligaments, and so forth, producing an elastic restoring force that is proportional to the amount of stretch (Fig. 122C). The restoring force can *assist* return motion in the opposite direction. Stiffness (rate at which restoring force increases with stretch) increases with actomyosin cross-bridge density.

Viscosity. Resistive viscous drag in the joint and attached tissues increases proportionally with movement *velocity*. Viscosity is also higher when cross-bridge density within the muscle fibers is high.

Inertia. Inertial impedance is the product of limb angular acceleration and the moment of inertia of the limb plus any external load. It is reduced by keeping the farthest moving point as close to the center of rotation as possible. Inertial properties sustain current limb momentum.

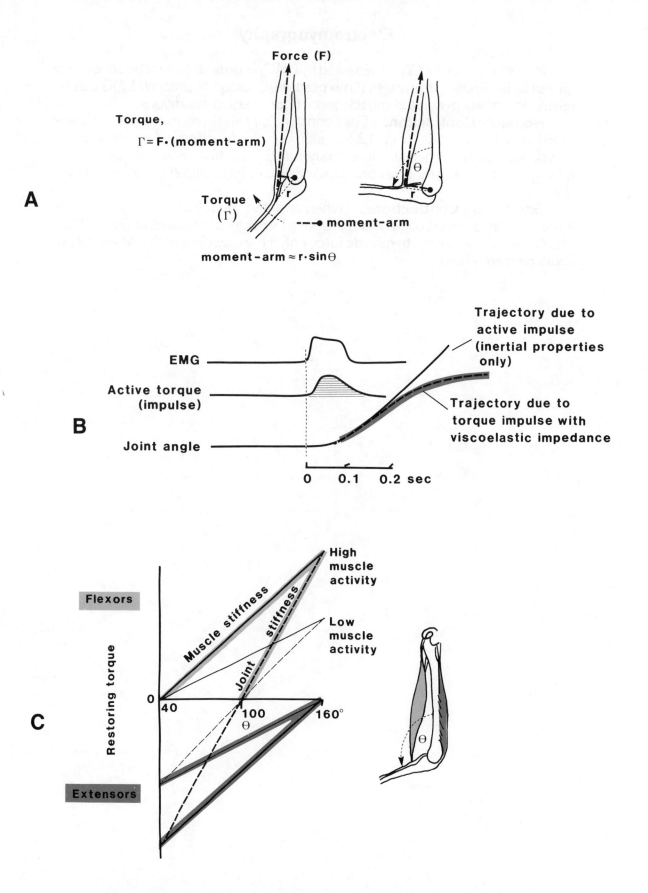

Figure 122 *A,* Muscle moment-arm. *B,* Impulse-momentum. *C,* Elasticity. *Figure continues.*

Electromyography

Motor output of the CNS, measured by EMG recording, cannot be adequately related to kinematic parameters (limb position, velocity) at present. EMG can be related to actively generated muscle *force* under certain conditions:

Isometric Contraction.   For a constant joint angle, muscle force is a linear function of EMG activity (Fig. 122D), although the function is time-dependent. Muscle force rises and decays more slowly than EMG activity. Also, for a given CNS driving signal (EMG), muscles produce maximum force at a specific length (see Unit 55).

Shortening Contractions.   When an active muscle shortens, the muscle force decreases hyperbolically with increased velocity of shortening (Fig. 122E). Thus EMG can be related to muscle force only if the muscle length and velocity of shortening are known.

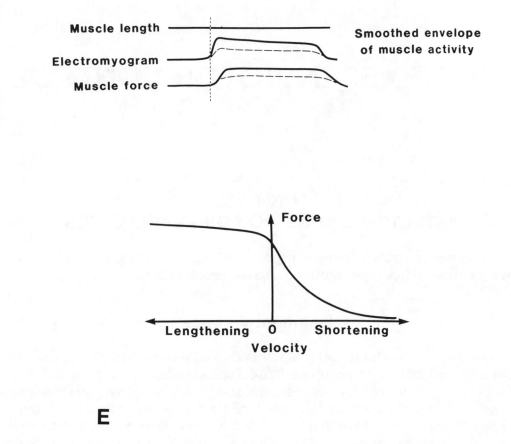

Figure 122 *(continued)*   *D*, Isometric contraction. *E*, Force-velocity relationship in active contraction.

17

LEXES IN MOTOR CONTROL

UNIT 123
STRETCH AND TENDON ORGAN REFLEXES

A **reflex** is a basic stimulus-response relationship: The *gain* (output/input) may be modified, but the output pattern is stereotyped.

Segmental Loops

Reflex networks for muscle spindle and Golgi tendon organ inputs (see Unit 67) are functionally tightly coupled. Muscle spindle afferents (Groups Ia, II) make direct synaptic contact with motoneurons, specifically **homonymous motoneurons** (projecting to the muscle whence come the spindle afferents). A **monosynaptic** loop (Fig. 123A) is thereby created, resulting in reflex contraction when a muscle is stretched or loaded. The latency is about 20 msec in arm muscles, 40 msec in leg.

The shortest reflex loop subserving **tendon organ** afferents (Group Ib) is **disynaptic**; i.e., an interneuron in the spinal intermediate zone is interposed between the afferent axon and motoneurons. Homonymous motoneurons are inhibited and motoneurons of antagonist muscles are excited. The reflex acts to reduce ongoing muscle contractions and facilitate opposing muscle activity (Fig. 123B).

In general, net motion about a joint involves active contraction of one or more muscle(s), the **agonist**, and passive stretch of the **antagonist** muscle(s). A tendon organ reflex would be elicited in the agonist, and stretch reflex in the antagonist. These functionally coupled reflexes produce the same output: activation of the stretched antagonist and silencing of the actively contracting agonist.

Function

Because this reflex system essentially *opposes* motion about a joint, it is particularly useful for stabilizing the joint, as in maintenance of steady posture against gravity. This is true within the normal range of tiny deviations from the desired position. Gross deviations cannot be adequately corrected by reflexes acting alone.

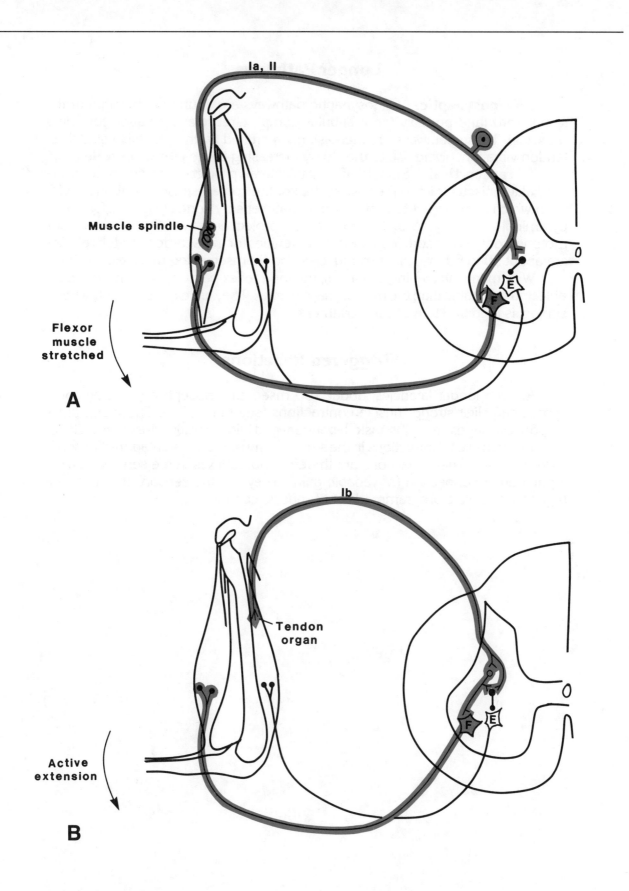

Figure 123 *A*, Stretch reflex (monosynaptic). *B*, Tendon organ reflex. *Figure continues.*

Longer Pathways

1. **Oligosynaptic.**   Oligosynaptic pathways are abundant throughout the spinal cord (and possibly the vestibular complex-reticular formation for some muscles). These pathways are increasingly recruited by the repetitive stretch of tendon vibration, giving rise to the slowly increasing **tonic vibration reflex**.

2. **Transcortical.**   Spindle afferent collaterals project up the dorsal column-medial lemniscus tract to the rostral shell of the somatosensory thalamus (VP), from which they project to motor and somatosensory cortex (Fig. 123C). Large pyramidal cells in layer V of the motor cortex project directly to the homonymous motoneurons via the corticospinal tract. Latencies for transcortical stretch reflexes are about 50 to 60 msec in arm muscles and 90 msec in leg muscles.

With many intervening synapses, the long reflex pathways are more modifiable and adaptable than the monosynaptic reflex. They are expressed only when a subject is prepared to make a movement.

Triggered Reactions

At even longer latencies, about 100 msec, proprioceptive (or cutaneous) stimuli can elicit strong muscle contractions (see Fig. 123C). These stimulus-response linkages are highly task-dependent and idiosyncratic. Muscle stretch, for example, can elicit contractions in the stretched muscle and its antagonist or some other muscles. These reactions are therefore not reflexes in the sense of a fixed input-output connection (of variable gain). They use the sensory stimulus as a trigger to release a programmed set of muscle contractions.

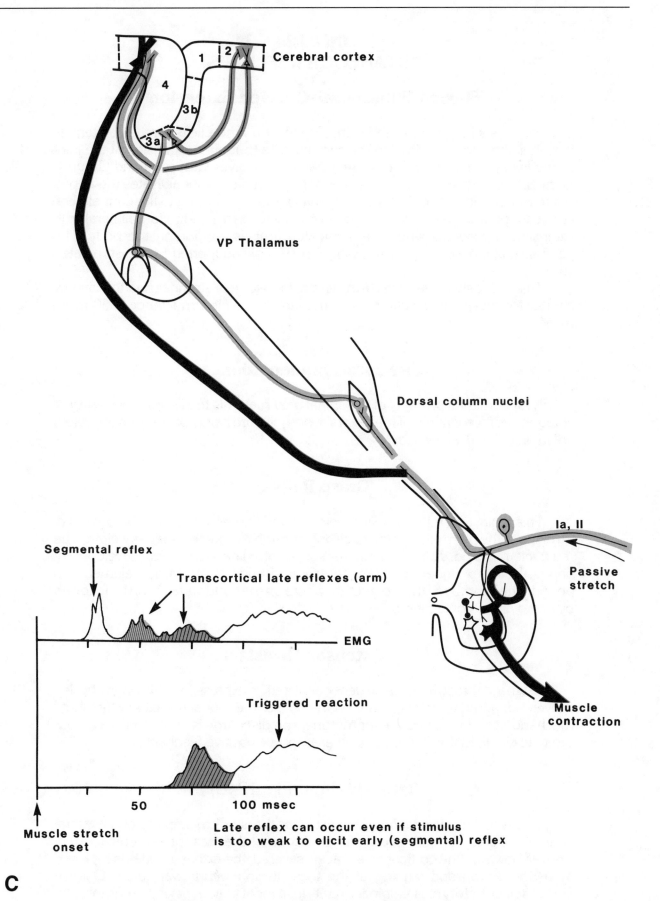

Cerebral cortex

1 2

4

3b

3a

VP Thalamus

Dorsal column nuclei

Ia, II

Passive stretch

Muscle contraction

Segmental reflex

Transcortical late reflexes (arm)

EMG

Triggered reaction

50   100 msec

Muscle stretch onset

Late reflex can occur even if stimulus is too weak to elicit early (segmental) reflex

C

Figure 123 *(continued)*   *C,* Late (transcortical) stretch reflex loops.

UNIT 124
CUTANEOUS REFLEXES

Flexion Withdrawal-Crossed Extension

Noxious stimulation of the skin on part of a limb elicits a reflex pattern of flexion at the joints proximal to the stimulus site (but often extension at the joint immediately distal to it). The afferent pathway involves Group Aδ and Group C nociceptors. Within the spinal cord, a polysynaptic network activates the appropriate motor nuclei (Fig. 124A). Segmental neurons crossing to the contralateral cord cause the activation of extensor motor nuclei on that side. Contralateral limb extension is essential when the stimulated limb is supporting the body. The contralateral limb must bear the weight previously supported by the stimulated limb.

This reflex shows **summation**: The response gets stronger and the latency shorter for more intense stimuli. For the leg, the minimum latency is 60 to 80 msec.

Reciprocal Innervation

A fundamental property of the spinal gray matter is the reciprocal pairing of antagonistic motor nuclei. If the flexors at one joint are being excited, the extensors are inhibited and vice versa.

Grasp Reflex

This brainstem reflex is fully developed and expressed in the newborn child. Stroking of the palm elicits a grasp strong enough to bear the infant's weight. The red nucleus is a possible site of the sensory-motor linkage. Cortical development brings the reflex under voluntary control and adds programmed elements to position the hand, such that contact anywhere on the hand surface can be followed by grasp of the contacting object.

Extensor Thrust

Extensor thrust is a phase-dependent reflex expressed only when the leg actively supports weight; pressure on the sole of the foot activates low-threshold mechanoreceptors. Leg extensor motoneuron discharge is reinforced via a polysynaptic circuit in the spinal cord, an example of positive feedback.

Babinski Sign (Fig. 124B)

This is a clinical variation of the extensor thrust: Firm stroking of the lateral edge of the sole normally elicits plantar flexion of the toes (physiological extension). If, however, the corticospinal tract is severed, the extensor reflex is replaced by a dorsiflexion and fanning of the toes (flexion withdrawal pattern). Tonic corticospinal activity biases spinal circuits in favor of plantar flexion, a component of normal posture.

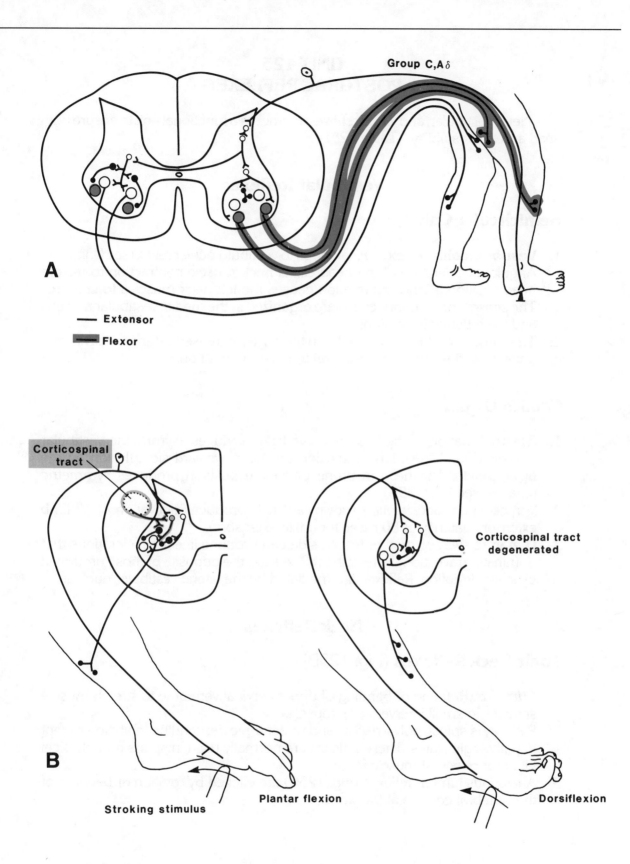

Figure 124 *A*, Flexion-crossed extension reflex. *B*, Babinski sign.

Group C,Aδ

A

— Extensor
— Flexor

Corticospinal tract

B

Stroking stimulus   Plantar flexion

Corticospinal tract degenerated

Dorsiflexion

UNIT 125
POSTURAL REFLEXES

Neck, vestibular, and visual reflexes interact as a functional unit to ensure both head and trunk stability (Table 125).

Vestibular Reflexes

Semicircular Canal

1. **Vestibulocollic reflex.** Analogous to vestibulo-ocular reflex (see Unit 126). Angular acceleration of the head elicits neck muscle contraction to restore head position. Rightward rotation causes the left neck muscles to contract. The sensorimotor connections are organized in the medial vestibular nucleus and the reticular formation.
2. The same stimulus elicits a reflex in the arms: increased extensor activity contralaterally, flexor activity ipsilateral to the head rotation.

Otolith Organs

1. **Static** deviation of the head from vertical produces asymmetric vestibular reflexes (Fig. 125A): limb extension on the downward side, flexion on the upward side. The head in prone or supine position produces symmetric reflexes (see Fig. 125A).
2. Vertical linear acceleration (downward fall) produces activation of all limb extensors (latency of 80 msec for ankle extensors).
3. **Dynamic** sway or motion to one side can produce linear accelerations that dominate gravitational effect; the reflexes are the opposite of those produced by static deviation. Reflexes are mediated by the lateral vestibular nucleus.

Neck Reflexes

Tonic Neck Reflexes (Fig. 125B)

1. *Stimulus:* Rotation or bending of upper cervical vertebrae to stretch muscle spindles in small intervertebral muscles.
2. Pathway is spinal, polysynaptic, and under tonic descending inhibition except in pathologic states. These reflexes are normally used in sports and physical labor for maximal muscle force.
3. Analogous lumbar reflexes (Fig. 125C) are elicited by rotation or bending of the vertebral column at the waist.

TABLE 125

Reflex	Rotation or Bending	Arm		Leg	
		L	R	L	R
Neck					
Symmetric	Forward	Flex	Flex	Flex	Flex
(swan dive)	Backward	Extend	Extend	Extend	Extend
Asymmetric (fencer)	Rightward	Flex	Extend	Flex	Extend
Waist					
Symmetric		(Same as neck)			
Asymmetric (golfer)	Rightward	Extend	Flex	Flex	Extend

Neck Righting Reflex

1. The neck righting reflex occurs in an animal lying on one side: If the head is passively raised, "reflex" activity brings the thorax into alignment with the head, and the lower body follows to put the entire body upright.
2. Postural *program* (see Unit 128) using proprioceptive and cutaneous input: neuraxis must be intact up to the mid-brain.

Visual Righting Reflex

1. *Stimulus:* Slow velocity motion of the visual field, even unperceived.
   Response: Increased postural sway in the direction of visual motion.
2. Pathway possibly via accessory optic system (see Unit 126).
3. Response to visual field motion accompanying postural disturbances facilitates stretch and vestibular reflexes.

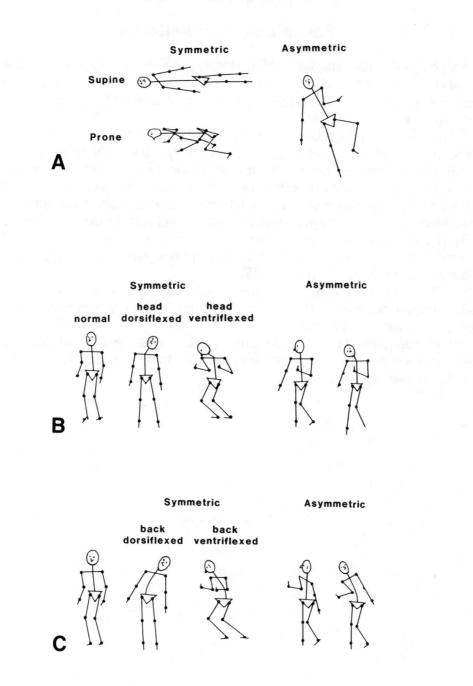

Figure 125 *A*, Tonic vestibular reflexes. *B*, Tonic neck reflexes. *C*, Tonic lumbar reflexes.

UNIT 126
OCULAR REFLEXES

Vestibulo-ocular Reflexes

Vestibulo-ocular reflexes (VORs) stabilize the visual image on the retina by causing compensatory changes in eye position as the head moves. Reflex eye movement is of the same magnitude as the head rotation (Fig. 126A), but in the opposite direction.

The afferent signal arises in semicircular canal hair cells (see Unit 69). Canal afferents fire in proportion to head angular velocity in a specific plane. This velocity signal is transmitted to the vestibular nuclei (superior and medial; see Unit 112) and from there to oculomotoneurons which move the eyes in the direction opposite the head movement. To regulate eye position, oculomotoneurons need a **position** signal (tonic **step**) as well as a phasic **velocity** (**pulse**) signal (see Unit 133). The vestibular velocity signal is therefore *integrated* over time in the adjacent pontine reticular formation to produce a position signal which is also transmitted to the oculomotoneurons (Fig. 126B).

VOR operates at a gain (eye movement/head movement) of about -0.9 over a wide frequency range (0.01 to 7 Hz). Its upper limit roughly corresponds to the limit of voluntary head rotation.

The adequate hair cell stimulus is really head **acceleration**. Hair cell responses die away when acceleration declines to zero (constant velocity). VOR then fades away in 15 to 20 sec.

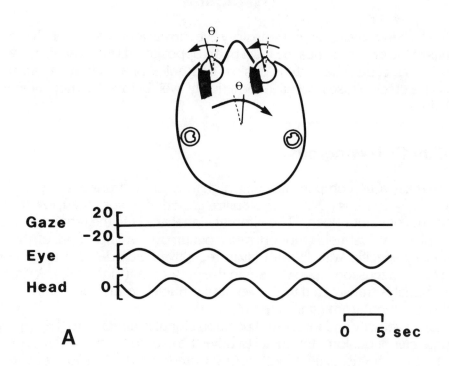

A

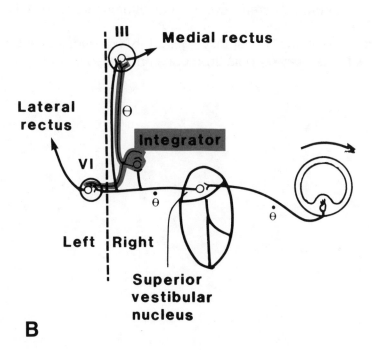

B

Figure 126 *A*, Vestibulo-ocular reflex. *B*, Vestibulo-ocular reflex circuit. *Figure continues.*

Nystagmus

During head rotation, compensatory eye movements can reach the mechanical limits of the orbit and must be reset by an oppositely directed quick movement, a primitive saccade. The pattern of slow and quick phases is **nystagmus** (Fig. 126C). The quick phases occur automatically, well before the mechanical limits are reached.

Optokinetic Nystagmus

Whereas VOR compensates for high-frequency, transient head rotation, optokinetic nystagmus (OKN) can stabilize gaze during sustained, low-frequency rotations at constant velocity. The afferent signal arises in the retina as a result of motion of the visual field; motion must occur over a large part of the retina. Directionally specific W cells with large receptive fields detect the motion and project to the accessory optic system in the pretectum (Fig. 126D). A visual field velocity signal is transmitted to the vestibular nuclei, to the same cells receiving head velocity input from canal afferents.

Again a velocity and integrated position signal is directed to the appropriate conjugate pair of oculomotor nuclei to drive the eyes in the same direction, at the same speed as the visual field motion. OKN latency is 100 to 130 msec. It follows velocities up to about 100 degrees per second. Eye velocity very quickly jumps to near-target velocity because of the **foveal smooth pursuit system** (see Unit 133). Without the pursuit system, eye velocity attains target velocity with a time constant of 6 sec.

During head rotation at constant velocity, OKN develops over the same time course as VOR fades away (cupula time constant is also 6 sec).

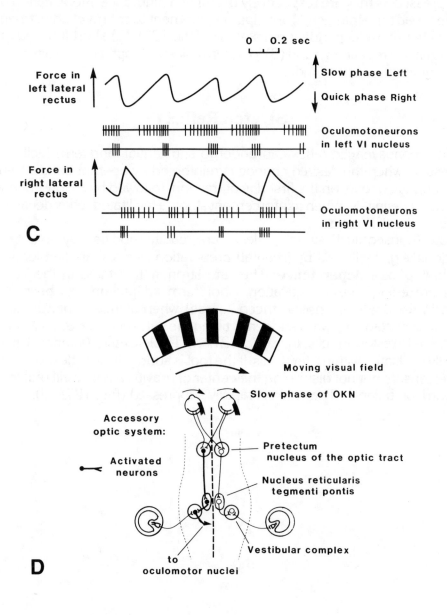

0   0.2 sec

Force in
left lateral
rectus

Slow phase Left

Quick phase Right

Oculomotoneurons
in left VI nucleus

Force in
right lateral
rectus

Oculomotoneurons
in right VI nucleus

C

Moving visual field

Slow phase of OKN

Accessory
optic system:

Activated
neurons

Pretectum
nucleus of the optic tract

Nucleus reticularis
tegmenti pontis

Vestibular complex

to
oculomotor nuclei

D

Figure 126 *(continued)*   *C*, Nystagmus. *D*, Optokinetic nystagmus.

UNIT 127
REFLEX MODIFIABILITY

Although their actions are basic and sterotyped, all reflexes can be facilitated or suppressed as they are respectively useful or a hindrance. Modification occurs in three broad time frames: (1) anticipatory, moment-to-moment adjustment (this includes the phase-dependent reflexes; see Unit 130); (2) short-term adaptation requiring a few repetitions; and (3) long-term plastic adaptations to altered conditions, requiring 1 week or more.

Stretch Reflex

The monosynaptic reflex can undergo substantial long-term facilitation or suppression when the desired change is reinforced by operant conditioning. An abrupt change occurs on the first day of training, followed by a slow change that continues indefinitely. When reinforcement stops, a facilitated reflex decays, with a half-life of about 17 days.

Late (transcortical) stretch reflexes are readily modified by voluntary task conditions, e.g., facilitated by (mental) preparation to resist applied loads. They also show **phase dependence**: They are strongly facilitated in the 100-msec period preceding muscle activation. Short-term adaptation has been demonstrated in the ankle extensors (triceps surae) when stance is perturbed. If the substrate is shifted backward suddenly, tilting the subject forward, ankle extensor reflex helps to restore erect stance (Fig. 127A, i). The late reflex (latency, 120 msec) is rapidly facilitated within a few trials. If the foot is suddenly dorsiflexed, stretching ankle extensors but not disturbing the center of gravity, a reflex will pull the body backward, off balance. The reflex is rapidly suppressed (Fig. 127A, ii).

i) Facilitation of long–latency stretch reflex
when it STABILIZES posture

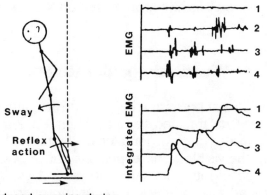

Sway

Reflex
action

**Induced swaying during
four consequtive trials**

ii) Suppression of long–latency stretch reflex
when it DESTABILIZES posture

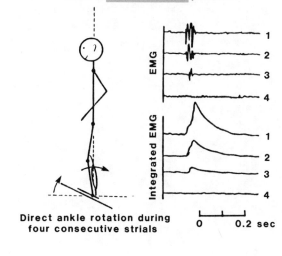

**Direct ankle rotation during
four consecutive strials**

0   0.2 sec

A

Figure 127   *A,* Rapid modification of the stretch reflex. *Figure continues.*

Flexion Withdrawal Reflex

In some situations the flexion withdrawal reflex fails to remove the limb from a noxious stimulus; it may even aggravate the stimulus. Knee flexion, for example, drives a pin further into the calf, rather than removing the leg from the pin. When such a stimulus occurs, the flexion pattern is rapidly altered within two or three trials. The basic reflex is suppressed and replaced by a longer latency (120 msec, possibly transcortical) response designed specifically to remove the limb from the stimulus. The later response is highly organized and varies with the initial position of the limb.

Vestibulo-ocular Reflex

VOR is automatically suppressed during large-amplitude eye–head saccades (see Unit 133) or in a visual tracking situation when it is desired that the eye move with the head. VOR can also undergo long-term adaptation. If 2 $\times$ telescopic lenses are worn constantly, the visible world appears to move twice as fast as the head. VOR adapts by increasing its gain: After about 5 days, VOR gain (eye movement–head movement) also doubles. If *reversing* prisms are worn, VOR gain gradually drops to about 25 percent of normal and the reflex is increasingly delayed (Fig. 127B). An approximate functional reversal is attained within 2 to 3 weeks.

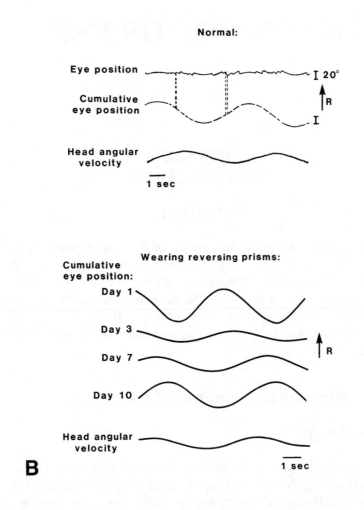

Figure 127 *(continued)*   *B,* Vestibulo-ocular reflex adaptation. (*A,* Adapted from Nashner LM. Adapting reflexes controlling the human posture. Exp Brain Res 1976; 26:62, 65, 66. *B,* Adapted from Gonshor A, Melvill Jones G. Extreme vestibulo-ocular adaptation induced by prolonged optical reversal of vision. J Physiol 1976; 256:386.)

18

MOTOR PROGRAMS

UNIT 128
INTRODUCTION

Definition

A motor program is an algorithm or set of rules that orders a sequence of input-output linkages. The input signals may be internally generated and/or elicited by peripheral stimuli; the outputs are directed to motor synergies.

A program is embodied within the CNS at several hierarchical levels from the general to the specific. At the general level a temporal sequence or goal may be specified; at the specific level exact muscle synergies are selected and dynamic parameters determined.

Structural Elements of a Program

Corollary Discharge

This is an internal loop transmitting descending motor signals back to sensory centers (Fig. 128A). Sensory centers can thereby distinguish externally imposed events (**exafference**) from those which are a consequence of self-motion (**reafference**).

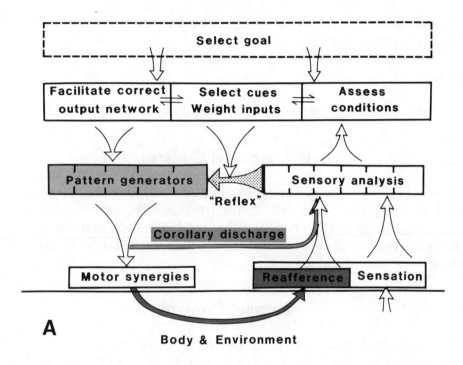

Figure 128 *A*, Program elements. *Figure continues.*

Central Pattern Generator

A central pattern generator (CPG) is a neuronal network responsible for autonomously timing and ordering a movement sequence; it requires an external trigger. Many CPGs may function in parallel, phase-linked to one another.

Motor Synergy

Motor synergies are co-activated sets of motor units, potentially in widely distributed muscles, which function together in the performance of a specific action. A synergy is task-dependent; it has no physical reality beyond the common task relationship. Synergies are selected by the convergent summation of numerous inputs to motor nuclei.

Reflexes

Reflexes regulate local parameters, simplifying the task of the CPG.

Hierarchical Control

Control of movement can be divided into many subtasks such as reflex regulations, postural support, and intended motion of a specific body part(s). Each task is served by different networks within the CNS, such that the motor goal is programmed at a high level which subjugates postural and reflex levels to serve the needs of the intended movement.

Parallel Control

Spinal, brainstem, and cortical subsystems are structured both hierarchically and in parallel (Fig. 128B). Networks performing similar functions, e.g., spinal and cortical stretch reflexes, may operate under different conditions. Spinal circuits handle common, stereotyped stimuli: cortical networks respond to more specialized and variable situations.

Temporal Ordering

The critical feature of motor programs is the recruitment of movement phases in a precise time sequence. Time intervals between successive motor outputs are generally in fixed proportion to one another, whether the overall speed of performance is fast or slow (Fig. 128C). The mechanisms of temporal ordering may involve oscillator networks and use of selected sensory cues. *Example*: Regularity of typing rhythms requires physical contact with the keys; cutaneous–proprioceptive reafference helps to trigger the succeeding stroke.

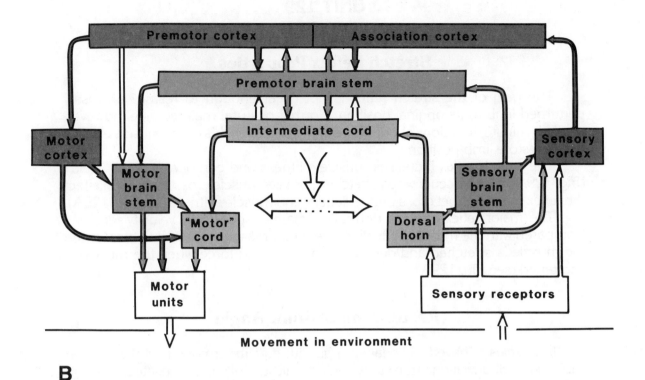

B

C

EN   CL   OSE   D   Fast

Slow

1 sec

Constant interval ratio is maintained between key strokes

Figure 128 *(continued)*   *B,* "Programming" networks of the central nervous system. *C,* Typing rhythm. (*C,* Modified after Terzuolo CA, Viviani P. Determinants and characteristics of motor sensory patterns used for typing. Neuroscience 1980; 5:1092.)

UNIT 129
POSTURE

Stretch Reflex Properties

The gain of the stretch reflex is not great enough to restore a grossly perturbed limb to its original position. Normal postural maintenance, however, involves minute deviations about desired joint angles. In this range muscle elasticity can restore limb position.

The stretch reflex increases muscle stiffness and compensates for "yield" (Fig. 129A), which occurs when stretching breaks muscle cross-bridges. In effect the reflex maintains net cross-bridge density and muscle stiffness (see Fig. 129A).

The major reflex effect is normally dynamic, specifically velocity-sensitive. Compared with the muscle by itself, the reflex increases the restoring force when the muscle is stretched and decreases the restoring force when the muscle is shortened (see Fig. 129A).

Restoration of Joint Angle

If muscles behaved as linear springs with equilibrium points at the desired joint angle, all deviations from that angle would be fully compensated. Position restoration would, however, involve oscillations around the equilibrium point, damped by system viscosity (Fig. 129B).

Oscillations are checked and position restoration facilitated by a program-regulated sequence of reflex (stretch and Golgi tendon organ) and triggered reactions to stop movement with minimal overshoot. Transient impulses accelerate the limb back toward the initial position, then decelerate it before the limb reaches that position (Fig. 129C).

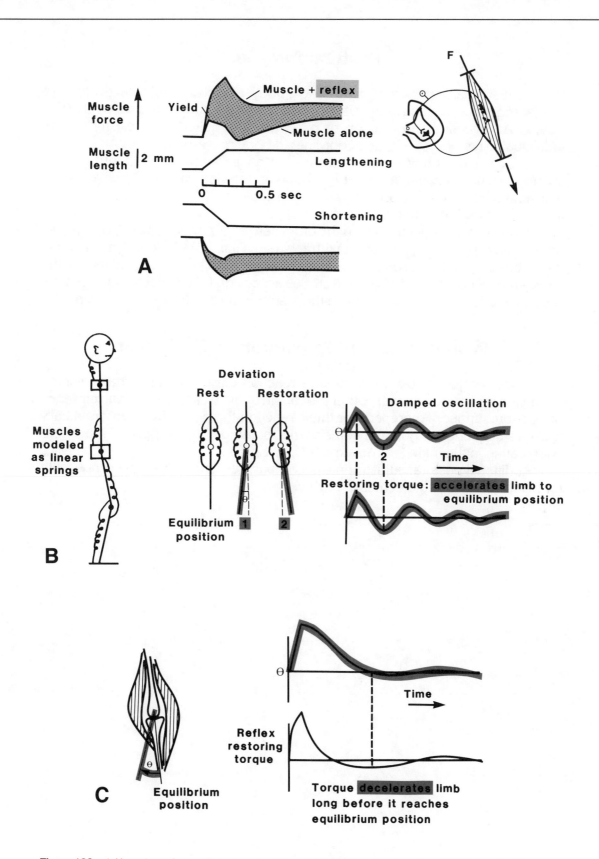

Figure 129 *A*, Viscoelastic forces: intrinsic and reflexive. *B*, Elastically restored posture. *C*, Reflexly restored posture. *Figure continues.*

Postural Program

To restore a posture across the whole body, muscles must be activated in a spatial sequence, starting at the site of contact with the supporting substrate (Fig. 129D). An overall plan of action or **program** is required because reflexes at individual joints do not produce coordinated body movement.

Body positions that deviate from erect stance can be lumped into regions sharing a common **synergy** (see Fig. 129D) or muscle combination which when activated accelerates the body toward metastable equilibrium, without crossing into another region (another synergy).

The synergy is selected within the brainstem and is imposed on motor nuclei by reticulospinal and vestibulospinal tracts (see Unit 121). The program subjugates the postural reflexes, which may play a modulatory role, adjusting the strength of activation of individual muscles according to the exact body position. Stretch and tendon reflexes regulate the restoring torque to prevent overshoot.

Postural Changes Preparatory to Movement

Movement of any body part creates reaction torques and mechanical interaction forces on virtually every other part of the body back to the inertial reference or support surface. To prepare for these reaction forces the body automatically makes a sequence of postural adjustments, starting at the support surface and culminating in the intended movement (Fig. 129E).

Additional postural adjustments accompany the movement to compensate for static changes in the center of gravity.

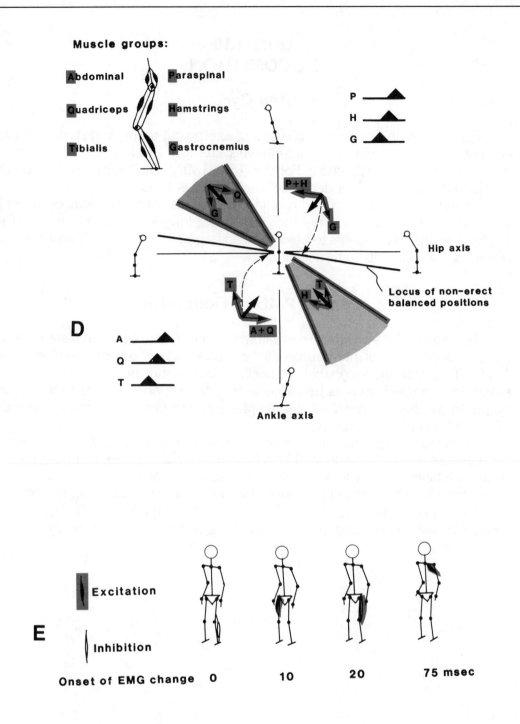

Muscle groups:

Abdominal

Paraspinal

Quadriceps

Hamstrings

Tibialis

Gastrocnemius

P

H

G

P+H

G

Q

G

Hip axis

Locus of non-erect balanced positions

D

A

Q

T

T

T

H

A+Q

Ankle axis

E

Excitation

Inhibition

Onset of EMG change   0   10   20   75 msec

Figure 129 *(continued)*   *D*, Synergies correcting anteroposterior sway. *E*, Postural adjustments preceding arm lift. (*A*, Modified after Nichols TR, Houck JC. Improvements in linearity and regulation of stiffness that results from actions of stretch reflex. J Neurophysiol 1976; 39:128. *D*, Adapted from Nasher LM, McCollum G. The organization of human postural movements: a formal basis and experimental synthesis. Behav Brain Sci 1985; 8:136, 139, 141.)

331

UNIT 130
LOCOMOTION

Step Cycle

For one leg, the step cycle consists of alternating swing and stance phases, each of which is subdivided into two intervals: *swing*, F (flexion) and E1 (extension in air) phases; *stance*, E2 and E3 phases (Fig. 130A). During E2 the load on the foot increases; during E3 it decreases as the heel is lifted.

For all rates of walking and running the F phase is remarkably constant in duration; the E phases are very modifiable, i.e., longer for slower speeds (Fig. 130B). The F phase appears to be controlled largely within the CNS and does not require sensory signals to turn itself off.

Central Pattern Generator

The step cycle is programmed within the spinal cord (intermediate zone) by an oscillator network of interneurons, the **central pattern generator** (CPG) (Fig. 130C). This network is capable, by itself, of producing the basic alternation of swing and stance, but relies heavily on sensory cues and reflexes to match the output to mechanical needs at the periphery and to phase-link one leg with the other and with the upper body.

The CPG incorporates reciprocal innervation. The flexor burst and extensor burst generators are mutually inhibitory (see Fig. 130C). The flexor burst generator is also capable of turning itself off (see discussion of early inspiratory burst generator, Unit 131), possibly through membrane accommodative properties.

The various joints move asynchronously with one another. The CPG must time each muscle contraction individually for a specific phase of the cycle.

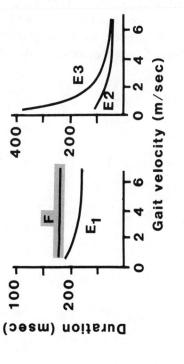

Figure 130 *A,* Step cycle. *B,* Duration of phases of step cycle. *Figure continues.*

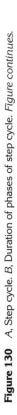

333

Phase-Dependent Reflexes

Many sensory inputs trigger or facilitate transitions to a new phase. These reflexive actions cannot be elicited at any other point in the cycle. Heel strike initiates the E2 phase and reinforces extensor activity through extensor thrust mechanisms. Stimulation of the foot during the swing phase tends to prolong flexion and has no effect on leg extensors. The flexion phase is not initiated until specific sensory cues are received: (1) the foot is unloaded; (2) the hip is extended (Fig. 130C)

Ankle Stretch Reflex

Heel strike mechanically unloads the ankle extensor muscles. They are not stretched until the center of gravity progresses past the heel. Stretch reflex gain (output/input) is progressively increased from early to late stance so that ankle extensor activity also increases markedly as the extensors are stretched (Fig. 130D). Reflex action thus adjusts extensor activity to the body load such that an adequate forward thrust is provided by the shortening contraction during E3.

Phase-Linking of the Limbs

Propriospinal tracts and commissural fibers link all of the individual CPGs for each limb and the trunk. Specific phases in one leg must take place in fixed relation to specific phases of the other and the rest of the body. This can be accomplished by requiring greater summation of signals before a phase is triggered; e.g., flexion phase would require conditions 1 and 2 above plus a third, the contralateral foot bearing weight.

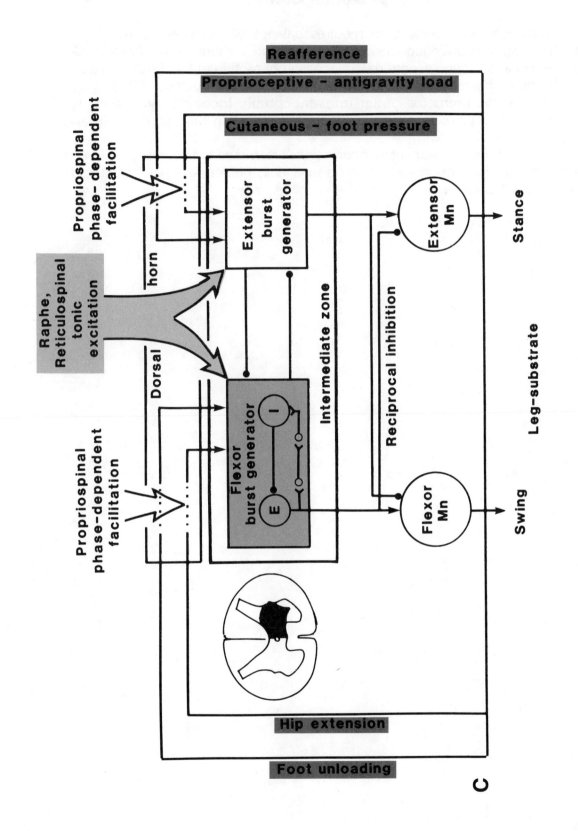

Figure 130 *(continued)* C, Spinal step pattern generator. *Figure continues.*

Supraspinal Control

Human bipedal locomotion requires balance of the trunk on top of the stepping legs, a coordination task that is impossible without the vestibular nuclei and reticular formation. Coordinated locomotory motion of the limbs and trunk needs the entire neuraxis up to the pedunculopontine nucleus (PPN), which functions as the premotor center (**mesencephalic locomotory region**) for locomotion. PPN projects to reticulospinal tract neurons in the gigantocellular and raphe nuclei (Fig. 130E).

Motor cortex involvement in locomotion is restricted to accurate positioning of the foot so that heel strikes first, and to visually guided foot placement (e.g., stairs, stepping stones).

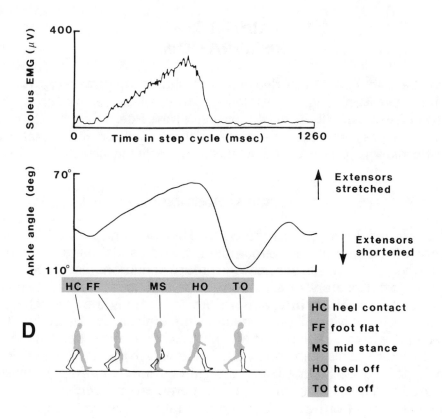

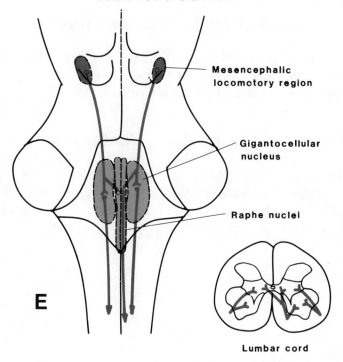

Figure 130 *(continued)* *D,* Ankle stretch reflex during stance phase. *E,* Brainstem controllers of locomotion. (*A,* Adapted from Murray MP. Gait as a total pattern of movement. Am J Phys Med 1967; 46:293. *B,* From Grillner S. Locomotion in vertebrates: central mechanisms and reflex interaction. Physiol Rev 1975; 55:250. With permission from The American Physiological Society. *D,* Adapted from Stein RB, Capaday C. The modulation of human reflexes during functional motor tasks. Trends Neurosci 1988; 11:332.)

UNIT 131
RESPIRATION

The respiratory cycle is divided into three phases: **inspiratory**, **postinspiratory**, and **expiratory** (Fig. 131A). Inspiration involves contraction of the diaphragm (increasing activity in the phrenic nerve) and external intercostal muscles. Expiration involves contraction of the internal intercostal and abdominal muscles. The postinspiratory phase is characterized by declining activity in the phrenic nerve.

Cycle Generator (Figure 131B)

The basic respiratory rhythm is produced by a neuronal network linking a few medullary nuclei, the nucleus retroambiguus, and caudal parts of the nucleus solitarius (Fig. 131C). Within this network, groups of neurons discharge during the inspiratory, postinspiratory, or expiratory phase and are actively inhibited for the rest of the cycle. **Inhibitory interactions** provide the only known mechanisms of generating cyclic activity. All of the neurons are tonically facilitated by CO_2 chemoreceptor discharge. Their phasic activity at a characteristic point in the cycle is due to inhibition and disinhibition by other elements in the "ring" network. Some neuronal types, e.g., early burst inspiratory neurons (inhibitory), rapidly cease firing once started as a result of accommodative membrane properties.

Efferent axons from expiratory and inspiratory cells project to respiratory motor nuclei or associated interneurons in the cervical (phrenic) and thoracic cord (intercostals).

Pulmonary Stretch Receptors

Stretch receptor afferents signaling lung inflation travel to the medulla in the vagus nerve. The slowly adapting receptors tend to excite expiratory neurons and inhibit inspiratory neurons (**Hering-Breuer reflex**).

Pneumotaxic Center

Two nuclei in the rostral pons—the medial parabrachial nucleus and the Kolliker-Fuse nucleus—exert a regulatory influence on the medullary respiratory pattern generator. The neurons receive pulmonary stretch receptor input and facilitate transitions from inspiration to expiration or vice versa.

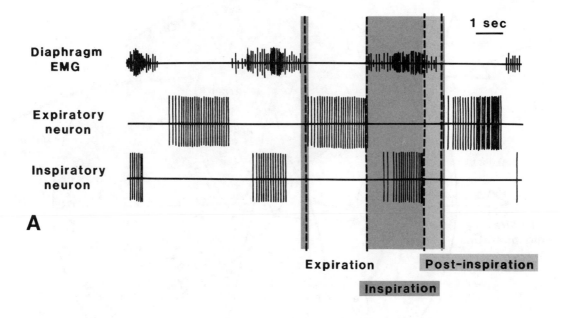

Figure 131 *A,* Respiratory activity in the medulla. *Figure continues.*

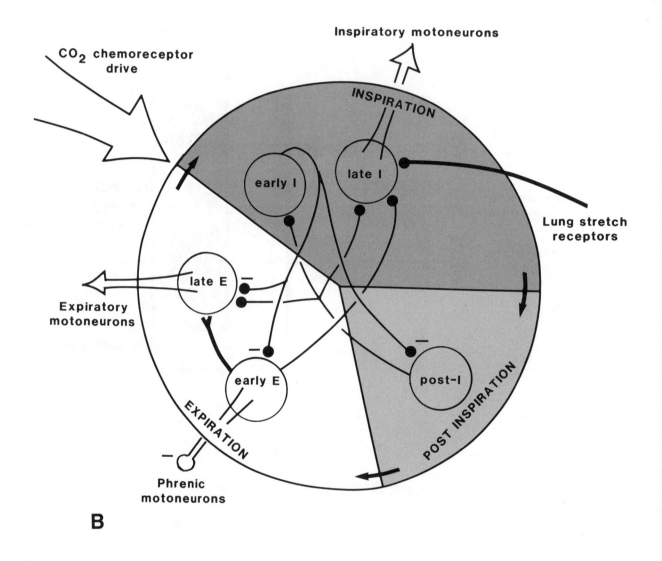

Figure 131 *(continued)* B, Known interactions within the cycle generator. *Figure continues.*

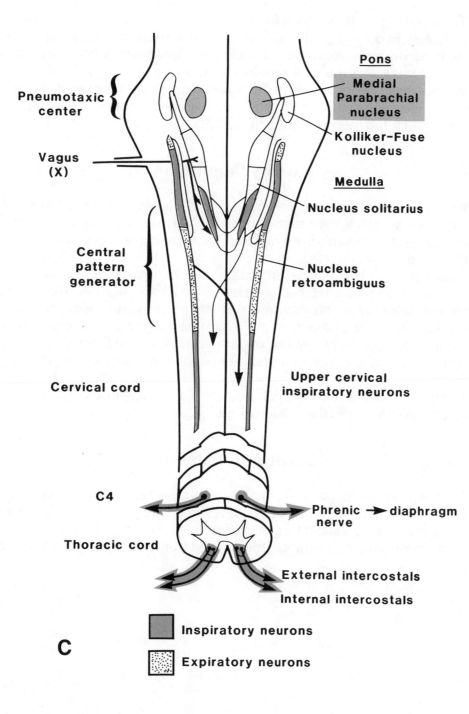

Pons

Pneumotaxic center {

Medial Parabrachial nucleus

Kolliker-Fuse nucleus

Vagus (X)

Medulla

Nucleus solitarius

Central pattern generator {

Nucleus retroambiguus

Cervical cord

Upper cervical inspiratory neurons

C4

Phrenic → diaphragm nerve

Thoracic cord

External intercostals

Internal intercostals

C

■ **Inspiratory neurons**

▦ **Expiratory neurons**

Figure 131 *(continued)* *C*, Respiratory nuclei. (*A*, Adapted from Graham K, Duffin J. Cross correlation of medullary expiratory neurons in the cat. Exp Neurol 1981; 73:460. *B*, Adapted from Long SE, Duffin J. The medullary respiratory neurons: a review. Can J Physiol Pharmacol 1984; 62:177.)

UNIT 132
MASTICATION

The chewing cycle is subdivided into three phases: opening, closing, and power strokes. In opening, the digastric muscle is active, and closer muscles are silent to lower the jaw a fixed amount. In closing, low-level activity in the temporalis and masseter (closer) muscles rapidly raises the jaw to engage food between molars. High-level closer activity in the power stroke raises the jaw to the point of maximum intercuspation of teeth. The central pattern generator is located in the pontine reticular formation (Fig. 132A, 132B).

Sensory Regulation

If food particles break, the jaw jerks upward, causing a transient reflex silencing of the closer muscles at a latency of about 10 msec ("unloading" reflex). The afferent signal arises mainly from high-threshold mechanoreceptors. Jaw opener muscles have no stretch reflex.

Closer muscle spindle afferents discharge maximally during the *opening* phase, when closers are stretched but silent (Fig. 132C). High firing rates occur in the power stroke only during attempts to crush hard food (isometric contraction). Both spindle afferents and periodontal ligament mechanoreceptors respond to the pressure and excite closer motoneurons (positive feedback). Thus spindle activity excites motoneurons in a phase-dependent manner, during closing, not opening.

Note: The spindle afferent cell bodies are located in the mesencephalic nucleus of nerve V, not in the gasserian ganglion.

Cortical Regulation

Chewing can be triggered from parts of the jaw representation in the motor and premotor cortex (see Fig. 135B). The cortex is very important in the coordination of the chewing cycle with tongue movements. The tongue works in a potentially lethal environment, pushing ground food from the teeth to the back of the mouth.

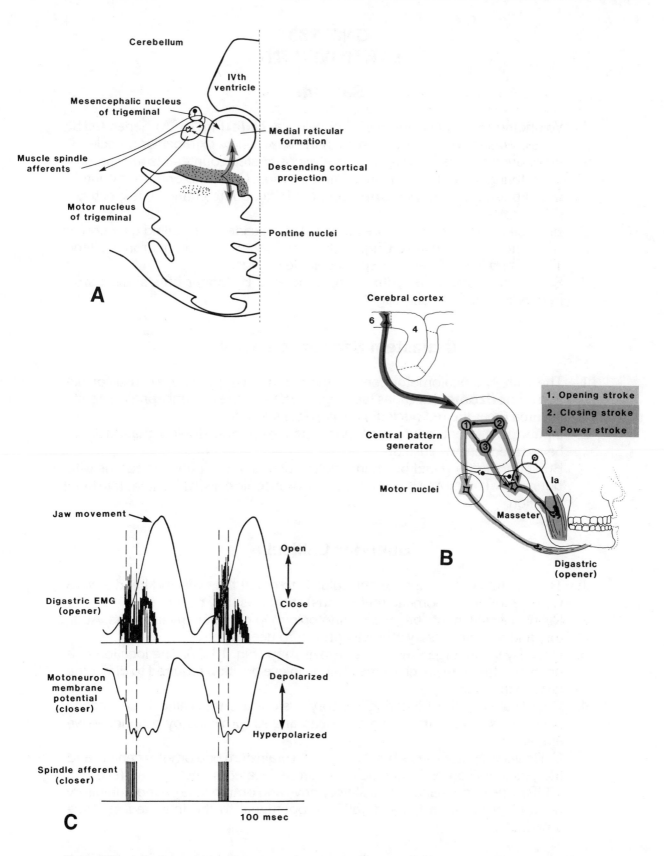

Figure 132 *A,* Pontine nuclei for mastication. *B,* Schematic of pattern generator interactions. *C,* Motor and sensory activity during the chewing cycle (with no food present). (*C,* Adapted from Goldberg LJ, Chandler SH. Evidence of pattern generator control of the effects of spindle afferent input during rhythmical jaw movements. Can J Physiol Pharmacol 1981; 59:710.)

UNIT 133
EYE MOVEMENT

Saccade

1. Voluntary movement of the eye is jumplike **saccade** (Fig. 133A), generated by phasic *pulse* and tonic *step* forces in the appropriate extraocular muscles.
2. Pulse during saccade overcomes eye viscosity; step counteracts muscle elastic restoring forces to maintain the new position. Oculomotoneurons contribute to pulse and step with **burst** and **tonic** firing rate changes, respectively (Fig. 133B).
3. Burst starts 5 to 8 msec before the onset of saccade if the pulling direction of the motor unit is suitable (Fig. 133C); otherwise, the motoneuron is silent. Tonic firing is maximal for a specific angle of gaze.
4. Saccades of greater amplitude are generated by longer bursts; discharge frequency increases only slightly.

Brainstem Saccade Generator

1. There are two oculomotor centers: the paramedian pontine reticular formation for **horizontal** saccades (see Fig. 133B), and the mesencephalic interstitial area (near the red nucleus) for **vertical** saccades.
2. Inputs to oculomotoneurons provide separate burst and tonic signals that can be independently adjusted.
3. Burst duration is gated by an interaction of inhibitory "pause" neurons with burst cells. Tonic input is postulated to arise in tonic cells, which integrate burst duration.

Superior Colliculus

1. The function of the superior colliculus is to orient the eyes and head toward visual, auditory, or somatic (cutaneous) stimuli as they occur.
2. Retinal (Y cell) inputs project a retinotopic map onto superficial layers. Auditory and somatosensory afferents project to deep layers.
3. Deep layers are organized into a **motor map** (Fig. 133D). The location of a neuron in the map specifies the change in eye position required to direct the gaze to the target.
4. Coordinates of the triggering sensory system are translated into saccade parameters given current eye and head angles (provided by proprioceptive afferents).
5. Collicular output activates burst neurons in brainstem oculomotor centers and triggers inhibition of "omnipause" neurons located at the midline (see Fig. 133B). The combination of excitatory drive and omnipause gating (inhibitory neuron) produces a burst duration proportional to the intended saccade amplitude.

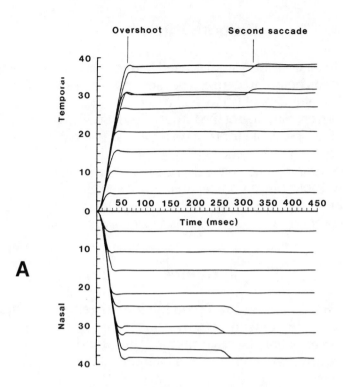

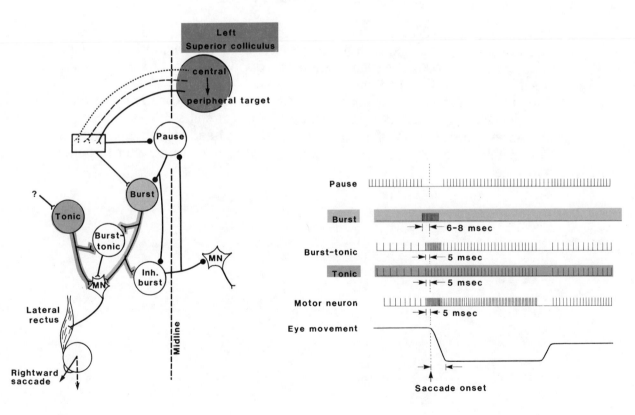

Figure 133 *A,* Saccade eye movements. *B,* Pontine saccade generator. *Figure continues.*

345

Smooth Pursuit

1. The smooth pursuit control system is used to track *moving* visual stimuli. It is accurate for speeds below 30 degrees per second. The onset of target motion evokes pursuit at latencies of 65 to 130 msec.
2. Retinal velocity error, slippage of the target away from the fovea, is detected in cortical area MT, responsible for motion analysis. The error is corrected by a proportional change in eye velocity (Fig. 133E).
3. New velocity is sustained automatically by the CNS model of target velocity in the visible world (possibly in cortical area MST; see Unit 137).
4. Inhibitory output from the flocculus of the cerebellar cortex adjusts activity in brainstem oculomotor centers to optimize pursuit movements.

Vergence

1. Conjugate eye movements are replaced by **convergence** or **divergence** of eyes for objects moving toward or away from eyes, respectively (Fig. 133F).
2. Vergence movements may be asymmetric. They are driven by signals from cortical areas involved in depth analysis (stereopsis).

Eye-Head Coordination

1. Target shifts of 2 to 20 degrees elicit saccades at latencies of about 200 msec. Saccade may be followed by a head movement during which VOR (see Unit 126) operates to rotate the eyes an equal and opposite amount. Gaze remains steadily on target (Fig. 133G).
2. Target shifts of more than 20 degrees elicit combined eye-head movements. Saccade latency is increasingly prolonged for larger shifts.
3. During large gaze shifts VOR is suppressed; eye and head movements interact to maintain gaze *velocity* roughly constant. VOR is restored after target is refoveated.

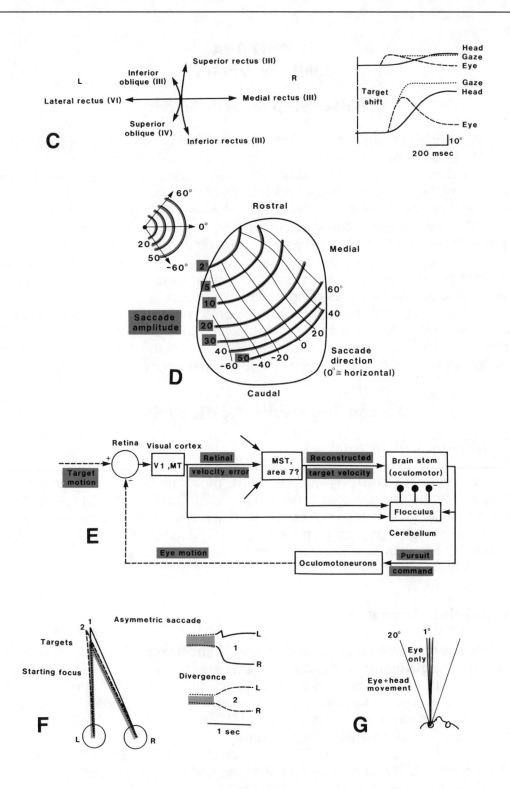

Figure 133 *(continued)* C, Extraocular muscle action (left eye). *D*, Motor map of the superior colliculus. *E*, Smooth pursuit control system. *F*, Vergence movements. *G*, Eye-head coordination. (*A*, Adapted from Fuchs AF. Saccadic and smooth pursuit eye movements in the monkey. J Physiol 1967; 191:615. *B, Right*, Adapted from Fuchs AF, Kanecko CRS, Scudder CA. Brainstem control of saccadic eye movements. Ann Rev Neurosci 1985; 8:319. *Left*, From Kandel ER, Schwartz JH. Principles of neural science. New York: Elsevier, 1985:581. With permission from Elsevier Science Publications. *C*, Adapted from Hering E. Der Raumsin und die Bewegungen des Auges. In: Handbuch der Physiologie. Vol. 3. Part I. FCW Vogel Verlag, 1879:515 and Uemura T, Arai Y, Shimazaki C. Eye head coordination during lateral gaze in normal subjects. Acta Otolaryngol 1980; 90:193. *D*, Adapted from Robinson DA. Eye movements evoked by collicular stimulation in the alert monkey. Vision Res 1972; 12:1800. *E*, Adapted from Lisberger SG, Morris EJ, Tychsen L. Visual motion processing and sensory-motor integration for smooth pursuit eye movements. Ann Rev Neurosci 1987; 10:103, 121.)

UNIT 134
LIMB MOVEMENT

Pulse-Step Muscle Activity

For single-joint limb movements, whether fast or slow or of large or small amplitude, the time to peak acceleration is quite constant (Fig. 134A). The fully expressed muscle *pulse* is triphasic. The magnitude of the **first agonist EMG burst** is scaled to the amplitude and velocity of the movement. It lasts 70 to 140 msec and serves to overcome limb inertia, driving the limb to peak momentum. An **antagonist muscle burst** occurs during the relative "silent period" of the agonist (see Fig. 134A) and serves to assist limb deceleration when it cannot be adequately accomplished by joint viscoelasticity and/or gravity. The **second agonist burst**, if required, "clamps" the limb at its target position, preventing backsliding due to elastic restoring forces.

Subsequent tonic *step* activity in the agonist muscle counteracts joint elastic forces and external loads. Except for the first agonist burst, which is mainly centrally produced from prior information, all parts of the pulse-step activity are strongly influenced by proprioceptive input from the moving limb.

Descending (Motor Cortical) Signals

Single Joint Movements

Motor cortical cells projecting to active motor nuclei have a variety of discharge patterns, usually phasic (see Fig. 135E). Tonic cortical firing is most common during isometric contraction against a load. The firing rate of any one cell will reflect some parts of the peripheral EMG pattern, but not all. The activity of muscle motor units is thus determined by a summation of many descending neurons and sensory afferents.

Multi-joint Movements

Muscle contractions are a combination of **shortening**, **isometric contraction**, and **lengthening**, with great variations in sensory reafference. Gravity can hinder and/or aid a given muscle. Muscle activity progresses in time from the support base, outward (generally axial to proximal to distal). Motor cortical units show the same temporal ordering (Fig. 134B). For an arm reach, shoulder and elbow units fire before wrist and finger units.

Like muscles, motor cortical units fire preferentially for a specific *direction* of limb movement. The direction of a trajectory, and proximity to limit of the work space, determine angular velocity relationships among successive joints.

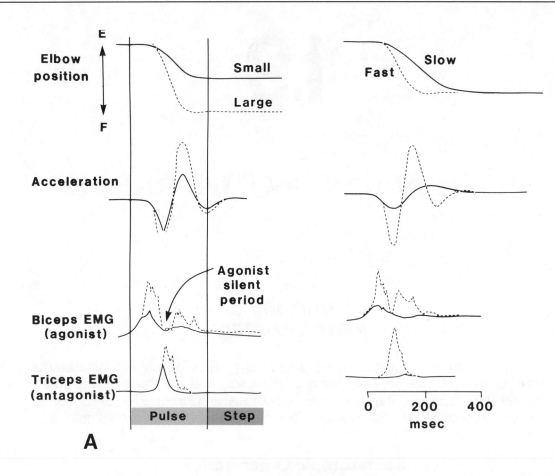

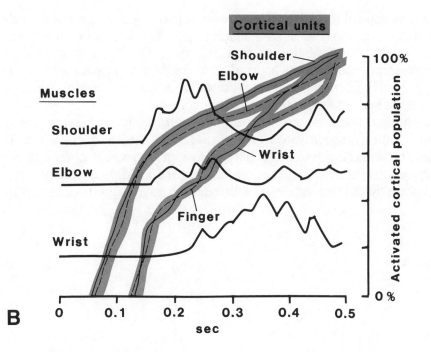

Figure 134 *A,* Single-joint movement (flexion): muscle activity. *B,* Multi-joint movement (pointing): recruitment order. (Adapted from Gielen CCAM, van den Oosten K, Pull ter Gunne F. Relation between EMG activation patterns and kinematic properties of aimed arm movements. J Motor Behav 1985; 17:426, 430. *B,* Adapted from Murphy JT, Wong YC, Kwan HC. Sequential activation of neurons in primate motor cortex during unrestrained forelimb movement. J Neurophysiol 1985; 53:436, 439.)

19

SPECIALIZED MOTOR AREAS

UNIT 135
MOTOR CORTEX

The motor cortex, located on the precentral gyrus, is the major cortical output center to all motor nuclei (excluding oculomotor) and the intermediate zone-reticular formation axis. It functions to select muscle synergies for *execution* of movements outside the basic posture-locomotion repertoire of the reticular axis.

Somatotopic Organization

From its medial to its lateral end, area 4 is divided into a lower body, upper body, and head region (Fig. 135A). Each region is individually organized according to a nested representation of joint movements. Stimulation of central foci produces discrete movements around distal joints, e.g., fingers in the upper body zone (Fig. 135B). Stimulation of surrounding (and overlapping) areas produces movements at successively more proximal joints.

Any single muscle, or small group of synergists, is *multiply represented* by "columns" within its own area (see Fig. 135B). At each columnar site, that particular muscle is adjacent to a different neighboring set of muscle columns, acting at the same and contiguous joints. Thus at each representation in the motor cortex, a given muscle is associated with a different synergy (muscle combination).

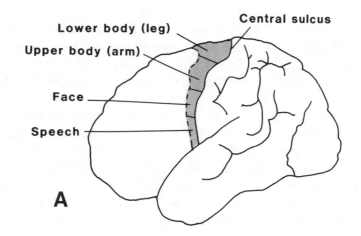

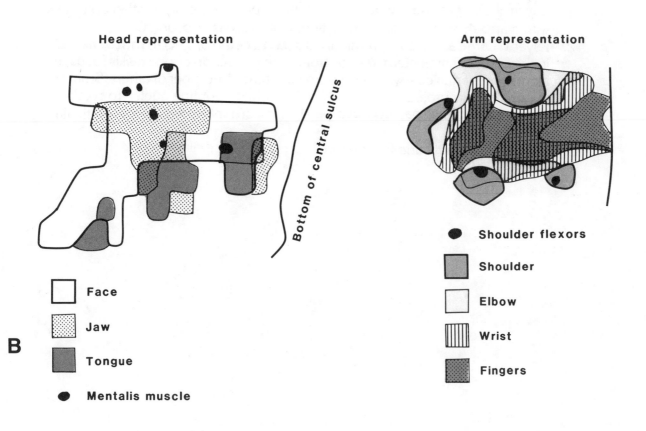

Figure 135 *A*, Somatotopy of area 4. *B*, Detailed motor maps. *Figure continues.*

Inputs

1. Somatosensory from cortical areas 1 and 2. **Proprioceptive** and **cutaneous** inputs project both to separate columns and converge on the same columns. Proprioceptive inputs to a **flexor** column usually arise from passive **extension** of the same joint, as in the stretch reflex. Cutaneous inputs can have a wide variety of relationships to the represented movement.
2. The **premotor** cortex, including the **supplementary motor area**, projects heavily into the motor cortex to regulate the flow of somatosensory input and to mediate conditioned signals (e.g., sight of doorknob) to initiate motor acts.
3. Thalamus. The **ventrolateral nucleus** (VL) conveys signals from all contralateral cerebellar nuclei to the motor cortex (Fig. 135C). Caudal VL also mediates spinothalamic sensory inputs. The rostral shell of the ventroposterior nucleus (VP) (see Unit 105) conveys lemniscal proprioceptive inputs.

Outputs (Fig. 135D)

1. Layers II-III. **Pyramidal cells** in one column project heavily to other columns within area 4; there are also projections out to areas 2, 5, and 6.
2. Layer V. Large and giant pyramidal cells (**Betz cells**) project to **motor nuclei** in the cord and brainstem. **Motor field**: The projection of one cell is focused on one motor nucleus, with fewer terminations on a number of others. Smaller pyramidal cells project to the striatum (putamen), pontine nuclei (to cerebellum), red nucleus (parvocellular part), and cord intermediate zone-reticular formation.
3. Layer VI. Pyramidal and fusiform cells project to VL thalamus.

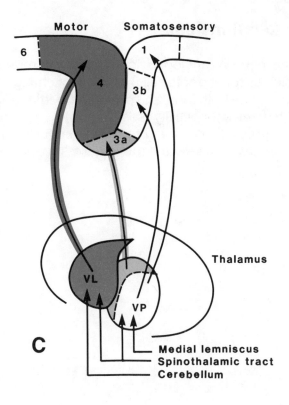

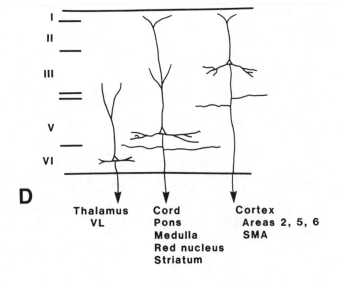

Figure 135 *(continued)* C, Thalamic inputs. D, Cortical outputs. *Figure continues.*

Motor Relationships

Discharge rates of motor cortical neurons are loosely correlated with muscle activity and dynamic parameters such as force (tonic cells) and rate of change of force (phasic cells). Many neurons combine both tonic and phasic properties (Fig. 135E). Some units may be related to fusimotor activity (see Unit 68).

Neurons in a specific muscle representation are not active every time that muscle is active (Fig. 135F). They participate in selected movements (synergies).

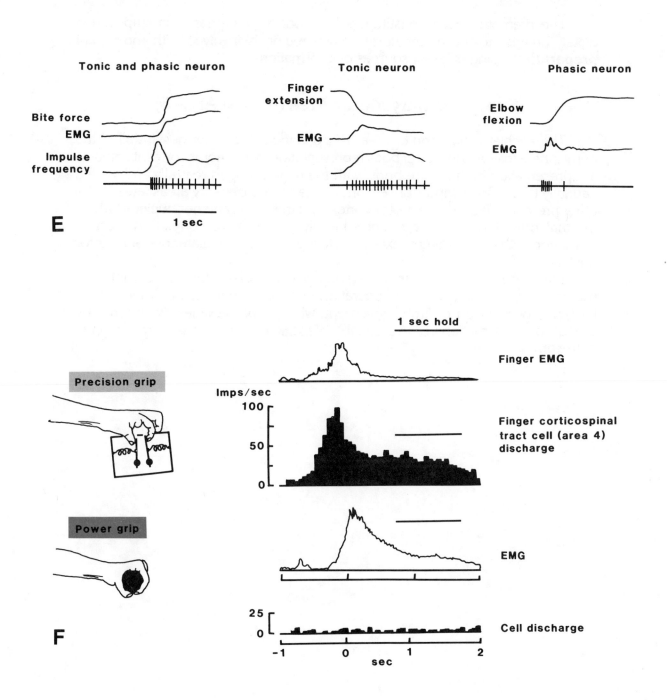

Figure 135 *(continued)* *E*, Activity patterns. *F*, Task (synergy) specificity. (*B*, Courtesy of B. Sessle and H. Kwan and Y.C. Wong, University of Toronto, Toronto, Canada. *E*, Adapted from Hoffman DS, Lushei ES. Responses of monkey precentral cortical cells during a controlled jaw bite task. J Neurophysiol 1980; 44:335 and Cheney PD, Fetz EE. Functional classes of primate corticomotoneuronal cells and their relation to active force. J Neurophysiol 1980; 44:787. *F*, Adapted from Muir RB, Lemon RN. Corticospinal neurons with a special role in precision grip. Brain Res 1983; 261:315.)

UNIT 136
PREMOTOR AREAS

The premotor areas constitute a functionally heterogeneous strip immediately anterior to the motor cortex. Each region is involved with movement **preparation**, using different sources of information.

Supplementary Motor Area (Medial Area 6)

The supplementary motor area (SMA) is located on the mesial wall of the hemisphere rostral to the lower body representation in the motor cortex. it contains a representation of the entire body, with the head mapped rostrally and the leg caudally (Fig. 136A). Inputs arise from all the somatosensory areas, area 7, the other premotor regions, the motor cortex, and the ventroanterior nucleus (VA) of the thalamus (Fig. 136B). It projects heavily to the motor cortex and reticular formation, with some efferents extending to the cord intermediate zone and motor nuclei.

Function. SMA appears to regulate the flow of somatosensory input to motor centers during program operation. It may be particularly important in bilateral coordination of limb movement, when opposite sides synchronously execute different motions. SMA is capable of blocking "mirror image" movements of the arms.

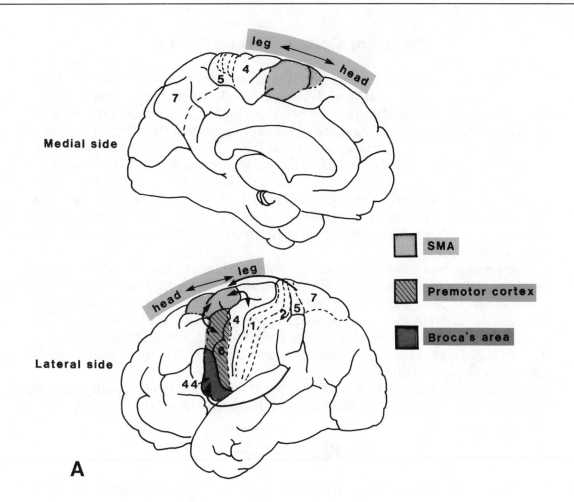

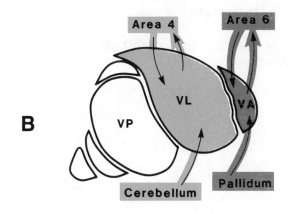

Figure 136   *A*, Premotor areas. *B*, Premotor thalamus. *Figure continues.*

Premotor Cortex (Lateral Area 6)

The premotor cortex is immediately anterior to the arm and head representations of area 4 (see Fig. 136A), and along its caudal edge it continues the motor representation of the axial parts of the body (see Unit 135). It projects heavily to the motor cortex and reticular formation, with some axons extending to the spinal cord. Only axial and proximal motor nuclei are innervated. Inputs arise from the fringe of the frontal eye field (see Unit 137), SMA, areas 5 and 7, and VA thalamus.

Function. The premotor cortex controls the activation of motor centers by visual (e.g., doorknobs) or auditory cues such that the motor response to an environmental stimulus is suppressed unless it is desired. Meaningful and expected visual stimuli elicit bursts in premotor cortical neurons at latencies as short as 50 msec.

Premotor neurons can *prepare* the motor cortex for specific movements in advance of their execution. If a WARNING signal is delivered, giving the direction of a movement to be performed (e.g., wrist extension), specific premotor neurons will gradually accelerate their discharge rate prior to the expected GO signal (Fig. 136C). The preparatory activity *facilitates* the subsequent GO response, which occurs sooner, as does the movement, than when preparatory activity is lacking (direction not specified).

Preparatory discharge can also *process* motor elements in advance, e.g., select a motor synergy when the intended movement direction is known.

Broca's Area

The caudal half of Broca's area (area 44 makes up the lateral end of the premotor strip in the left hemisphere (see Fig. 136A). It receives inputs from the rostral half of Broca's area (area 45) and the language centers of the temporal lobe (Wernicke's area, angular gyrus). It projects to the premotor cortex, the SMA, and the motor cortex.

Function. Broca's area is essential for organizing speech and writing movements in grammatical patterns.

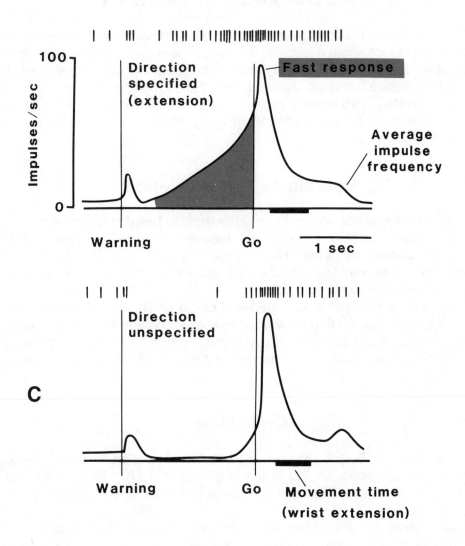

Figure 136 *(continued)* C, Area 6 preparatory facilitation. (A, Adapted from Nieuwenhuys R, Voogd J, van Huijzen C. The human central nervous system. Heidelberg: Springer-Verlag, 1981:10. B, Adapted from Jones EG. Connectivity of the primary sensory-motor cortex. In: Jones EG, Peters A, eds. Cerebral cortex. Vol. 5. New York: Plenum Press, 1986:121. C, Courtesy of A. Richle and J. Requin, Marseille, France.)

UNIT 137
VISUAL GUIDANCE OF MOVEMENT

The use of visual information to guide body movements in space requires coding of target location in relation to the body. The visual system codes stimuli in **retinotopic** coordinates, which vary with angle of gaze. Transformation into head and trunk reference frames is done partly in the superior colliculus and partly in the cerebral cortex. Two cortical regions are critically involved in relating retinotopic information to body coordinates (Fig. 137A): the parietal area 7 and the frontal eye field (FEF).

Coordinate Transformation

The first stage of conversion from retinotopic to **head reference** mapping is done by a subset of area 7 cells. They have a retinotopic receptive field, but response magnitude varies greatly with angle of gaze (Fig. 137B). A maximum is reached when eyes point to a specific direction so that the stimulus has a unique position with respect to the head.

Sensitivity to position about the head could be made independent of eye position if many cells, coding for the same spatial position but for different gaze angles, converged on a common neuron. Such convergence may occur in anterior area 6, where some neurons respond to specific locations regardless of eye position.

Optic Flow

Many area 7 cells are very sensitive to visual motion in radially oriented vectors, toward or away from the center of gaze (Fig. 137C). Receptive fields are usually very large but tend to spare the fovea; a few are very restricted. Speed of motion is not coded.

Again, angle of gaze modulates the response. Looking straight ahead strongly facilitates sensitivity to motion along the vertical and horizontal meridians. Objects coming toward or leaving the body tend to follow the meridians when gaze is centered. This motion detection system appears to be important in the guidance of the fast initial projection of limbs in space, not the final approach.

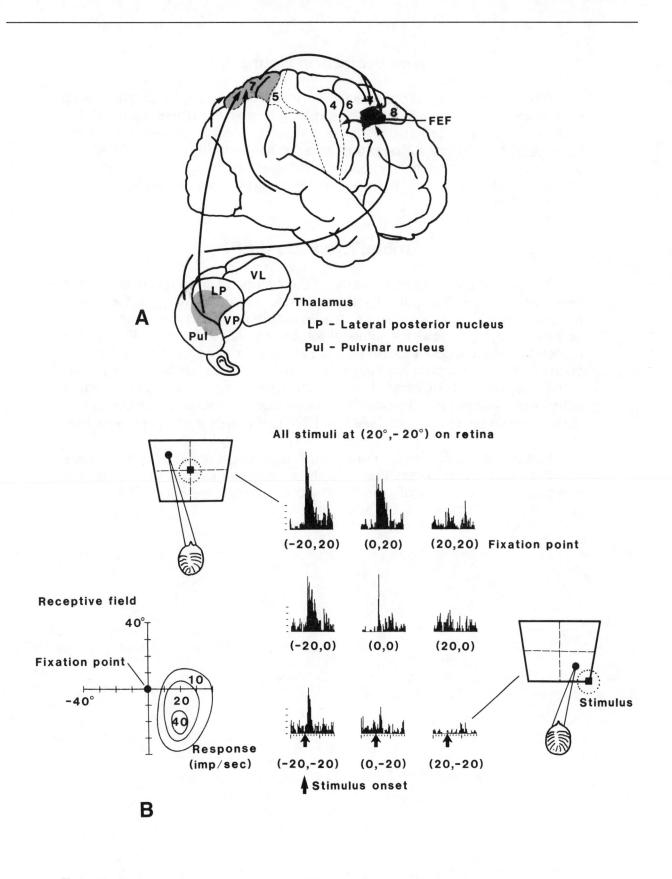

Figure 137 *A*, Thalamocortical regions for visual guidance. *B*, Retina to head reference transformation (area 7). *Figure continues.*

Arm Projection Neurons

Also in area 7 are neurons specifically related to reaching for targets. **Visual** cells respond to the appearance of the target, provided a reach toward it is intended; they are often specific for a particular location relative to the head (latency, 60 to 160 msec). **Movement** cells discharge during the reach. They can be very specific for a spatial location or arm trajectory toward that location (Fig. 137D). Both cell types could be important for controlling approach of the arm to a specific target.

Frontal Eye Field (FEF)

The posterior zone of FEF has direct connections with the pontine saccade network (see Unit 133) in parallel with the superior colliculus. Whereas the colliculus automatically drives eye-head saccades to foveate visual (or auditory) stimuli as they occur, FEF allows for greater flexibility in the use of targets. **Visual** cells respond to target appearance (Fig. 137E) within a broad receptive field (latency, 50 to 120 msec): response is greatly enhanced if a saccade is subsequently made to the receptive field. **Movement** cells discharge in a burst, starting immediately before a saccade in a specific direction. They trigger the saccade even after a long delay since target appearance (see Fig. 137E), or even if the target is imagined (Fig. 137F).

Visuomovement cells fire continuously from target appearance to saccade onset; an extra burst occurs immediately prior to the saccade, i.e., when the ever-present stimulus is finally made the saccade target (see Fig. 137E).

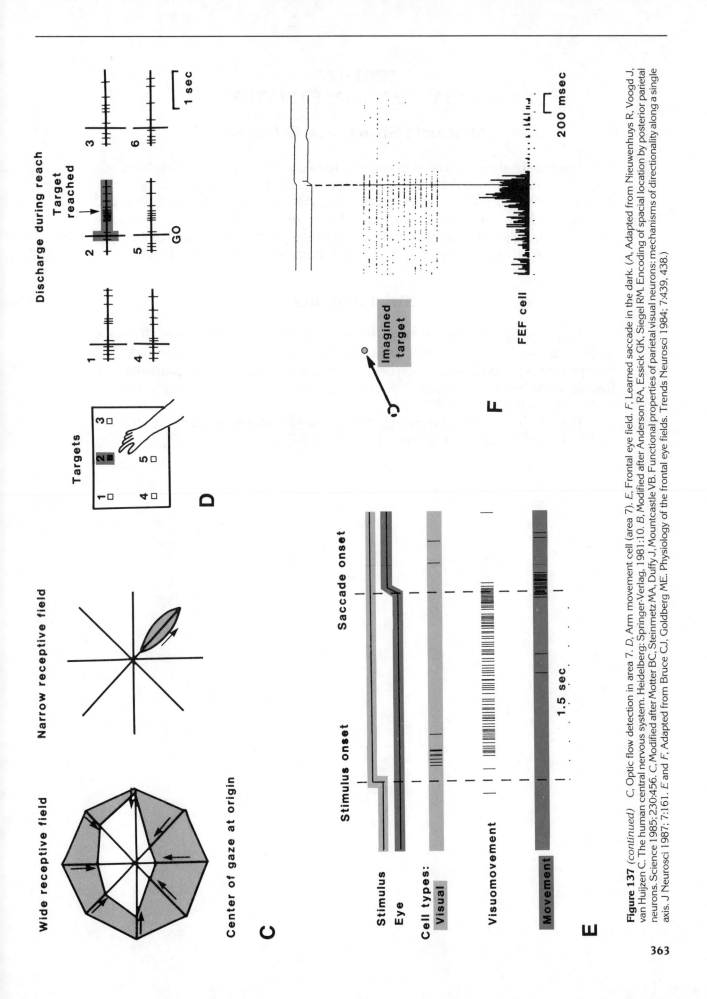

Figure 137 *(continued)* *C,* Optic flow detection in area 7. *D,* Arm movement cell (area 7). *E,* Frontal eye field. *F,* Learned saccade in the dark. (*A,* Adapted from Nieuwenhuys R, Voogd J, van Huijzen C. The human central nervous system. Heidelberg: Springer-Verlag, 1981:10. *B,* Modified after Anderson RA, Essick GK, Siegel RM. Encoding of spacial location by posterior parietal neurons. Science 1985; 230:456. *C,* Modified after Motter BC, Steinmetz MA, Duffy J, Mountcastle VB. Functional properties of parietal visual neurons: mechanisms of directionality along a single axis. J Neurosci 1987; 7:161. *E* and *F,* Adapted from Bruce CJ, Goldberg ME. Physiology of the frontal eye fields. Trends Neurosci 1984; 7:439, 438.)

363

UNIT 138
BASAL GANGLIA: STRIATUM

Anatomic Structures: Overview

The basal ganglia can be subdivided into two levels — input, or **striatum**, and output, or **pallidum**. The nuclei comprising the striatum are the putamen, caudate, and accumbens. The globus pallidus, substantia nigra pars reticulata, and ventral pallidum make up the pallidum. Each level is influenced by a specific modulatory nucleus: the striatum by the dopaminergic cells of the substantia nigra pars compacta, and the pallidum by the subthalamic nucleus (Fig. 138A).

Striatal Inputs

Afferents to the striatum arise from most of the cerebral cortex (layer V pyramidal cells) and from the centromedian nucleus of the thalamus (CM). Roughly three parallel streams can be distinguished — **motor**, **associational**, and **limbic** — originating from sensorimotor, association, and limbic regions of the cortex, respectively (Fig. 138B).

The afferents are excitatory to both cholinergic interneurons of the striatum and GABAergic projection neurons (see Fig. 138B).

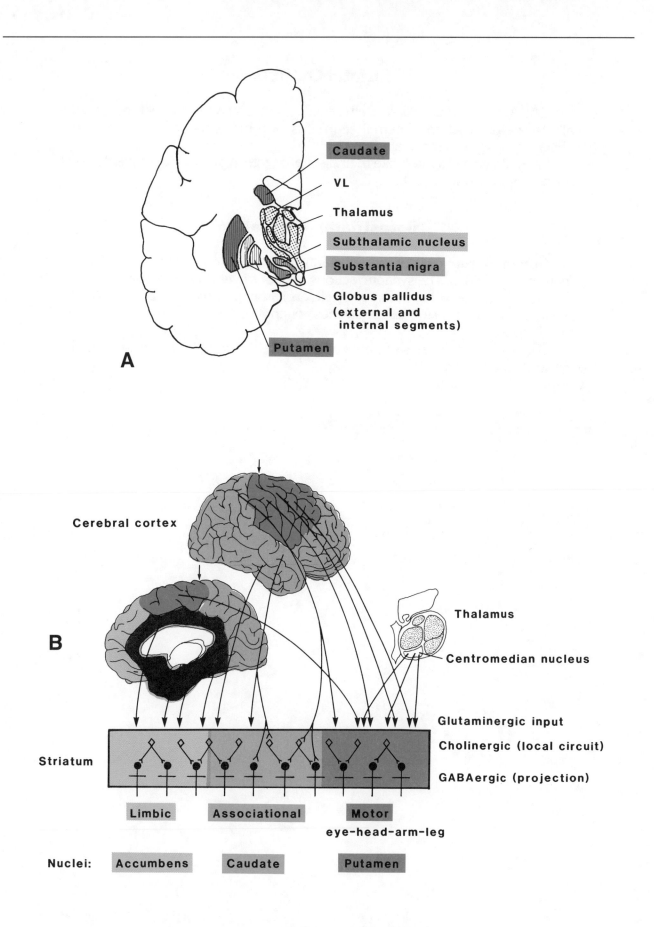

Figure 138 *A*, Anatomical structures. *B*, Striatal inputs. *Figure continues.*

Striatal Outputs

GABAergic and peptidergic efferents from the striatum project topographically to the external and internal segments of the globus pallidus and to the substantia nigra pars reticulata (Fig. 138C).

Many striatal cells modulate their discharge rate in phase with movements of part of the body (Fig. 138D).

Nigrostriatal Modulation

Dopaminergic cells of the substantia nigra pars compacta project to the striatum (Fig. 138E). The synaptic actions are controversial and probably numerous, including a facilitation of cholinergic excitatory postsynaptic potentials. The net effect enhances (?) the responsiveness of cholinergic and GABAergic cells to striatal inputs.

Changes in firing rates of pars compacta cells during limb movements are slow and long-lasting.

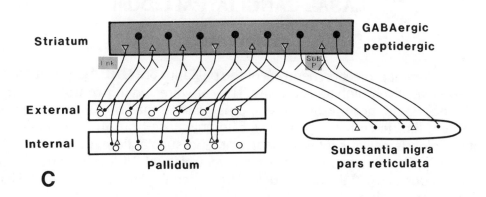

C

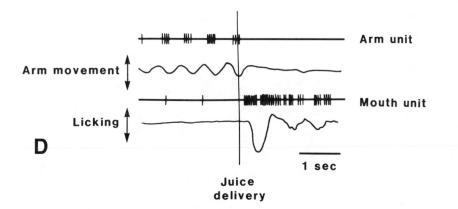

D

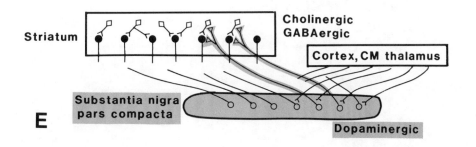

E

Figure 138 *(continued)* *C*, Striatal efferents. *D*, Striatal activity during movement. *E*, Nigrostriatal (dopaminergic) modulation. (*B*, Adapted from Nieuwenhuys R, Voogd J, van Huijzen C. The human central nervous system. Heidelberg: Springer-Verlag, 1981:10. *D*, Adapted from Evarts EV, Kimura M, Wurtz RH, Hikosaka O. Behavioral correlates of activity in basal ganglia neurons. Trends Neurosci 1984; 7:451.)

UNIT 139
BASAL GANGLIA: PALLIDUM

Efferents

The efferent projection neurons of the pallidum are **GABAergic** (inhibitory) and have a relatively high tonic activity. They are directed to **premotor** (program organizing) areas, not motor centers, plus (via the thalamus) frontal **associational** and **limbic** cortex (Fig. 139A). Efferents arise from the ventral pallidum (limbic), globus pallidus internal segment, and substantia nigra pars reticulata (Fig. 139B). The target zones include the ventrolateral (VL), ventroanterior (VA), and mediodorsal (MD) thalamic nuclei, the habenula (H), the superior colliculus (SC), the pedunculopontine nucleus (PPN) and the reticular formation (RF).

Within the premotor division, eye-head programs are controlled by the substantia nigra pars reticulata, and trunk-limb movements by the globus pallidus.

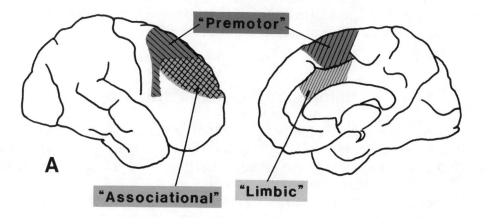

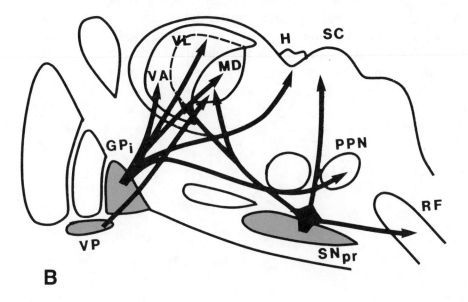

Figure 139 *A*, Cortical targets (via the thalamus). *B*, Pallidal outputs. *Figure continues.*

Subthalamic Nucleus

Pallidal output is modulated by the subthalamic nucleus, which appears to have a net excitatory effect (transmitter possibly glutamate). Topographic inhibitory input from the pallidal **external** segment makes the subthalamic nucleus a negative image (?) of pallidal activity that can be used with modification to regulate the relative weighting of excitation and inhibition in the pallidal **internal** segment (Fig. 139C).

Pallidum as Program Facilitator

The pallidum tonically inhibits premotor nuclei such as the superior colliculus. In order to initiate premotor activity, and thereby a specific motor program, a selected group of pallidal neurons must *stop* firing (Fig. 139D). Suppression of pallidal activity *disinhibits* premotor networks.

Function. Strong dynamic stimuli can always trigger motor programs without basal ganglia. Much voluntary movement, however, proceeds in a "static" sensory environment. Relevant sensory cues and motor outputs need to be selected by premotor centers. The process is triggered by internal, motivational signals, originating in limbic-frontal regions, which pass through the basal ganglia "filter" in order to inhibit unwanted and disinhibit appropriate networks.

Without dopaminergic enhancement at the striatal level, the signal is stopped. If it passes to the pallidal level, the degree of pallidal inhibition is modulated by the subthalamic nucleus. This may roughly determine the general speed or force of the released movement.

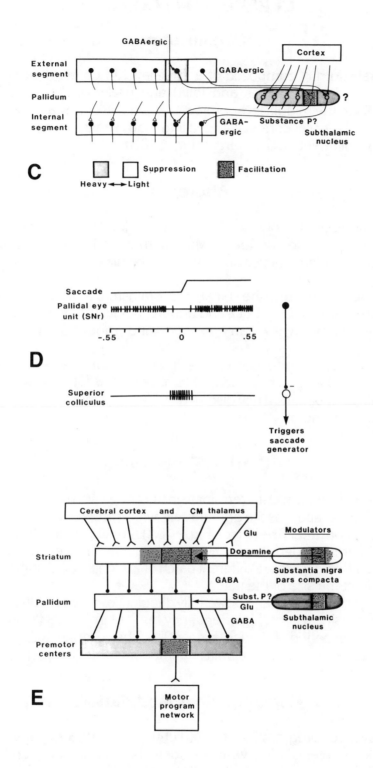

Figure 139 *(continued)* C, Pallidosubthalamic interactions. D, Pallidal silence during movement. E, Program facilitation. (B, Adapted from Anderson ME, Crill WE. Basal ganglia and cerebellum. In: Ruch T, Patton HD, eds. Physiology and biophysics. The brain and neural function. 20th ed. Philadelphia: WB Saunders, 1979:128.)

371

UNIT 140
CEREBELLUM: CORTEX

Organization

The cerebellum is composed of a three-layered cortex (heavily folded into mediolaterally oriented lobules and folia) and underlying nuclei (Fig. 140A). **Purkinje cells** in the middle layer project to the nuclei. They are *GABAergic* and inhibitory. The cerebellar cortex is divided into many sagittally oriented zones, each projecting to a different nuclear target (Fig. 140B).

Afferents

Cerebellar afferents convey signals from all levels of the CNS (Fig. 140C). There are two types: **mossy fibers**, which terminate in the granular layer, and **climbing fibers**, which synapse directly onto Purkinje cell dendritic trees (see Fig. 140A).

Mossy fibers originate in the spinal cord, brainstem reticular nuclei, vestibular nuclei, red nucleus (see Unit 121), and pontine nuclei (conveying input from the sensorimotor cortex). They carry sensory and motor (corollary discharge) information.

Climbing fibers originate from the inferior olivary nucleus in the ventral medulla (see Fig. 140C). They usually fire at very slow rates (1 per second) in a characteristic burst pattern. They discharge when *unexpected* sensory inputs are received in a given motor setting.

Cortical Processing

Cerebellar afferents mostly terminate in the cortex with sparse collaterals sent to the nuclei. Mossy fibers excite granule cells which project to the molecular layer and bifurcate as **parallel fibers** (see Fig. 140A). Purkinje cell activity is facilitated at the locus of greatest density of active parallel fibers. Thus each combination of excited afferents will facilitate a different patch of Purkinje cells. Inhibitory interneurons also restrict the size of the patch.

Climbing fibers directly and powerfully depolarize Purkinje cells in a functional sagittal strip, causing a short high-frequency burst of impulses **(complex spike)** followed by a brief period of silence (Fig. 140D). The complex spike may enhance Purkinje cell responsiveness to parallel fiber inputs for a finite period.

Climbing Fiber Modulation

When a motor program fails to predict the sensory effect of a given movement (error), the inferior olivary nucleus detects the mismatch and discharges complex spikes to specific cerebellar strips. The change in complex spike activity modulates Purkinje cell firing rates and thus causes a compensatory change in output activity from the cerebellar nuclei.

Example: Increased load imposed on an accurate hand movement degrades the performance (Fig. 140E). Complex spike rate increases in particular cerebellar regions until the performance returns to normal. The complex spike modulation is associated with a sustained reduction in selected Purkinje cell simple spikes (Fig. 140E). The exact mechanisms by which modulation of Purkinje cell activity by climbing fibers helps to correct motor outputs is unknown.

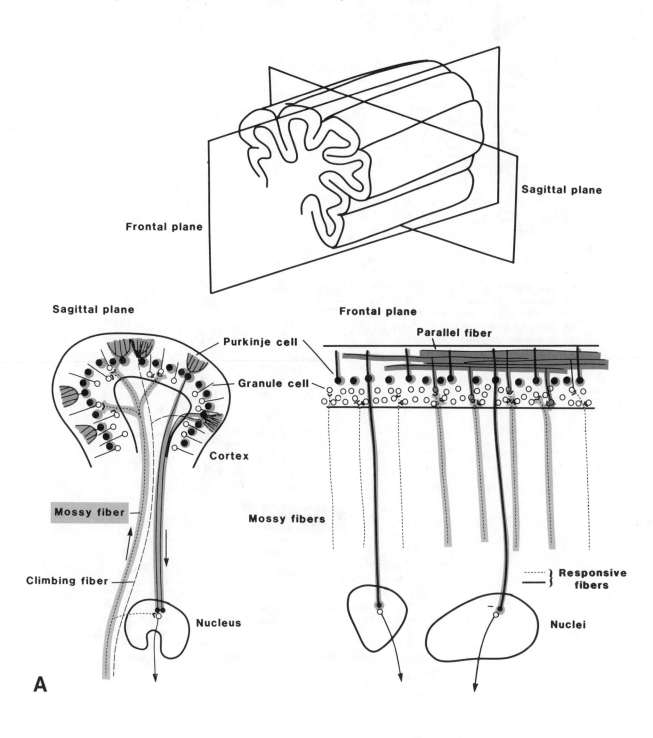

Figure 140 *A*, Cerebellar cortical structure. *Figure continues.*

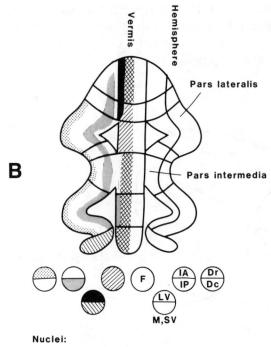

B

Vermis

Hemisphere

Pars lateralis

Pars intermedia

F | IA/IP | Dr/Dc

LV

M,SV

Nuclei:

F fastigial
LV lateral vestibular
M,SV medial and superior vestibular
IA anterior interpositus
IP posterior interpositus
Dr rostral dentate
Dc caudal dentate

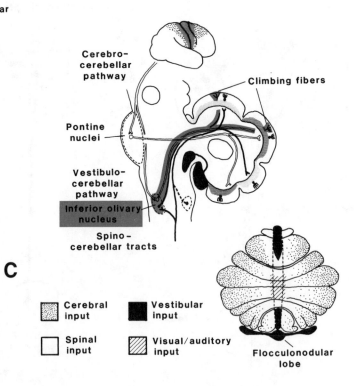

Cerebro-
cerebellar
pathway

Climbing fibers

Pontine
nuclei

Vestibulo-
cerebellar
pathway

Inferior olivary
nucleus

Spino-
cerebellar tracts

C

Cerebral input

Vestibular input

Spinal input

Visual/auditory input

Flocculonodular lobe

Figure 140 *(continued)* B, Cortical projections to nuclei. C, Cerebellar afferents. *Figure continues.*

374

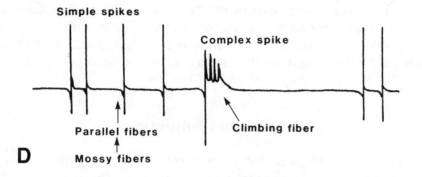

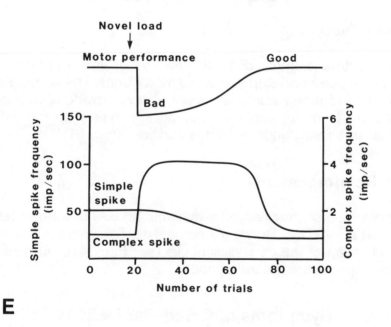

Figure 140 *(continued)* D, Purkinje cell climbing fiber response. *E*, Change in complex spike frequency during unprepared conditions of movement. (*B*, Adapted from Groenewegen HJ, Voogd J. The longitudinal zonal arrangement of the olivocerebellar climbing fiber projection in the cat. An autoradiographic and degeneration study. Exp Brain Res 1976; Suppl 1:69. *C*, Adapted from Nieuwenhuys R, Voogd J, van Huijzen C. The human central nervous system. Heidelberg: Springer-Verlag, 1981:157. *E*, Adapted from Thach WT. Complex spikes, the inferior olive, and natural behavior. In: Courville J, de Montigny C, Lamarre Y, eds. The inferior olivary nucleus: anatomy and physiology. New York: Raven Press, 1980:355.)

UNIT 141
CEREBELLUM: NUCLEI

Efferents

Cerebellar efferents arise from the deep nuclei (Fig. 141A); they tonically *facilitate* all of the **brainstem motor centers** and the **VL thalamus** (projects to motor cortex). Some output is also directed to premotor regions, e.g., superior colliculus, parvicellular red nucleus, pedunculopontine nucleus, and VA thalamus (projects to premotor cortex), and to autonomic motor regions, e.g., periaqueductal gray matter, hypothalamus (see Fig. 141A).

Motor Signal Adjustment

Cerebellar output adjusts activity in all motor centers to achieve a finely tuned balance. Adjustment may be **predictive** for transient environmental conditions of a frequent nature, or may serve as long-term **compensation** in cases of chronic injury or altered peripheral conditions.

Examples of Adjustment

Pulse-Step Matching

The accurate attainment of targets for eye or limb movements requires matching of the pulse and step signals to motor units. The summated input to motor centers and motor nuclei does not always provide a balanced match. Cerebellar input to motor centers automatically makes up the difference by predicting the imbalance under existing conditions (Fig. 141B, i).

Dynamic Reinforcement

Cerebellar output may reinforce dynamic phases of limb acceleration or deceleration (Fig. 141B, ii). Bursts of neuronal discharge enhance fast reactions. Transient inhibition of the cerebellar nuclei (see Fig. 141B, ii) reinforces limb deceleration to prevent target overshoot.

Symptoms of Cerebellar Deficits

1. Limb or eye movements overshoot their target (see Fig. 141B); pulse signal is too long or intense (**dysmetria**).
2. Static (postural) muscle contractions are poorly maintained: continuously corrected giving tremor of about 3 cycles per second.

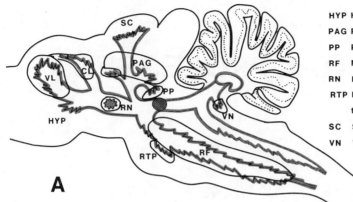

HYP Hypothalamus
PAG Periaqueductal gray
PP Pedunculopontine nucleus
RF Medial reticular formation
RN Red nucleus
RTP Nucleus reticularis
    tegmenti pontis
SC Superior colliculus
VN Vestibular nuclei

Thalamus:

VL Ventrolateral nucleus
CL Centrolateral nucleus

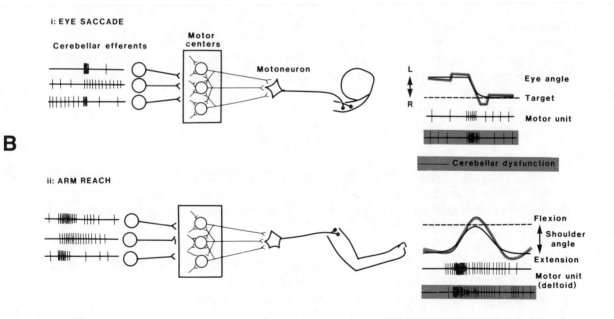

Figure 141 *A*, Cerebellar efferents. *B*, Cerebellar adjustment. (*A*, Adapted from Faull RLM. The cerebellofugal projections in the brachium conjunctivum of the rat. II. The ipsilateral and contralateral descending pathways. J Comp Neurol 1978; 178:530.)

20

MENTAL PROCESSES

UNIT 142
PREFRONTAL CORTEX

The cortex anterior to the premotor strip (Fig. 142A) extends preparatory motor functions to general planning of behavioral strategy and social interaction.

Frontal-Parietal Antagonism

The parietal lobe discriminates sensory cues for specific motor responses or guidance. If unopposed, parietal signals would reflexly drive motor outputs whether the movement was currently appropriate or not. Prefrontal cortex regulates parietal access to the motor regions. It thereby controls environmental drives within a larger behavioral context — the doorknob is not grasped unless you want to open the door.

Personality

The behavioral rules and sets of priorities programmed by the prefrontal cortex define individual personality. Prefrontal damage is often impossible to measure objectively, although personality and behavioral changes are obvious. These changes can include

1. "Utilization" and "imitation" behavior (patient makes compulsive use of visible objects and automatically mimics gestures of others).
2. Loss of attentive power (patient is easily distracted and impulsive).
3. Inability to plan goal-directed strategies over an extended period; loss of motivation.

Correlates in Unit Activity

1. Prefrontal activity is shaped to facilitate behavioral goals. Automatic "reflexive" responses to stimuli are lacking. Many neurons discharge specifically in response to stimuli that are goal-related and ignore identical stimuli (visual, auditory,) when they are irrelevant to the goal (Fig. 142B).
2. Many prefrontal neurons fire over extended periods (seconds to a minute) during a period of waiting for an expected, goal-related signal (Fig. 142C). The discharge may embody a type of short-term memory, maintaining attention for the intended goal so that competing stimuli do not interfere.

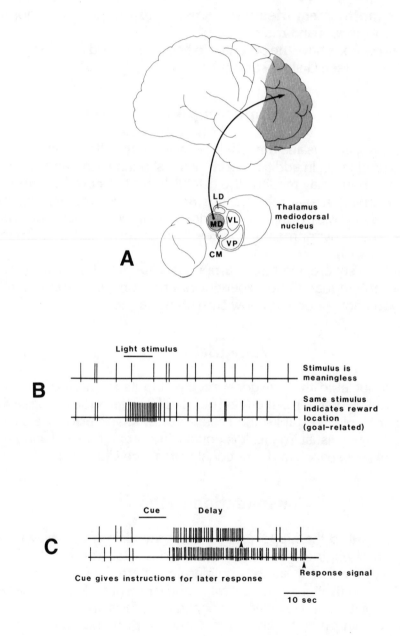

Figure 142 *A*, Prefrontal cortex. *B*, Prefrontal discrimination of goal-related stimuli. *C*, Prefrontal activity while planned behavior is prepared. (*A*, Adapted from Nieuwenhuys R, Voogd J, van Huijzen C. The human central nervous system. Heidelberg: Springer-Verlag, 1981:10.)

UNIT 143
MEMORY

Two classes of memory are recognized: cognitive (declarative) and habit (reflexive). Although the final cellular mechanisms of memory "storage" may be the same for both, the acquisition process differs.

Cognitive memory requires the participation of the **limbic system** (see Unit 146), specifically the hippocampus, amygdala, anterior thalamus, and mamillary bodies (Fig. 143A). Cognitive memory requires limbic areas only for consolidation; storage is probably in the same cortical areas where sensory perception occurs.

Habits or **motor memories** (programs) simply require repetition of the associated sensory inputs and motor outputs.

Possibly all neurons have the potential to become altered by activity and thus to store "memories" (see Units 49 and 50).

Hippocampus

Both the hippocampus and amygdala serve equally well to establish recognition memories of objects. In addition, each has distinct specializations.

The hippocampus may mediate the establishment of **cognitive maps**. It is necessary for learning spatial relationships among environmental objects with respect to the body. Single pyramidal neurons in the hippocampus (cornu ammonis) discharge when environmental "places," which form part of a "map," are recognized (Fig. 143B).

In the left hemisphere, the hippocampus is important for establishing relationships between language and experiences and concepts. It is essential for knowing that you know or do not know something (a memory directory).

Amygdala

Various subnuclei in the amygdala receive inputs from all of the sensory systems, olfaction being the most direct (Fig. 143C). This is the substrate for the amygdala's critical role in establishing **cross-modal associations**, e.g., a smell eliciting an associated visual image. It is equally important for mediating the link between sensory perceptions and emotional states (see Unit 146).

Consolidation Paths

Processed input to the hippocampus and amygdala must "play back" on sensory areas to strengthen neuronal associations. Both project to the basal forebrain where they can activate the cholinergic system directed to the cerebral cortex (Fig. 143D). Activation of cortical muscarinic receptors leads to membrane protein phosphorylation and facilitated synaptic transmission.

Cognitive learning may be limited to stimuli with behavioral or emotional significance. The amygdala has an enkephalinergic projection to sensory "perceptual" areas which is activated in conjunction with the associated emotional state and reinforces memory consolidation.

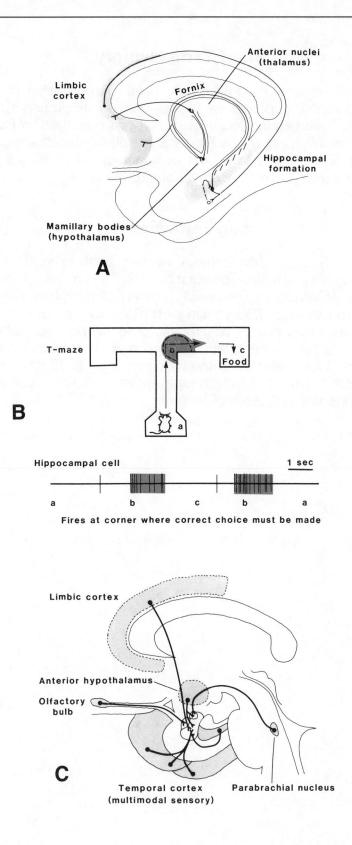

Figure 143 *A*, Hippocampal memory circuit (circuit of Papez). *B*, Hippocampal "place" cells. *C*, Afferents of the amygdala. *Figure continues.*

Short-Term Memory

Lasting a maximum of 1 to 2 hours, initial memory relies on presynaptic facilitation and inhibition processes. It does not require protein synthesis. Sustained activity in "reverberatory loops" (e.g., hippocampal circuit of Papez; see Fig. 143A) is one possible mechanism. Post-tetanic potentiation of synaptic transmission (see Unit 50), which has a time constant of about 90 sec, provides a mechanism for short-term enhancement of neural circuits.

Long-Term Memory

Maintained synaptic enhancement involves **protein synthesis**, which is triggered presumably by activity in neural circuits. The protein synthesis results in modified synaptic structures: increased numbers of receptors, changes in dendritic spines, and so forth. **Long-term potentiation** (see Unit 51) is a related process that can develop after post-tetanic potentiation, especially if repeated several times. It is prominent in hippocampal granule cells and pyramidal cells (Figs. 143E and 143F), where it is known to persist up to 13 days. This provides long-lasting enhancement of transmission in active nerve circuits—a possible requirement for some processes of memory.

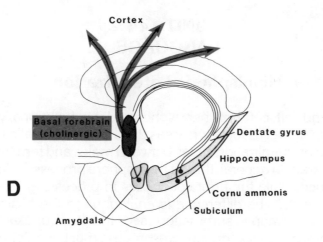

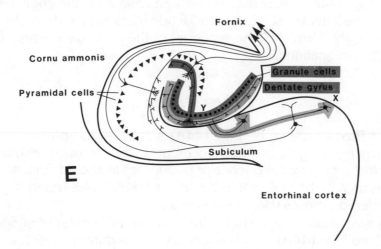

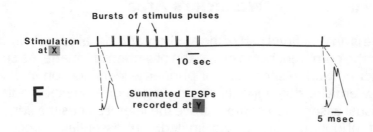

Figure 143 *(continued)* *D,* Cholinergic memory consolidation. *E,* Internal hippocampal network. *F,* Long-term potentiation in the hippocampus. (*A, B,* and *D,* Adapted from Nieuwenhuys R, Voogd J, van Huijzen C. The human central nervous system. Heidelberg: Springer-Verlag, 1981:214, 209, 214.)

UNIT 144
LANGUAGE

Hemispheric Lateralization

The right and left cerebral hemispheres differ functionally, especially in homologous higher-level association areas that have dense callosal interconnections. The degree of lateralization varies between males and females and between dextrals and sinistrals. In general, the left hemisphere processes signals in precise temporal sequence, while the right specializes in processing "spatial" relations among parallel inputs. The difference is analogous to the basic dichotomy of temporal and spatial synaptic summation (see Unit 49). For exact interpretation within the temporal or spatial domain, one process must be minimized in favor of the other.

Language analysis and production is very demanding of temporal sequence precision. The key areas serving language function are usually located in the left hemisphere (Fig. 144A), where they are enlarged relative to their right hemisphere homologues. The latter subserve the production (right Broca's homologue) or the interpretation (right Wernicke's homologue) of the prosodic element of speech, i.e., the affective intonations.

Broca's Area

Much of Broca's area (see Fig. 144A) serves as the premotor cortex for speech and writing. It regulates the flow of inputs to the motor cortex oral (or hand) region such that a prepared sequence of phonemes is uttered. Patients who have lesions in this area of the brain can utter only monosyllables (often meaningless) instead of ordered phrases (Broca's aphasia).

Broca's area shares its premotor function with the anterior supplementary motor area (see Fig. 144A), which is equally active during speech and may be essential for the voluntary initiation of speech.

Wernicke's Area

This zone is an ill-defined part of the auditory and visual association cortex. It is necessary for the comprehension of spoken or written language. As such it forms part of a larger network responsible for phoneme identification and sequencing (Fig. 144B). Wernicke's area identifies language components mediated by the auditory or visual association cortex. Above the lateral sulcus the somatosensory correlates of phonemes are discriminated, an essential aspect of speech production.

Similarly, the rostral part of Broca's area, to which Wernicke's area projects, maps phonemes in terms of motor output patterns. Bracketing the phoneme identification network are two multimodal cortical territories that serve as a short-term memory buffer for sets of phonemes prior to sequencing (see Fig. 144B).

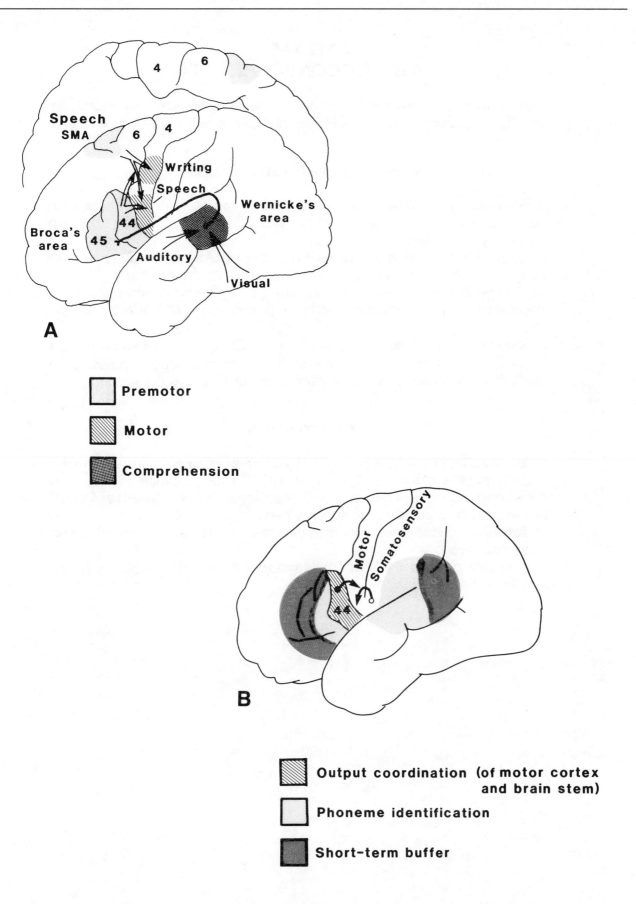

Figure 144 *A*, Areas of the brain involved in language analysis and production. *B*, Functional organization.

UNIT 145
STATES OF CONSCIOUSNESS

Levels of consciousness are monitored by scalp-recorded electroencephalograms (EEGs). Specific patterns of CNS activity may be responsible for each state.

Awake: Desynchronized EEG

1. There is little synchrony of discharge among cortical units, and hence, no summation of potentials in the EEG, which is of low amplitude and high frequency (Fig. 145A).
2. Supported by the **reticular activating system (RAS)** originating in cholingergic cells of the mid-brain and upper pontine tegmentum (Fig. 145B).
3. RAS projects to the cortex via cholinergic basal forebrain and peptidergic caudolateral hypothalamus (topographic projection to cortical laminae I and VI).
4. **Alpha rhythm** (large amplitude synchronized EEG) occurs when the brain is idling ("day-dreaming"). Thalamic oscillators entrain large populations of cortical neurons into an activity rhythm of about 10 cycles per second.

Circadian Clock

1. Sleep-waking periodicity is controlled by internal oscillators: (a) the suprachiasmatic nucleus of the hypothalamus (see Fig. 145B), entrained to light-dark cycles by direct retinal afferents; and (b) the pineal body, entrained to nightfall by sympathetic input from the superior cervical ganglion.
2. **Melatonin** secreted by the pineal in darkness *resets* circadian rhythms and facilitates sleep.
3. The preoptic nucleus of the hypothalamus (see Fig. 145B) may also be necessary for sleep induction.

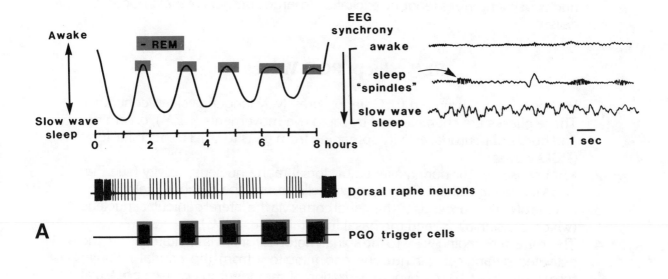

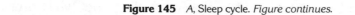

Figure 145 *A*, Sleep cycle. *Figure continues.*

Slow-Wave Sleep: Synchronized EEG

1. Various sleep stages are characterized by increasing degrees of EEG synchronization (see Fig. 145A).
2. Large potential waves of deep **slow-wave sleep** are due to synchronized thalamocortical volleys depolarizing populations of cortical neurons together. Waves occur at a frequency of 3 per second ("δ rhythm").
3. The sleeper cycles through sleep stages repeatedly during the night (see Fig. 145A).
4. The thalamic reticular nucleus (see Fig. 145B) may be partly responsible for degree of synchronized rhythmic firing: Rhythmic inhibition from the reticular nucleus synchronizes rebound excitation in large numbers of thalamocortical cells.

REM Sleep: PGO Waves

1. Phases of desynchronized EEG get progressively longer as sleep continues. These phases are characterized by rapid eye movements (REM), dreaming, and bursts of neuronal activity spreading from pons to LGN to occipital lobe (**PGO waves**).
2. REM phases occur during silence of dorsal raphe nucleus activity (see Fig. 145A), causing disinhibition of trigger cells around the parabrachial nuclei.
3. A wave of activity ascends to the visual cortex via the lateral geniculate nucleus (which is disinhibited) and the basal forebrain (Fig. 145C).
4. There is a descending wave to the spinal motoneurons; it is excitatory from the activated gigantocellular nucleus and inhibitory from the caudal reticular formation. A net 10 mV hyperpolarization of motoneurons causes **postural atonia** (see Fig. 145C).

Note: Somnambulism occurs during slow-wave sleep, not while dreaming. Body movement is impossible during REM motoneuron hyperpolarization.

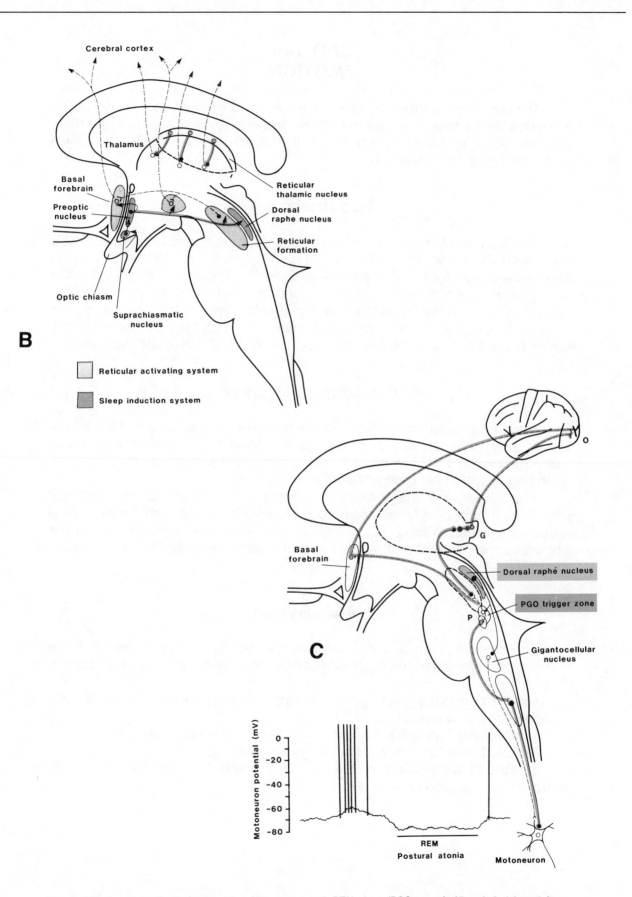

Figure 145 *(continued)* *B*, Sleep and waking systems. *C*, REM sleep (PGO waves). (*B* and *C*, Adapted from Nieuwenhuys R, Voogd J, van Huijzen C. The human central nervous system. Heidelberg: Springer-Verlag, 1981:151.)

UNIT 146
EMOTION

The brain areas subserving emotional states and expression — limbic cortex, amygdala, hypothalamus — are in part the same as those involved in memory consolidation (Fig. 146A). In general, it is the experiences which elicit emotional reactions that are remembered.

Hypothalamus

The basic emotional states — fear, anger, pleasure, and so forth — are closely associated with autonomic behaviors organized by the hypothalamus and periaqueductal gray matter. The amygdala tonically suppresses these behaviors through inhibition of the hypothalamus. When circumstances are appropriate, the amygdala removes the inhibition from a particular hypothalamic circuit and the behavior is released. The perceived emotional correlate of the behavior is dependent on parallel activity in the limbic cortex, specifically the orbitofrontal cortex.

Orbitofrontal Cortex

The cortex surrounding the eye sockets on the ventral surface of the frontal lobe is closely interconnected with the hypothalamus and amygdala. Removal of this region causes a blunting of feeling. Even intense chronic pain loses its agonizing aspect to become just another sensation.

Most neurons in this region respond selectively to attractive or aversive stimuli (Fig. 146B). Some cells will respond preferentially to the sight or taste of a particular (desirable) food. For many cells the response depends not on the physical appearance of a stimulus but on the associated aversive or attractive quality.

Limbic System

The limbic system is a network interconnecting the limbic cortex, basal ganglia, basal forebrain, diencephalon, amygdala, hypothalamus, and olfactory bulb.

Limbic cortex: cingulate gyrus and hippocampal region ("border" of hemispheres) and orbitofrontal cortex.

Limbic basal ganglia: nucleus accumbens and ventral pallidum.

Limbic basal forebrain (cholinergic): septal nuclei.

Limbic diencephalon: anterior nucleus of the thalamus (see Unit 100), mamillary bodies, and habenula (see Unit 139).

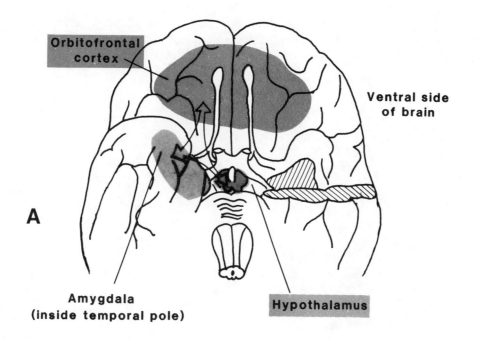

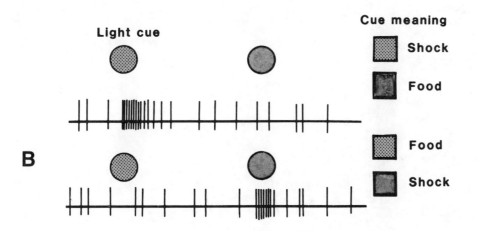

Figure 146   *A,* Emotion-related areas of the brain. *B,* Aversive cell of the orbitofrontal cortex.

GLOSSARY

Throughout this book, a number of terms are introduced in one unit and reappear in others. We have listed them here to enable the reader to follow material throughout the book. Major terms which form chapter headings are not included here.

Accommodation: (a) Ability of the lens of the eye to adjust its focal length to sight objects at different distances. (b) Decrease in firing rate of a neuron during maintained depolarization (usually involves inactivation of membrane sodium channels).

Afferent: Axon projecting *toward* a given CNS locus, especially primary sensory axons entering spinal cord.

After-potential: Voltage change following an action potential.

Adenohypophysis: The anterior part of the pituitary (hypophysis), containing secretory cells that secrete and release hormones into the circulation. (These secretory cells are acted on by releasing and release-inhibiting hormones of the hypothalamus).

Agonist: Muscle(s) acting as prime mover in a given movement.

Alpha-adrenergic receptor: Receptor for noradrenaline (and adrenaline) coupled to an ion channel and preferentially blocked by certain pharmacological agents, e.g., phentolamine.

Alpha motoneuron: Motoneuron innervating extrafusal muscle fibers.

Antagonist: Muscle(s) acting to *oppose* prime mover and thus to decelerate a given movement.

Association cortex: All neocortex which is neither primary/secondary sensory or motor.

Astrocyte: Glial cell with many processes, found in the central nervous system, and providing structural support to neurons and capillaries.

Autoreceptor: Receptor on a transmitter-releasing neuron responsive to the transmitter released by the neuron.

Basilar membrane: Membranous structure of the cochlea containing the hair cells responsible for sound detection.

Beta-adrenergic receptor: Receptor for noradrenaline (and adrenaline) to a second messenger system (adenylate cyclase) and preferentially blocked by certain pharmacological agents, e.g., propranolol.

Capacitance: Measure of ability of a structure (such as a membrane) to store electrical charge. Ratio of charge stored per unit of applied voltage.

Carotid body: Chemosensory structure at the carotid bifurcation of the arterial system; sensitive to blood levels of pH, O_2, and CO_2.

Central pattern generator: CNS neuronal network which autonomously produces a motor output sequence when suitably triggered.

Cochlea: The portion of the inner ear that detects sound.

Collateral: Side-branch of an axon projecting to a different target zone than main axon.

Column: In cerebral cortex, a cylinder, block or slab of gray matter extending through all of the cortical layers: several subtypes with different dimensions. In spinal cord, either a longitudinal string of white matter ("funiculus") extending the length of the cord, or an elongated nucleus extending through many segments of gray matter.

Conductance: A measure of the electrical permeability of a membrane or channel: ratio of current flowing across the membrane or channel to the applied voltage. (Reciprocal of electrical resistance).

Cupula: Gelatinous mass overlying hair cells in the semicircular canals of the inner ear (detects angular acceleration of the head).

Depression: Decrease in postsynaptic potential with repeated release of transmitter (firing of presynaptic neuron).

Desensitization: Loss of receptor-mediated response during prolonged presence of an agonist at the receptor.

Dorsal columns: Tracts of sensory axons, all mechanoreceptors, ascending the spinal cord in the dorsal white matter divided into 2 columns, the gracile serving the lower body and the cuneate serving the arms and chest.

Efferent: Axon projecting *away* from a given CNS locus, especially motor axons leaving spinal cord.

End-plate potential: The voltage response at the end-plate of a muscle fiber produced by action of released transmitter substance on available ligand-specific receptors.

Enteric nervous system: System of neurons in the walls of the intestine; possessed of intrinsic activity, but regulated by the autonomic nervous system.

EPSP: Excitatory postsynaptic potential: The potential change created by release of transmitter substance from an excitatory neuron through its action on receptors of the receiving (postsynaptic) neuron.

Equilibrium potential: For a given ionic species, the potential at which there is no net transmembrane current carried by that ion. (Diffusional and electrical forces acting on the ionic species are equal at the equilibrium potential).

Exocytosis: The process by which materials are released from cells through fusion of vesicles with the plasma membrane and consequent liberation of vesicular contents.

Extrafusal muscle fiber: Muscle fibers located outside the muscle spindles (forming the majority of fibers in almost all muscles).

Facilitation: (a) Enhanced synaptic transmission resulting from previous impulse activity in a presynaptic (transmitting) neuron. (b) "Spatial facilitation" is increased likelihood of impulses occurring in a neuron receiving two or more synaptic inputs at different locations but close together in time.

Gamma motoneuron: Motoneuron innervating intrafusal muscle fibers.

Gap junction: A contact between two cells characterized by a narrow gap traversed by periodic transjunctional particles which join the two cells together and permit electrical currents and small molecules to pass between them.

Gating: The process by which membrane particles associated with ionic channels control the movement of ions through the channel. Channels may be "gated open" or "gated shut" by transmembrane voltage or appropriate ions or ligands.

Glandotropic hormone: Hormone released by the pituitary and acting on one or more endocrine glands elsewhere in the body.

Group I afferents: Large-diameter nerve axons derived from muscle spindles (Group Ia) or tendon organs (Group Ib); typically include the most rapidly conducting axons in peripheral nerves.

Group II afferents: Intermediate-diameter nerve axons derived from secondary sensory endings in muscle spindles.

Hypercolumn: A unit of cerebral cortex, about 1 mm^2 in area, whose neurons share a common receptive field, response property, or motor output.

Hypophysiotropic zone: The region of the hypothalamus containing neurons which release hormones that regulate pituitary (hypophyseal) hormone-secreting activity.

Inactivation: The process by which membrane channels lose their ability to conduct ions, in spite of maintained activating voltage.

Intermediate zone: Middle layers of the spinal cord gray matter between dorsal and ventral horns.

Intrafusal muscle fibers: Muscle fibers within a muscle spindle.

Intramural ganglion: Ganglion (cluster of neurons) embedded in an effector organ (often supplied by parasympathetic innervation).

Ionophore: Transmembrane channel capable of conducting ions across the membrane (often controlled in its opening and closing by a receptor).

IPSP: Inhibitory postsynaptic potential: The potential change created by release of transmitter substance from an inhibitory neuron through its action on receptors of the receiving (postsynaptic) neuron.

Isometric contraction: Tension produced by a muscle (or motor unit) contracting without shortening.

Isotonic contraction: Shortening of a muscle made to contract while lifting a constant load.

Kinase: An enzyme (often activated by a second messenger) which catalyzes a reaction involving a substrate protein, usually by phosphorylating it.

L cone: Cone retinal receptor containing a pigment selectively sensitive to long wavelengths (red light).

Lemniscus: Refers to *medial* lemniscus, large, phylogenetically recent tract of axons conveying mechanoreceptive signals from dorsal column nuclei to thalamus.

Limbic: Phylogenetically old parts of brain associated with control of autonomic behaviors, emotions, and memory consolidation.

M cone: Cone retinal receptor containing a pigment selectively sensitive to middle wavelengths (green light).

Magnocellular: Large-celled region of gray matter.

Motor program: Multi-level processing scheme for transforming ongoing neuronal activity into purposeful body movement.

Motor unit: The group of muscle fibers innervated by a single motor axon.

Muscarinic receptor: Receptor for acetylcholine preferentially reacting with muscarine (e.g., postganglionic sympathetic neurons).

Neurohypophysis: The posterior part of the pituitary (hypophysis), containing endings of neurons located in the hypothalamus that secrete and release hormones (vasopressin and oxytocin) into the circulation.

Nicotinic receptor: Receptor for acetylcholine preferentially reacting with nicotine (e.g., at the neuromuscular junction).

Oligodendrocyte: Glial cell in the central nervous system responsible for creating the myelin sheath around processes of central neurons.

Operculum: Part of cerebrum forming upper and lower banks of the lateral fissure.

Orbitofrontal cortex: Cerebral cortex in ventral frontal lobe surrounding the eye sockets.

Otolith: Gelatinous structure with minute calcite inclusions overlying hair cells in the macula, or statolith organs of the inner ear (detects linear acceleration).

Parvocellular: Small-celled region of gray matter.

Periaqueductal gray: Cylinder of gray matter in midbrain which surrounds the cerebral aqueduct linking third and fourth ventricles.

Phasic: Pertaining to rapidly changing rates of neuronal or muscular activity.

Postganglionic neuron: Neuron with cell body in a sympathetic ganglion (where it synapses with preganglionic neurons) and with axon leading to an effector organ.

Post-tetanic potentiation: Enhanced synaptic transmission following a rapid train of impulses in a presynaptic (transmitting) neuron; lasts seconds to minutes.

Preganglionic neuron: Neuron leading from the central nervous system to a sympathetic ganglion, where it forms synapses with peripheral (postganglionic) neurons.

Presynaptic inhibition: Reduction of transmitter release from a presynaptic terminal due to the action of an inhibitory transmitter substance on receptors of the terminal.

Ramus communicans: Short axonal pathway joining the sympathetic chain to peripheral nerve trunks near the spinal cord.

Receptive field: Peripheral or environmental territory from which an adequate stimulus elicits a sensory response in a given neuron.

Receptor potential: Voltage change occurring in a sensory receptor in response to an appropriate stimulus.

Refractory period: The short period of time following an action potential during which the nerve axon or muscle fiber is unable to respond to a voltage stimulus with a second action potential.

Release-inhibiting hormone: Hormone carried from the hypothalamus to the adenohypophysis by the hypophyseal portal circulation, acting on secretory cells to prevent release of a pituitary hormone.

Releasing hormone: Hormone carried from the hypothalamus to the adenohypophysis by the hypophyseal portal circulation, acting on secretory cells to cause release of a pituitary hormone.

Reticular formation: Network of neuronal somata and axonal tracts extending through the core of the brainstem from medulla to midbrain.

Retinotopy: Spatial organization of visual neurons such that the pattern of responses in the retina is represented in the same relative order.

Reversal potential: The membrane potential at which net current flow through activated transmembrane channels is zero (i.e., inward flow of current is equal and opposite to outward flow of current).

S cone: Cone retinal receptor containing a pigment selectively sensitive to short wavelengths (blue light).

Schwann cell: Glial cell responsible for generating the myelin sheath around nerve axons in the peripheral nervous system.

Somatotopy: Spatial organization of sensory neurons which represent body parts such that body order is maintained.

Summation: Addition of postsynaptic potentials occurring close together in time due either to rapid firing of a single presynaptic neuron, or the near-simultaneous arrival of impulses from two or more presynaptic neurons.

Synergy: A set of muscles functionally acting together to perform a specific task.

Tectorial membrane: Membrane structure overlying hair cells of the cochlear basilar membrane; responsible for detection of sound.

Tetanic contraction: The contraction produced in a motor unit (or entire muscle) by a train of impulses in the motor axon (or by closely spaced stimuli to the motor nerve).

Tonic: Pertaining to maintained neuronal or muscle discharge.

Tonotopy: Spatial organization of auditory neurons such that individual (sound) frequency bands are represented in sequential order.

Twitch contraction: The contraction produced in a motor unit by one nerve impulse, or the contraction of a whole muscle produced by one stimulus to the motor nerve.

INDEX